Radiographic Positioning AND Related Anatomy Workbook AND Laboratory Manual

VOLUME 1

FIFTH EDITION

Radiographic Positioning AND Related Anatomy

Workbook AND Laboratory Manual

VOLUME 1
Chapters 1-13

Kenneth L. Bontrager, MA, RT(R)
John P. Lampignano, M.Ed., RT(R) (CT)

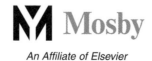

Mosby

An Affiliate of Elsevier

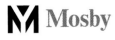
Mosby

An Affiliate of Elsevier

Executive Editor: Jeanne Wilke
Developmental Editor: Jennifer Moorhead
Project Manager: Linda McKinley
Production Editor: Rich Barber
Designer: Julia Ramirez
Cover Art: Amy Buxton

Mosby, Inc.
An Affiliate of Elsevier
11830 Westline Industrial Drive
St. Louis, Missouri 63146

Printed in the United States of America

International Standard Book Number
0-323-0143-56

04 GW/KPT 9 8 7 6 5

Acknowledgments

I am pleased to acknowledge and recognize those persons who have made significant contributions to the fifth edition of this student workbook and laboratory manual.

I first want to thank **John P. Lampignano,** MS, RT(R) (CT), who as coauthor expanded the objectives for each chapter and submitted first drafts of additional questions for the new sections of the textbook. John is a very qualified and effective educator and has put a lot of effort and energy into this project. Thank you, John, for your excellent contributions.

I want to thank **David Hall,** MS, RT(R) for his careful and meticulous review and proofing of all chapters of this manuscript. Not only did he make corrections, but he also made valuable suggestions for improving the clarity of the information being presented.

I also thank **Jeanne Rowland, Jennifer Moorhead,** and **Rich Barber** of the Mosby staff for their help and support in the preparation of this manuscript.

David Hall and **Cindy Murphy,** ACR, also reviewed, made suggestions, and proofed the more than 1200 questions in the computerized test bank, which is available as an ancillary to these workbooks and the textbook. Thank you, Dave and Cindy, for the significant time and effort you invested in this project. Both John Lampignano and I greatly appreciate your valuable contributions.

Last and most important, I want to thank my wife, **Mary Lou,** for organizing our rough composition of questions and answers, along with the associated illustrations, into an orderly and easy-to-follow format.

KLB

I would like to thank **Ken Bontrager** for his patience and dedication in developing my skills as a writer. I've been honored to work with him over the past two editions. **Jennifer Moorhead,** our developmental editor, deserves praise for her dedication and vision in coordinating this project. She kept us on task and focused but always with a smile and a gentle word.

I would like to thank the diagnostic medical imaging faculty and clinical instructors at GateWay Community College who provide a shining example of excellence each and every day for our students and community. To my students—past, present, and future—you have made teaching a rewarding experience! Without you, I would never have had the courage to write a single word. Finally, to my close friend, **Jerry Olson,** who taught me everything about radiography and many things about life—you have made my life richer and more worthwhile.

My family—**Deborah, Daniel,** and **Molly**—provide me with the greatest joy of all. I look at each of you and realize that I'm the luckiest person alive. Thank you for your love and support for the past 25 years. This book is dedicated to each of you.

JPL

Preface

The success of the first four editions of this workbook and the accompanying textbook, along with the associated audiovisual materials, is demonstrated by the many schools of radiologic technology throughout the United States, Canada, and other countries that have been using all or parts of these instructional media for more than 25 years.

New to This Edition

New illustrations and **expanded questions** have been added to reflect all the new content added to the fifth edition of *Textbook of Radiographic Positioning and Related Anatomy.* The use of visuals in these review exercises not only increases comprehension but also increases retention, because most individuals retain information most effectively through visual images.

The **detailed laboratory activities** have been updated, and the positioning question and answer exercises have been expanded with less emphasis on rote memory recall. More **situational questions** involving **clinical applications** have been added. These questions aid in the understanding of positioning principles and of which anatomical structures are best demonstrated on which projections. The clinical situational questions added to each chapter require students to think through and understand how application of this positioning information relates to specific clinical examples.

Pathology questions have been added to help students understand why they are performing specific exams and how exposure factors may be affected.

Critique exercises have been reorganized to be consistent with the new format of radiographic critique descriptions in the textbook.

Included in the positioning chapters of both the textbook and these workbooks are new sections on **geriatric** and **pediatric considerations, alternative modalities and procedures,** and **pathologic indications.** As in the textbook, entirely new sections added to the workbook include **venipuncture, digital radiography, bone densitometry, sialography,** and **hysterosalpingography.** Introductions to **nuclear medicine, radiation oncology,** and **ultrasound imaging** have also been added.

How to Work with the Textbook and the Workbook and Laboratory Manuals

This fifth edition of the student workbook and laboratory manual is organized to be in complete agreement with the fifth edition of the *Textbook of Radiographic Positioning and Related Anatomy.* Each chapter in the textbook has a corresponding chapter in the workbook-manuals to reinforce and supplement the information presented in the main text.

The most effective way to use this workbook-manual is for the student to complete the workbook chapter exercises immediately after reading and studying corresponding chapters in the textbook. To use both the student's and the instructor's time most effectively, this study should be done **before** the classroom presentation. The instructor can therefore spend more time in both the classroom and laboratory on problem areas and answering questions and less time on the fundamentals of anatomy and positioning, which students should already have learned.

Ancillaries

A **computerized test bank** (CTB) is available to instructors who use the textbook in their classrooms. The test bank features 1890 questions and 23 images. Some of these questions originally appeared as the Final Evaluation Exams in the Instructor's Manual in previous editions, but they have been expanded and fully revised into registry-type questions for the test bank. These questions can be used as final evaluation exams for each chapter, or they can be used to create custom exams.

Also available for the first time is an **electronic image collection** (EIC), which features more than 2000 images that are fully coordinated with the fifth edition textbook and workbooks. The fourth edition slide set contains 1780 slides and includes the two-volume Instructor's Manual with lecture notes and thumbnail prints of each slide.

Contents

Volume 1

Volume 2

Student Instructions

The following information will show you how correctly using this workbook and the accompanying textbook will help you master radiographic anatomy and positioning.

This course becomes the core of all your studies and your work as a radiographer. **This is one course that you must master.** You cannot become a proficient radiographer by marginally passing this course. Therefore please read these instructions carefully **before** beginning Chapter 1.

Objectives

Study the list of objectives carefully so that you will understand what you must know and be able to do after you complete each chapter.

Learning Exercises

These exercises are the focal point of this workbook-laboratory manual. Using them correctly will help you learn and remember the important information presented in each chapter of the textbook. To maximize the benefits from each exercise, **follow the correct six-step order of activities** as outlined next:

Chapter 1   Textbook and Workbook

Chapter 1 is a comprehensive introduction that prepares you for the remaining chapters of this positioning course. It is divided into six sections in both the textbook and this workbook. Your instructor may assign specific sections of this chapter at various times during your study of radiographic positioning and/or procedures. Read and study these sections in the textbook first, and then complete the corresponding review exercise in this workbook before taking that portion of the self-test.

Chapters 2 to 24

PART I

Step 1. **A. Textbook:** Carefully read and learn the **radiographic anatomy** section of each chapter. Include the anatomic reviews on labeled radiographs provided in each chapter of the textbook. Pay particular attention to those items in **bold type** and to the **summary review boxes** where provided.

Step 2. **B. Workbook:** Complete **Part I** of the review exercises on **radiographic anatomy.** Do **not** look up the answers in the textbook or look at the answer sheet until you have answered as many of the questions as you can. Then refer to the textbook and/or the answer sheet and correct or complete those questions you missed. Reread those sections of the textbook in which you could not answer questions. Textbook page numbers are provided next to each review exercise in this workbook.

PART II

Step 3. **A. Textbook:** Carefully read and study Part II on **radiographic positioning.** Note the general **positioning considerations, alternate modalities,** and **pathologic indications** for each chapter. This is followed by the specific positioning pages, which include **pathology demonstrated; technical factors;** and the **dose ranges** of skin, midline, and specific organ doses where provided. Pay particular attention to dose comparisons between different techniques, or anteroposterior (AP) versus posteroanterior (PA) projections. Learn the **specific positioning steps,** the **central ray location and angle,** and the four-part **radiographic criteria** for each projection or position.

Step 4. **B. Workbook:** Complete **Part II** of the review exercises, which include **technical considerations and positioning.** Also included is a section on **problem solving for technical and positioning errors.** As before, complete as many of the questions as you can before looking up the answers in the textbook or checking the answers on the answer sheet.

The last review exercise covers **radiographic critique questions** in the workbook. This challenging section is based on the critique radiographs at the end of chapters in the textbook. These important exercises will help you make the transition from factual knowledge to application and will help you prepare for clinical experience. **Compare each critique radiographs that demonstrate errors with correctly positioned radiographs in that chapter of the textbook** and see if you can determine which radiographic criteria points could be improved and which are repeatable errors. Students who complete these exercises successfully will be ahead of those students who don't attempt them before coming to the classroom. The instructor will then explain and clarify those repeatable and nonrepeatable errors on each radiograph.

PART III

Step 5. **Workbook – Laboratory Activity:** These exercises must be performed in a radiographic laboratory using a phantom and/or a student (without making exposure) with an energized radiographic unit and illuminators for viewing radiographs. Arrange for a time when you can use your radiographic laboratory or a diagnostic radiographic room in a clinic setting.

This is one of the most important aspects of this learning series and should not be neglected or underemphasized. Students frequently have difficulty transferring the information they have learned about positioning to effective use in a clinical setting. Therefore you must carry out the laboratory activities as described in each chapter. Your instructors and/or lab assistants will assist you as needed in these exercises.

Each radiograph taken of the phantom and/or other radiographs provided by your instructor should be evaluated as described in your lab manual. Critique and evaluate each radiograph for errors of less-than-optimal positioning or exposure factors based on radiographic criteria provided in the textbook. Also, with the help of your instructor, learn how to discriminate between less-than-optimal, but passable radiographs, and those that need to be repeated. This generally requires additional experience and practice before you can make these judgments without assistance from a supervising technologist or radiologist.

Step 6. Self-Test

You should **take the self-test only after you have completed all of the preceding steps.** Treat the self-test like an actual exam. After you have completed it, compare your answers with the answer sheet at the end of this workbook. If your score is less than 90% to 95%, you should go back and review the textbook again; pay special attention to the areas you missed before you take the final chapter evaluation exam provided by your instructor.

Warning: Statistics prove that students who diligently complete all the exercises described in this section will invariably get higher grades in their positioning courses and will perform better in the clinical setting than those who don't. **Avoid the temptation of taking shortcuts.** If you bypass some of these exercises or just fill in the answers from the answer sheets, your instructors will know by your grade and by your clinical performance that you have taken these shortcuts. Most importantly, you will know that you are not doing your best and you will have difficulty competing with better prepared technologists in the job market when you graduate.

Go to it and enjoy the feeling of satisfaction and success that only comes when you know you're doing your best!

Radiographic Positioning AND Related Anatomy Workbook AND Laboratory Manual

VOLUME 1

Principles, Terminology, and Radiation Protection

CHAPTER OBJECTIVES

After you have successfully completed the activities in this chapter, you will be able to:

A. GENERAL, SYSTEMIC, AND SKELETAL ANATOMY AND ARTHROLOGY

_____ 1. List the four basic types of tissues.

_____ 2. List the 10 systems of the body.

_____ 3. Match specific bodily functions to their correct anatomic system.

_____ 4. List the four general classifications of bone.

_____ 5. Identify specific characteristics and aspects of bone.

_____ 6. Classify specific joints by their structure and function.

_____ 7. Classify specific synovial joints by their movement.

B. RADIOGRAPHIC TERMINOLOGY

_____ 1. Define general radiographic and anatomic relational terminology.

_____ 2. Define the imaginary planes, sections, and surfaces of the body used to describe central ray angles or relationships among body parts.

_____ 3. Distinguish among a radiographic projection, position, and view.

_____ 4. Given various hypothetical situations, identify the correct radiographic projection.

_____ 5. Given various hypothetical situations, identify the correct radiographic position.

_____ 6. List the antonyms (terms with opposite meanings) of specific terms related to movement.

C. BASIC IMAGING PRINCIPLES

_____ 1. Identify the criteria for evaluating a radiograph for positioning accuracy and image quality.

_____ 2. Identify the importance of collimation, anatomic side markers, and proper radiograph identification.

_____ 3. List the four image quality factors of a radiograph.

_____ 4. Define _radiographic density_ and identify its controlling factors.

_____ 5. Given a hypothetical situation, select the correct factor to improve radiographic density.

_____ 6. Define _radiographic contrast_ and identify its controlling factors.

_____ 7. Distinguish between long- and short-scale radiographic contrast.

_____ 8. Given a hypothetical situation, select the correct factor to improve radiographic contrast.

_____ 9. Define _radiographic detail._

_____ 10. List the three geometric factors that influence image sharpness.

_____ 11. Identify the best ways of controlling voluntary and involuntary motion.

_____ 12. Given a hypothetical situation, select the correct factor to improve radiographic detail.

_____ 13. Define _radiographic distortion_ and identify its controlling factors.

_____ 14. Given a hypothetical situation, select the correct factor to minimize radiographic distortion.

_____ 15. Define the _anode heel effect._

_____ 16. Identify how the application of the anode heel effect can affect radiographic quality.

D. POSITIONING PRINCIPLES

_____ 1. Given a hypothetical clinical situation, identify the response as required in the professional code of ethics.

_____ 2. Identify the correct sequence of steps taken to perform a routine radiographic procedure.

_____ 3. Given a set of circumstances, apply the two general rules of radiography concerning the minimal number of projections required for specific regions of the body.

_____ 4. Match the correct vertebral level to specific topographical landmarks.

_____ 5. List the four types of body habitus.

_____ 6. Identify the correct way to view a conventional radiograph, computed tomography (CT) image, and magnetic resonance (MR) image.

E. DIGITAL IMAGING

_____ 1. Define the acronym _PACS._

_____ 2. Identify general differences and similarities between CT and digital fluoroscopy.

_____ 3. Identify the major components of a digital fluoroscopy system.

_____ 4. Identify the components of the computed radiography (CR) image plate.

_____ 5. Identify the steps required to process an image produced with CR.

_____ 6. Identify the impact of correct centering, collimation, use of lead masking, and use of grids on the overall quality of the CR image.

_____ 7. Identify specific differences and similarities between computed radiography (CR) and digital radiography (DR).

_____ 8. Identify specific differences between conventional and digital chest radiography.

_____ 9. List advantages and disadvantages of digital mammography.

F. RADIATION PROTECTION

_____ 1. List and define the traditional units and International System of Units (SI units) of radiation measurement and the conversion factors used to convert between systems.

_____ 2. List the specific annual dose limiting recommendations of _whole body effective dose_ for the general population and occupationally exposed workers.

_____ 3. Define _ALARA._

_____ 4. Apply the principles of ALARA to any given hypothetical situation.

_____ 5. Define _skin entrance exposure (SEE)_ and _effective dose (ED)._

_____ 6. Identify specific methods to reduce exposure to the radiographer during fluoroscopic and radiographic procedures.

_____ 7. Identify specific methods to reduce exposure to the patient during radiographic procedures.

_____ 8. Identify the major types of area and gonadal shields and the minimum lead equivalent thickness requirements of these shields.

_____ 9. Define the *10-day rule* and describe its limitations.

_____ 10. Define patient dose terminology for specific regions of the body.

Learning Activity Exercises

The following review exercises should be completed only after careful study of the associated pages in the textbook as indicated by each exercise. Because certain topics may be too advanced for the entry-level student, the review exercises for Chapter 1 are divided into sections A through F. Students can complete specific sections of review exercises as directed by their instructor, to best meet their learning needs.

After completing each of these individual exercises, check your answers with the answers provided at the end of the review exercises.

REVIEW EXERCISE A: General, Systemic, and Skeletal Anatomy and Arthrology (see textbook pp. 2 to 13)

1. The lowest level of the structural organization of the human body is the _____ .

2. List the four basic types of tissues of the body:

   A. _____   C. _____

   B. _____   D. _____

3. List the ten systems of the human body:

   A. _____   F. _____

   B. _____   G. _____

   C. _____   H. _____

   D. _____   I. _____

   E. _____   J. _____

4. Match the following functions to the correct body system:

   _____ 1. Eliminate solid waste from the body   A. Skeletal system

   _____ 2. Regulate fluid and electrolyte balance and volume   B. Circulatory system

   _____ 3. Maintain posture   C. Digestive system

   _____ 4. Regulate body activities with electrical impulses   D. Respiratory system

   _____ 5. Regulate bodily activities through various hormones   E. Urinary system

   _____ 6. Eliminate carbon dioxide from blood   F. Reproductive system

   _____ 7. Receive stimuli such as temperature, pressure, and pain G. Nervous system

   _____ 8. Reproduce the organism   H. Muscular system

   _____ 9. Helps regulate body temperature   I. Endocrine system

   _____ 10. Store calcium   J. Integumentary system

5. True/False: One of the six functions of the circulatory system is to protect against disease.

6. List the two divisions of the human skeletal system:

   A. _____   B. _____

7. True/False: The adult skeleton system contains 256 separate bones.

8. True/False: The scapula is part of the axial skeleton.

9. True/False: The skull is part of the axial skeleton.

10. True/False: The pelvis is part of the appendicular skeleton.

11. List the four classifications of bones:

    A. _____   C. _____

    B. _____   D. _____

12. The outer covering of a long bone, which is composed of a dense, fibrous membrane, is called what?

    A. Spongy or cancellous bone   C. Medullary aspect

    B. Compact bone   D. Periosteum

13. Which aspect of long bones is responsible for the production of red blood cells?

    A. Spongy or cancellous bone   C. Medullary aspect

    B. Compact bone   D. Periosteum

14. Which aspect of the long bone is essential for bone growth, repair, and nutrition?

    A. Medullary aspect   C. Periosteum

    B. Compact bone   D. Articular cartilage

15. What are the primary and secondary growth centers for long bones?

    A. Primary growth center: _____   B. Secondary growth center: _____

16. True/False: Epiphyseal fusion of the long bones is complete by the age of 16 years.

17. The study of joints or articulations is called _____ .

18. List the three *functional* classifications of joints:

    A. _____

    B. _____

    C. _____

19. List the three *structural* classifications of joints:

    A. _____

    B. _____

    C. _____

20. Match the following joints to the correct structural classification:

———— 1. First carpometacarpal of thumb   A. Fibrous joint

———— 2. Roots around teeth   B. Cartilaginous joint

———— 3. Proximal radioulnar joint   C. Synovial joint

———— 4. Skull sutures

———— 5. Epiphyses

———— 6. Interphalangeal joints

———— 7. Distal tibiofibular joint

———— 8. Intervertebral disk space

———— 9. Symphysis pubis

———— 10. Hip joint

21. List the six types of movement for synovial joints. (List both the preferred terms and the synonyms.):

A. _____   D. _____

B. _____   E. _____

C. _____   F. _____

22. Match the following synovial joints to the correct type of movement:

———— 1. First carpometacarpal joint   A. Plane

———— 2. Elbow joint   B. Ginglymus

———— 3. Shoulder joint   C. Trochoid

———— 4. Intercarpal joint   D. Ellipsoid

———— 5. Wrist joint   E. Sellar

———— 6. Third metacarpophalangeal joint   F. Spheroid

———— 7. First and second cervical vertebra joint

———— 8. Second interphalangeal joint

———— 9. Distal radioulnar joint

———— 10. Ankle joint

REVIEW EXERCISE B: Radiographic Terminology (see textbook pp. 14 to 29)

1. A _____ is an x-ray film containing an image of an anatomic part of a patient.

2. An upright position with the arms abducted, palms forward, and head and feet directed straight ahead describes the _____ position.

3. The vertical plane that divides the body into equal right and left parts is the _____ plane.

4. The vertical plane that divides the body into equal anterior and posterior parts is the _____ plane.

5. A plane taken at right angles along any point of the longitudinal axis of the body is the _____ plane.

6. True/False: *Reid's base line* is a plane located between the infraorbital margin of the orbit and the external auditory meatus.

7. True/False: Reid's base line is also referred to as *the anthropological plane.*

8. The direction or path of the central ray of the x-ray beam defines the following positioning term:

   A. Projection   C. Position

   B. View   D. Perspective

9. The positioning term that describes the general and specific body position is:

   A. Projection   C. Position

   B. View   D. Perspective

10. True/False: Oblique positions are described according to the side of the body closest to image receptor.

11. True/False: Decubitus positions always utilize a horizontal x-ray beam.

12. What is the name of the position in which the body is turned 90° from a true anteroposterior (AP) or posteroanterior (PA) projection? _____

13. **Situation:** A patient is erect with the back to the image receptor. The left side of the body is turned 45° toward the image receptor. What is this position? _____

14. **Situation:** A patient is recumbent facing the image receptor. The right side of the body is turned 15° toward the image receptor. What is this position? _____

15. **Situation:** The patient is lying on the back. The x-ray beam is directed horizontally and enters the right side of the body. An image receptor is placed against the left side of the patient. Which specific position has been used? _____

16. **Situation:** The patient is erect with the right side of the body against the image receptor. The x-ray beam enters the left side of the body. Which specific position has been used? _____

17. **Situation:** A patient is placed lying on the left side on a cart. The x-ray beam is directed horizontally and enters the posterior aspect of the body. The image receptor is against the anterior surface. Which specific position has been used? _____

18. Match the following definitions to the correct term (using each term only once):

    _____ 1. Palm of the hand   A. Posterior

    _____ 2. Lying on the back facing upward   B. Anterior

    _____ 3. An upright position   C. Plantar

    _____ 4. Lying down in any position   D. Dorsum

    _____ 5. Front half of the patient   E. Trendelenburg

    _____ 6. Top or anterior surface of the foot   F. Erect

    _____ 7. Position in which head is higher than the feet   G. Supine

    _____ 8. Posterior aspect of foot   H. Palmar

    _____ 9. Position where head is lower than feet   I. Recumbent

    _____ 10. Back half of patient   J. Fowler

19. What is the name of the projection in which the central ray enters the anterior surface and exits the posterior surface? _____

20. A projection directed parallel to or at an angle along the long axis of the body or a part is called a/an _____ projection.

21. The specific position that demonstrates the apices of the lungs, without superimposition of the clavicles, is called a _____ .

22. True/False: The radiographic view is the radiographic image seen from the vantage point of the image receptor.

23. True/False: The term *varus* describes the bending of a part outward.

24. Match the following:

    _____ 1. Anteroposterior   A. Position

    _____ 2. Lying on abdomen   B. Projection

    _____ 3. Trendelenburg

    _____ 4. Left posterior oblique

    _____ 5. Left lateral chest

    _____ 6. Mediolateral ankle

    _____ 7. Apical AP

    _____ 8. Lordotic

    _____ 9. Transthoracic

    _____ 10. Left lateral decubitus

25. List the term that has the **opposite** meaning for each term that follows:

    A. Flexion: _____

    B. Ulnar deviation: _____

    C. Dorsiflexion: _____

    D. Eversion: _____

    E. Lateral (external) rotation: _____

    F. Abduction: _____

    G. Supination: _____

    H. Retraction: _____

    I. Depression: _____

26. Match the following relationship terms to the correct definition (using each term only once):

    _____ 1. Near the source or beginning   A. Caudad or inferior

    _____ 2. On the opposite side   B. Deep

    _____ 3. Toward the center   C. Distal

    _____ 4. Toward the head end of the body   D. Contralateral

    _____ 5. Away from the source or beginning   E. Cephalad or superior

    _____ 6. Outside or outward   F. Proximal

    _____ 7. On the same side   G. Medial

    _____ 8. Near the skin surface   H. Superficial

    _____ 9. Away from the head end   I. Ipsilateral

    _____ 10. Farther from the skin surface   J. Exterior

27. Moving or thrusting the jaw forward from the normal position is an example of _____ .

28. To turn or bend the wrist toward the radius side is called _____ .

REVIEW EXERCISE C: Basic Imaging Principles (see textbook pp. 30 to 38)

1. The restriction of the x-ray beam to include only essential anatomy being recorded on the image receptor (IR) is called:

    A. Central ray placement   C. Beam restriction

    B. Milliamperage seconds   D. Collimation

2. Which two identification markers must be placed and seen on all radiographs?

    A. _____   B. _____

3. True/False: A radiograph taken without the two necessary identification markers visible on the radiograph may need to be repeated (see previous question).

4. List the four image quality factors of a radiograph:

   A. _____ C. _____

   B. _____ D. _____

5. Which specific exposure factor controls the quality or penetrating ability of the x-ray beam? _____

6. The amount of blackness seen on a processed radiograph is called _____ .

7. The controlling factor for the overall blackness on a radiograph is _____ .

8. If the distance between the x-ray tube and image receptor is increased from 40 to 80 inches, what specific effect will it have on the radiographic density if other factors are not changed?

   A. Increase density to 50%   C. No effect on density

   B. Decrease density to 25%   D. Decrease density to 50%

9. Which term is used to describe a radiograph that has too little density? _____

10. **Situation:** A radiograph of the foot is produced using conventional film-screen cassettes. The resulting radiograph demonstrates too little density and must be repeated. The original exposure was 5 mAs. What milliamperage seconds is needed to correct the density on this radiograph?

    A. 5 mAs   C. 20 mAs

    B. 7.5 mAs   D. 10 mAs

11. True/False: The use of digital radiography systems does not give the radiographer the ability to manipulate image density once it is recorded.

12. The difference in density between two adjacent areas of the radiograph defines _____ .

13. List the two scales of radiographic contrast, and identify which is high and which is low contrast:

    A. _____ B. _____

14. Which scale of contrast is produced with a 110 kVp technique? _____

15. True/False: A 50 kVp technique produces a **high** contrast image.

16. True/False: A **low** contrast image demonstrates more shades of gray on the radiograph.

17. What is the primary controlling factor for radiographic contrast? _____

18. What percent increase in the original kilovoltage peak (kVp) is needed to double the density on a radiograph?

    _____

19. **Situation:** A radiograph of the hand is underexposed and must be repeated. The original technique used was 55 kVp with 2.5 mAs. The technologist decides to keep the mAs at the same level but change the kVp to increase radiographic density. How much of an increase is needed in kilovoltage peak to double the density?

    A. 3 to 5 kVp increase   C. 10 to 15 kVp increase

    B. 8 to 10 kVp increase   D. 15 to 20 kVp increase

20. Which one of the following set of exposure factors will result in the least patient exposure and produce long scale contrast for a PA chest radiographic image?

    A. 50 kVp, 800 mAs   C. 80 kVp, 100 mAs

    B. 70 kVp, 200 mAs   D. 110 kVp 10 mAs

21. The visible sharpness of structures or objects on the radiograph defines _____ .

22. The lack of visible detail is called _____ .

23. List the three **geometric** factors that control or influence image sharpness:

    A. _____

    B. _____

    C. _____

24. What is the best mechanism to control involuntary motion during an exposure?

    A. Use of the small focal spot   C. Decrease object image-receptor distance (OID)

    B. Use of a grid   D. Shorten exposure time

25. Which one of the following changes will improve recorded detail?

    A. Decrease OID   C. Use a large focal spot

    B. Decrease source image-receptor distance (SID)   D. Use a higher kilovoltage peak

26. **Situation:** The radiographer is performing an elbow series on a young pediatric patient. It is essential that the radiographs reflect the highest degree of recorded detail possible. Which one of the following set of factors will produce that level of detail?

    A. 0.3 mm focal spot and 30-inch SID   C. 0.5 mm focal spot and 40-inch SID

    B. 1 mm focal spot and 45-inch SID   D. 0.3 mm focal spot and 40-inch SID

27. The misrepresentation of an object size or shape projected onto a radiographic recording medium defines _____ .

28. True/False: Through careful selection and control of exposure and geometric factors, it is possible to eliminate all image distortion.

29. List the four controlling factors for distortion:

    A. _____   C. _____

    B. _____   D. _____

30. True/False: A decrease in SID reduces distortion.

31. True/False: An increase in OID reduces distortion.

32. True/False: Distortion is reduced when the central ray is kept perpendicular to the film.

33. The SID for general radiographic procedures resulting in the least patient exposure and maximum recorded detail is:

    A. 40 inches (100 cm)   C. 44 inches (110 cm)

    B. 72 inches (180 cm)   D. 48 inches (120 cm)

34. **Situation:** A chest x-ray on a patient with an enlarged heart has been requested. Which one of the following SIDs is recommended for this study?

    A. 40 inches (100 cm)   C. 44 inches (110 cm)

    B. 72 inches (180 cm)   D. 48 inches (120 cm)

35. True/False: Every radiographic image reflects some degree of penumbra or unsharpness, even if the smallest focal spot is used.

36. True/False: As the distance of between the object and the image receptor is increased, magnification is reduced.

37. True/False: Image distortion increases as the angle of divergence increases from the center of the x-ray beam to the outer edges.

38. According to the anode heel effect, the x-ray beam is less intense at the (cathode or anode) end of the x-ray tube _____.

39. To best utilize the anode heel effect, the thicker part of the anatomic structure should be placed under the (cathode or anode) end of the x-ray tube. _____

REVIEW EXERCISE D: Positioning Principles (see textbook pp. 39 to 47)

1. True/False: Radiographers have the right to refuse to perform an examination on a patient whom they find offensive.

2. True/False: Radiographers are responsible for the professional decisions they make during the care of the patient.

3. True/False: The radiographer has the responsibility of communicating with the patient to obtain pertinent clinical information.

4. True/False: The radiographer is expected to provide a preliminary interpretation of radiographic findings to the referring physician.

5. True/False: The radiographer may reveal confidential information pertaining to a patient who is less than 18 years of age to the patient or guardian.

6. A *PBL* collimator refers to:

    A. Positive beam limiting   C. Patient based life-saving

    B. Power beam limiting   D. Penumbra biased limiting

7. True/False: PBL collimators are required for all x-rays units manufactured after 1995.

8. Which one of the following steps should be performed first during a positioning routine?

    A. Film centering   C. Placing anatomic side markers on cassette

    B. Placing gonadal shielding as needed   D. Patient and part positioning

9. What is the final step taken before making the exposure during a positioning routine?

    A. Image receptor centering   C. Collimation

    B. Placing anatomic markers on cassette   D. Ensuring correct gonadal shield placement

10. List the two rules or principles for determining positioning routines as they relate to the maximum number of projections required in a basic routine:

    A. _____   B. _____

11. Indicate the minimum number of projections required for the following anatomic regions:

    A. Foot _____   F. Fifth toe _____

    B. Chest _____   G. Postreduction of wrist (image of wrist in cast) _____

    C. Wrist _____   H. Left hip _____

    D. Tibia/fibula _____   I. Knee _____

    E. Humerus _____

12. **Situation:** A young child enters the emergency room with a fractured forearm. After one projection is completed, which confirms a fracture, the child refuses to move the forearm for any additional projections.

    A. What is the minimum number of projections that should be taken for this forearm study?

        (a) One   (c) Three

        (b) Four   (d) Two

B.   If additional projections are required for a routine forearm series, what should the radiographer do with the patient described in this situation?

(a) Because only one projection is required fora fractured forearm, the radiographer is not required to take additional projections.

(b) With the help of a parent or guardian, gently but firmly move the forearm for each additional projection required.

(c) Rather than move the forearm for a second projection, place the cassette and x-ray tube as needed for a second projection 90° from the first projection.

(d) Ask the emergency room physician to move the forearm for a second projection. This eliminates any liability for the radiographer in case the patient is injured further.

13. Match the metric measurements for image receptor sizes to the nearest equivalent traditional size:

        METRIC   *TRADITIONAL (ENGLISH)*

____   1. 24 × 30 cm   A.   14 × 17 inches

____   2. 18 × 24 cm   B.   14 × 36 inches

____   3. 35 × 43 cm   C.   12 × 14 inches

____   4. 30 × 35 cm   D.   10 × 12 inches

____   5. 24 × 24 cm   E.   8 × 10 inches

____   6. 35 × 90 cm   F.   8 × 8 inches

14. Match the following topographical landmarks to the corresponding vertebral level:

____   1. Sternal angle   A.   T9-10

____   2. Anterior superior iliac spine   B.   L2-3

____   3. Xiphoid process   C.   T4-5

____   4. Iliac crest   D.   S1-2

____   5. Jugular notch   E.   T2-3

____   6. Inferior costal margin   F.   L4-5

15. The physical localization of bony landmarks on a patient is called _____ .

16. The greater trochanter is located on the:

A. Proximal femur   B. Cervical spine   C. Sternum   D. Lower pelvis

17. The ischial tuberosity corresponds with the vertebral level of:

A. T9-10   C. S1-2

B. L4-5 interspace   D. 1 to 2 inches inferior to distal coccyx

18. List the four types of body habitus:

A. _____   C. _____

B. _____   D. _____

19. Which type of body habitus is described as being "average?" _____

20. What percentage of the population has this "average" body type? _____

Questions 21 to 24 refer to Figs. A and B:

21. Which body habitus type is represented by Fig. A ? _____

22. Which body habitus type is represented by Fig. B? _____

23. What percentage of the population has the body habitus type in Fig. A?

   _____

24. What percentage of the population has the body habitus type in Fig. B?

   _____

25. True/False: Always place a radiograph for viewing as the x-ray tube "sees" the patient. (The patient's left is to the viewer's left on PA projections.)

26. True/False: CT images are viewed so that the patient's right is to the viewer's left.

A   B

REVIEW EXERCISE E: Digital Imaging (see textbook, pp. 48-52)

1. True/False: Digital imaging requires that images still be chemically processed.

2. True/False: CT has been used since the late 1970s.

3. True/False: The visible image produced with digital imaging is called the *analog* image.

4. True/False: Direct capture digital imaging does not require the use of an image intensifier.

5. True/False: PACS automatically transport conventional x-rays films to the chemical processor after they have been exposed.

6. Define the acronym *PACS:*

   P : _____

   A : _____

   C : _____

   S : _____

7. Which of the following imaging modalities is/are *not* part of a PACS network?

   A. Nuclear medicine   D. Digital fluoroscopy

   B. Ultrasound   E. Digital mammography

   C. Conventional film/screen radiography F. Computed radiography

8. Which one of the following devices is *not* required in the design of the digital fluoroscopy system?

   A. X-ray tube   C. Video camera

   B. Optics   D. Cassette filming device

9. What is the name of the device found in advanced digital fluoroscopy systems that eliminates the need for the image intensifier, video camera, and the analog-to-digital converter? _____

10. With CR, the IR plate:

    A. Must be kept in a light tight cassette

    B. Must be used in conjunction with light-sensitive film

    C. Must be used in conjunction with intensifying screens

    D. None of the above

11. When using a CR image plate, patient data can be recorded by use of a/an:

    A. Bar code reader   C. Laser

    B. White light source   D. Ultraviolet light source

12. True/False: Once the CR image plate has had an image recorded on it, it must be discarded.

13. True/False: The latent or recorded image on a CR image plate is read line by line by a laser.

14. True/False: A special double emulsion film is used to print actual hard copy of CR images.

15. True/False: It takes approximately 20 seconds to process a CR image and reload the cassette with a clean imaging plate.

16. CR permits exposure factor compensation even with over exposures of _____ when automatic exposure control (AEC) is not used.

    A. 10%   C. 30%

    B. 85%   D. 500%

17. What is the only indicator that the ideal exposure factors were utilized with a CR system?

    A. Kilovoltage peak and millamperage seconds used   C. Outcome of actual image

    B. Exposure index number   D. Laser read out index

18. True/False: If careful collimation is used for multiple images placed on the same image plate, the use of lead masking is not necessary.

19. True/False: Because of the sensitivity of the CR image plate, part centering is not as critical as it is with film-screen systems.

20. True/False: The use of aggressive collimation is discouraged with CR.

21. True/False: The use of grids is not required with CR, even when radiographing a thick anatomic part.

22. True/False: The images produced with digital chest radiography still require chemical processing.

23. A common detector size for digital chest radiography units is:

    A. 27.9 × 35.6 cm   C. 43 × 43 cm

    B. 43 × 49 cm   D. 19 × 23 cm

24. In direct capture digital radiography:

    A. A CR image plate is required.

    B. Image plates are not required.

    C. Visible images must be chemically processed.

    D. The kilovoltage peak and milliamperage seconds for each exposure must be manually set.

25. A common size for the new type of digital detector table Bucky is:

    A. 43 × 43 cm (17 × 17 inches)   C. 35 × 43 cm (14 × 17 inches)

    B. 35 × 90 cm (14 × 36 inches)   D. 30 × 35 cm (12 × 14 inches)

26. True/False: A drawback with digital mammography units is a significant loss in image quality as compared to film-screen systems.

27. Sending images to remote locations through high-speed telephone lines or by satellite is:

    A. Teleradiology   C. Image reconstruction

    B. Impossible   D. Computed radiography

28. True/False: The major disadvantage of digital mammography is the initial equipment cost.

29. True/False: PACS provide the ability to view images at multiple sites simultaneously.

30. True/False: PACS still require storage of hard-copy images for medicolegal reasons.

31. True/False: Existing radiographic equipment (x-ray tubes) must be modified when using a CR system.

32. True/False: One of the disadvantges of using a CR system is the possibility of excessive exposure to the patient when using manual techniques.

33. True/False: The shortage of qualified installation and service personnel has limited the widespread use of DR.

34. Write the complete term for the following digital imaging acronyms:

    A. DICOM _____

    B. DF _____

    C. DR _____

    D. CT _____

    E. RIS _____

    F. HIS_____

REVIEW EXERCISE F: Radiation Protection (see textbook pp. 53-61)

1. Which traditional unit is used to measure radiation exposure in air? _____

2. Which traditional unit of measurement is used to describe patient dose? _____

3. What does the acronym *ED* stand for? _____

4. What is the **whole body effective** dose limit per year for a radiographer (in traditional and International System (SI) units)_____

5. What is the cumulative lifetime dose for a 35-year-old radiographer (in traditional and SI units)?
   _____

6. List the SI units of radiation measurement and its symbol for the following traditional units:

TRADITIONAL UNIT	*SI UNIT*
A. Roentgen (R)	_____
B. Radiation absorbed dose (rad)	_____
C. Radiation equivalent man (rem)	_____

7. Convert the following doses, stated in traditional units, into the appropriate SI units:

   A. 3 rad = _____ Gy   C. 38 rem = _____ Sv

   B. 448 mrad = _____ mGy   D. 15 rem = _____ mSv

8. What is the maximum dose limit for a pregnant radiographer?

    A. Per month: _____

    B. For the entire gestational period: _____

9. The acronym **ALARA** stands for _____ .

10. **Situation:** A young child comes to radiology for a skull series. The child is combative and will not hold still for the procedure. Which one of the following individuals should be asked to restrain the patient?

    A. A family member (if not pregnant)   C. The oldest radiographer

    B. A student radiographer   D. A nuclear medicine technologist

11. True/False: With accurate and close collimation, area shields do not need to be used.

12. True/False: Skin entrance exposure (SEE) has the highest numerical value of all patient doses.

13. True/False: In radiography, SEE carries the least biological significance.

14. True/False: Effective dose (ED) describes gonadal dose levels only for each radiographic procedure.

15. What is the best method of reducing scatter to a worker's eyes and neck during fluoroscopy?

    _____

16. Which of the following is the best place for a radiographer to stand during fluoroscopy to reduce occupational exposure?

    A. Head end of table   C. Behind the radiologist

    B. Foot end of table   D. Next to the radiologist

17. What is the federal standards set limit for exposure rates for intensified fluoroscopy units?

    A. 1 R/min   C. 3 to 4 R/min

    B. 6 to 8 R/min   D. 10 R/min

18. With most modern fluoroscopy equipment, the average exposure rate is:

    A. 0.5 R/min   C. 1 R/min

    B. 3 to 4 R/min   D. 10 R/min

19. What is one of the **primary** causes for repeat radiographs? (Select the best answer.)

    A. Excessive kilovoltage peak   C. Poor communication between radiographer and patient

    B. Wrong film selection   D. Distortion caused by incorrect SID

20. In addition to the primary cause identified in the previous question, what two other factors often lead to repeat exposures?

    A. _____

    B. _____

21. Refer to the Patient Dose chart on p. 55 of the textbook to answer these questions (A to G)

    A. Which chest projection, AP or PA, provides the greatest ED for females? _____

    B. Which gender receives a greater ED for an AP hip? With or without gonadal shielding? _____

C. List the gonadal dose for male and female patients for an AP abdomen projection using 70 kVp:

Male, shielded: _____   Female, unshielded: _____

Male, unshielded: _____

D. Which specific organ in each gender receives the greatest dose in AP, PA, and lateral upper GI projections: lungs, testes, ovaries, thyroid, marrow, or breast?_____

E. List the gonadal doses for an AP hip projection with and without shielding:

Male without shielding (testes): _____   Female without shielding (ovaries): _____

Male with shielding: _____   Female with shielding: _____

F. Which radiographic procedure listed on this chart provides the **least amount of SEE** for males and females? (Note the correlation among kilovoltage peak, milliamperage seconds and dose.)_____

G. Which procedure on the chart provides the **greatest amount** of ED for a **male** patient? _____ For a **female** patient? _____

22. If a radiographer receives 3.3 to 6.7 mR/min standing 1 foot from a fluoroscopy unit, what will the dose be if the radiographer moves to a distance of 4 feet (see Exposure Levels chart on p. 56)?

A. Less than 0.25 mR/min   C.   0.8 to 1.7 mR/min

B.   0.4 to 0.8 mR/min   D.   1.7 to 3 mR /min

23. List the two major forms of filtration found in x-ray tubes that affect the quality of the primary x-ray beam:

A. _____

B. _____

24. What is the most common metal used in filters for diagnostic radiology equipment? _____

25. List the two ways collimation will reduce patient exposure:

A. _____

B. _____

26. True/False: Safety standards require that collimators be accurate to within 10% of the selected SID.

27. True/False: Positive beam limitation (PBL) collimators restrict the size of the exposure field to the size of the cassette in a Bucky tray.

28. True/False: PBL collimators became optional on new equipment manufactured after May, 1993, because of a change in Food and Drug Administration (FDA) regulations.

29. List the two general types of area shields:

A. _____

B. _____

30. The minimum thickness of a gonadal shield placed within the primary x-ray field should be:

A. 0.1-mm lead equivalent   C.   1-mm lead equivalent

B.   0.25-mm lead equivalent   D.   0.5-mm lead equivalent

31. If placed properly, gonadal shields absorb _____ of the primary beam in the 50 to 100 kVp range.

    A. 95% to 99%   C. 70% to 80%

    B. 80% to 90%   D. 50% to 70%

32. An area shield should be used when radiation-sensitive tissues lie within _____ inches or _____ cm of the primary beam.

33. According to the 10-day rule, when is the safest time for a female of child-bearing age to have a radiographic examination of the lower abdomen and pelvis?

    A. 10 days before beginning of menses   C. First 10 days of each month

    B. 10 days after onset of menses   D. Last 10 days of each month

34. True/False: The 10-day rule is considered by the International Commission on Radiological Protection (ICRP) and American College of Radiology as being obsolete and no longer valid.

35. **Situation:** A 20-year-old female enters the emergency room with a possible fracture of the pelvis. What should the technologist do in regard to gonadal shielding?

    A. Use it for all projections   C. Ask the patient whether she is pregnant

    B. Use it for the AP projections only   D. Do not use shielding for initial pelvis projection

36. What is the disadvantage of using faster-speed screens for all film-screen radiographic procedures?

    _____

37. List the complete term for the following abbreviations used in patient dose icon boxes (in positioning pages of text):

    A. Sk: _____

    B. ML: _____

    C. Gon: _____

    D. NDC: _____

38. True/False: Area shields must be used for all radiographic procedures with all patients.

Answers to Review Exercises

Review Exercise A: General, Systemic, and Skeletal Anatomy and Arthrology

1. Chemical level
2. A. Epithelial
   B. Connective
   C. Muscular
   D. Nervous
3. A. Skeletal
   B. Circulatory
   C. Digestive
   D. Respiratory
   E. Urinary
   F. Reproductive
   G. Nervous
   H. Muscular
   I. Endocrine
   J. Integumentary
4. 1. C
   2. E
   3. H
   4. G
   5. I
   6. D
   7. J
   8. F
   9. B
   10. A
5. True
6. A. Axial skeleton
   B. Appendicular skeleton
7. False (206)
8. False (part of appendicular)
9. True
10. True
11. A. Long bones
    B. Short bones
    C. Flat bones
    D. Irregular bones
12. D. Periosteum
13. C. Medullary aspect
14. C. Periosteun
15. A. Body (midshaft or diaphysis)
    B. Epiphyses
16. False
17. Arthrology
18. A. Synarthrosis
    B. Amphiarthrosis
    C. Diarthrosis
19. A. Fibrous
    B. Cartilaginous
    C. Synovial
20. 1. C
    2. A
    3. C
    4. A
    5. B
    6. C
    7. A
    8. B
    9. B
    10. C
21. A. Plane (gliding)
    B. Ginglymus (hinge)
    C. Trochoid (pivot)
    D. Ellipsoidal (condyloid)
    E. Sellar (saddle)
    F. Spheroid (ball and socket)
22. 1. E
    2. B
    3. F
    4. A
    5. D
    6. D
    7. C
    8. B
    9. C
    10. B

Review Exercise B: Radiographic Terminology

1. Radiograph
2. Anatomic
3. Median or midsagittal plane
4. Midcoronal plane
5. Transverse or axial
6. True
7. True
8. A. Projection
9. C. Position
10. True
11. True
12. Lateral position
13. Left posterior oblique (LPO)
14. Right anterior oblique (RAO)
15. Dorsal decubitus (left lateral)
16. Right lateral
17. Left lateral decubitus (PA)
18. 1. H
    2. G
    3. F
    4. I
    5. B
    6. D
    7. J
    8. C
    9. E
    10. A
19. Anteroposterior (AP)
20. Axial
21. Lordotic position
22. True
23. False (inward, toward midline)
24. 1. B
    2. A
    3. A
    4. A
    5. A
    6. B
    7. B
8. A
9. B
10. A
25. A. Extension
    B. Radial deviation
    C. Plantar flexion
    D. Inversion
    E. Medial (internal) rotation
    F. Adduction
    G. Pronation
    H. Protraction
    I. Elevation
26. 1. F
    2. D
    3. G
    4. E
    5. C
    6. J
    7. I
    8. H
    9. A
    10. B
27. Protraction
28. Radial deviation

Review Exercise C: Basic Imaging Principles

1. D. Collimation
2. A. Patient identification
   B. Anatomic side marker
3. True
4. A. Density
   B. Contrast
   C. Recorded detail
   D. Distortion
5. Kilovoltage peak (kVp)
6. Density
7. Milliamperage seconds (mAs)
8. B. Decrease density to 25%
9. Underexposed
10. D. 10 mAs (double mAs)
11. False
12. Radiographic contrast
13. A. Long-scale contrast (low contrast)
    B. Short-scale contrast (high contrast)
14. Long-scale contrast (low)
15. True
16. True
17. Kilovoltage peak (kVp)
18. 15%
19. B. 8 to 10 kVp increase
20. D. 110 kVp 10 mAs
21. Detail or definition
22. Blur or unsharpness
23. A. Focal spot size
    B. Source image-receptor distance (SID)
    C. Object image-receptor distance (OID)

24. D. Shorten exposure time
25. A. Decrease OID
26. D. 0.3 mm focal spot and 40 inch SID
27. Distortion
28. False (There is always some magnification and distortion caused by OID and divergence of the x-ray beam.)
29. A. Source-image distance (SID)
    B. Object image distance (OID)
    C. Object film alignment
    D. Central ray placement
30. False (increase distortion)
31. False (decrease distortion)
32. True
33. C. 44 inches (110 cm)
34. B. 72 inches (180 cm)
35. True
36. False
37. True
38. Anode
39. Cathode

Review Exercise D: Positioning Principles

1. False
2. True
3. True
4. False
5. False
6. A. Positive beam limiting
7. False
8. D. Patient and part positioning
9. D. Ensuring correct gonadal shielding
10. A. A minimum of two projections 90° from each other
    B. A minimum of three projections when joints are in the prime interest area
11. A. 3
    B. 2
    C. 3
    D. 2
    E. 2
    F. 3
    G. 2
    H. 2
    I. 3
12. A. (d) Two
    B. (c) Rather than move the forearm for additional projections, place the cassette and x-ray tube as needed.
13. 1. D
    2. E
    3. A
    4. C
    5. F
    6. B
14. 1. C
    2. D
    3. A

4. F
5. E
6. B
15. Palpation
16. A. Proximal femur
17. D. 1 to 2 inches inferior to distal coccyx
18. A. Hypersthenic
    B. Sthenic
    C. Hyposthenic
    D. Asthenic
19. Sthenic
20. 50%
21. A. Hypersthenic
22. B. Asthenic
23. 5%
24. 10%
25. False (Place as if radiographer were facing the patient; patient's right to radiographer's left.)
26. True

Review Exercise E: Digital Imaging

1. False
2. True
3. True
4. True
5. False
6. P: Picture
    A: Archiving
    C: Communication
    S: System
7. C. Conventional radiography
8. D. Cassette filming device
9. Direct conversion digital detector
10. D. None of the above
11. A. Bar code reader
12. False
13. True
14. False
15. True
16. D. 500%
17. B. Exposure index number
18. False
19. False
20. False
21. False
22. False
23. B. 43 × 49 cm
24. B. Image plates are not required.
25. A. 43 × 43 cm (17 × 17 inches)
26. False
27. A. Teleradiology
28. True
29. True
30. False
31. False
32. True
33. True
34. A. Digital imaging comunications in medicine
    B. Digital fluoroscopy

C. Direct digital radiography
D. Computed tomography
E. Radiology information system
F. Hospital information system

Review Exercise F: Radiation Protection

1. Roentgen
2. Rad
3. Effective dose
4. 5 rem (50 mSv) per year
5. 35 rem or 350 mSv
6. A. Coulombs per kilogram (C/kg) of air
    B. Gray (Gy)
    C. Seivert (Sv)
7. A. 0.03 Gy
    B. 4.48 mGy
    C. .38 Sv
    D. 150 mSv
8. A. 0.05 rem or (0.5 mSv)
    B. 0.5 rem or (5 mSv)
9. As low as reasonably achievable
10. A. Family member (if not pregnant)
11. False (still need to be used)
12. True
13. True
14. False (considers dose levels to all organs, see p. 38)
15. Keep the image intensifier tower as close as possible to the patient
16. C. Behind the radiologist
17. D. 10 R/min
18. B. 3 to 4 R/min
19. C. Poor communication between radiographer and patient
20. A. Carelessness in positioning
    B. Selection of incorrect exposure factors
21. A. AP (more than double because of increased thyroid and breast doses)
    B. Male (from greater dose to gonads because of proximity of testes to primary beam)
    C. Male, shielded: 2 mrad
       Male, unshielded: 6 mrad
       Female, unshielded: 80 mrad
    D. Lungs
    E. Male, unshielded: 322 mrad
       Male, shielded: 42 mrad
       Female, unshielded: 59 mrad
       Female, shielded: 14 mrad
    F. PA chest
    G. Male: AP hip projection without shielding
       Female: AP T spine on 14 × 17
22. B. 0.4 to 0.8 mR/min
23. A. Inherent
    B. Added
24. Aluminum
25. A. Reduces the volume of tissue irradiated

   B. Reduces the accompanying scatter radiation, which adds to patient dose
26. False (2%, not 10%)
27. True
28. True
29. A. Shadow shields
    B. Contact shields

30. C. 1-mm lead equivalent
31. A. 95% to 99%
32. 2 inches, 5 cm
33. B. 10 days after the onset of menses
34. True
35. D. Do not use it (for initial total pelvis projection).

36. Results in some loss of recorded detail
37. A. Skin dose
    B. Midline dose
    C. Gonadal dose
    D. No detectable contribution
38. False (only if it doesn't cover pertinent anatomic parts for that exam)

SELF-TEST

My Score = _____%

This series of self-tests should be taken only after completing all of the readings, review exercises, and laboratory activities for a particular section. This self-test is divided into six sections. The purpose of this test is not only to provide a good learning exercise but also to serve as a strong indicator of what your final evaluation grade will cover. It is strongly suggested that if you do not get at least a 90% to 95% grade on each self-test, you should review those areas in which you missed questions before going to your instructor for the final evaluation exam.

SELF-TEST A: General, Systemic, and Skeletal Anatomy and Arthrology

1. Which of the following are **not** one of the four basic types of tissue in the human body?

   A. Integumentary   D. Osseous

   B. Connective   E. Muscular

   C. Nervous   F. Epithelial

2. How many separate bones are found in the adult human body?

   A. 180   C. 206

   D. 243   D. 257

3. Which one of the following systems distributes oxygen and nutrients to the cells of the body?

   A. Digestive   C. Skeletal

   B. Circulatory   D. Urinary

4. Which one of the following systems maintains the acid-base balance in the body?

   A. Digestive   C. Reproductive

   B. Urinary   D. Circulatory

5. Which one of the following systems involves the skin and all structures derived from the skin?

   A. Muscular   C. Skeletal

   B. Endocrine   D. Integumentary

6. The two divisions of the human skeleton include:

   A. Bony and cartilaginous   C. Vertebral and extremities

   B. Axial and appendicular   D. Integumentary and appendicular

7. Which portion of the long bones is responsible for the production of red blood cells?

   A. Spongy or cancellous   C. Hyaline

   B. Periosteum   D. Compact aspect

8. What type of tissue covers the ends of the long bones?

   A. Spongy or cancellous   C. Hyaline or articular cartilage

   B. Periosteum   D. Compact aspect

9. The narrow space between the inner and outer table of the flat bones in the cranium is called the:

   A. Calvarium   C. Medullary portion

   B. Periosteum   D. Diploe

10. What is the primary center for endochondral ossification in long bones?

    A. Diaphysis (shaft)   C. Epiphyses

    B. Epiphyseal plate   D. Medulla

11. What is the name of secondary growth centers of endochondral ossification found in long bones?

    A. Diaphysis (shaft)   C. Epiphyses

    B. Epiphyseal plate   D. Medulla

12. A skull suture has the structural classification of a _____ joint.

    A. Fibrous   C. Synovial

    B. Cartilaginous   D. Diarthrosis

13. The symphysis pubis has the structural classification of a _____ joint.

    A. Fibrous   C. Synovial

    B. Cartilaginous   D. Synarthrosis

14. Which specific joint(s) is(are) the only true syndesmosis, amphiarthrodial, fibrous joint(s)?

    A. Joints between the roots of teeth and adjoining bone   C. Distal tibiofibular joint

    B. First carpometacarpal joint   D. Proximal and distal radioulnar joints

15. Match the following bones to their correct classification:

    _____ 1. Sternum   A. Long bone

    _____ 2. Femur   B. Short bone

    _____ 3. Tarsal bones   C. Flat bone

    _____ 4. Pelvic bones   D. Irregular bone

    _____ 5. Scapulae

    _____ 6. Humerus

    _____ 7. Vertebrae

    _____ 8. Calvarium

16. The three structural classifications of joints include synovial, cartilaginous, and:

    A. Amphiarthrodial   C. Diarthrodial

    B. Ellipsoid   D. Fibrous

17. Classify the following synovial joints based on their type of movement:

    _____ 1. First carpometacarpal joint   A. Plane (gliding)

    _____ 2. Intercarpal joint   B. Ginglymus (hinge)

    _____ 3. Hip joint   C. Trochoid (pivot)

    _____ 4. Proximal radioulnar joint   D. Ellipsoid (condyloid)

    _____ 5. Interphalangeal joint   E. Sellar (saddle)

    _____ 6. Fourth metacarpophalangeal joint   F. Spheroid (ball and socket)

    _____ 7. Knee joint

    _____ 8. Wrist joint

SELF-TEST B: Radiographic Terminology

1. Which plane divides the body into equal anterior and posterior parts?

   A. Sagittal   B. Transverse   C. Midcoronal   D. Longitudinal

2. True/False: The terms *radiograph* and *x-ray film* refer to the same thing.

3. A longitudinal plane that divides the body into right and left parts is the:

   A. Coronal plane   C. Sagittal plane

   B. Horizontal plane   D. Oblique plane

4. Match the following definitions to the correct term:

   _____ 1. Near the source or beginning   A. Eversion

   _____ 2. Away from head end of the body   B. Circumduction

   _____ 3. Nearer to the center   C. Pronation

   _____ 4. Increasing the angle of a joint   D. Contralateral

   _____ 5. Outward stress of the foot   E. Proximal

   _____ 6. Movement of an extremity away from the midline F. Medial

   _____ 7. Turning palm downward   G. Interior

   _____ 8. A backward movement   H. Retraction

   _____ 9. To move around in the form of a circle   I. Caudad

   _____ 10. Toward the center   J. Extension

   _____ 11. Away from the source or beginning   K. Abduction

   _____ 12. On the opposite side of the body   L. Distal

5. Match the following definitions to the correct term:

    ____ 1. Lying down in any position   A. Reid's base line

    ____ 2. Head lower than the feet position   B. Plantar

    ____ 3. Upright position, palms forward   C. Palmar

    ____ 4. Top of the foot   D. Fowler's position

    ____ 5. Frankfort horizontal plane   E. Lithotomy position

    ____ 6. A plane at right angles to sagittal or coronal planes   F. Anatomic position

    ____ 7. Head higher than feet position   G. Trendelenburg position

    ____ 8. Palm of hand   H. Horizontal plane

    ____ 9. Sole of foot   I. Midcoronal plane

    ____ 10. Front half of body   J. Dorsum

    ____ 11. A plane that divides body into anterior and posterior halves   K. Anterior

    ____ 12. A recumbent position with knees and hips flexed with   L. Recumbent
              support for legs

6. The direction or path of the central ray of the x-ray beam defines the positioning term:

    A. Position   C. Perspective

    B. View   D. Projection

7. **Situation:** A patient is placed in a recumbent position facing downward. The left side of the body is turned 30° toward the film. Which specific position has been used?

    A. LAO   C. LPO

    B. Left lateral decubitus   D. RAO

8. **Situation:** A patient is placed into a recumbent position facing downward. The x-ray tube is directed horizontally and enters the left side of the body. A film is placed against the right side of the patient. Which position has been used?

    A. Dorsal decubitus   C. Ventral decubitus

    B. Left lateral decubitus   D. Right lateral decubitus

9. **Situation:** A patient is erect with the back to the film. The central ray enters the anterior aspect and exits the posterior aspect of the body. Which projection has been used?

    A. Posteroanterior   C. Ventral decubitus

    B. Tangential   D. Anteroposterior

10. What is the name of the projection in which the central ray merely skims a body part?

    A. Tangential   C. Axial

    B. Decubitus   D. Trendelenburg

SELF-TEST C: Basic Imaging Principles

1. Which of the following is not one of the four primary image quality factors?

   A. Density   D. Detail

   B. Contrast   E. Distortion

   C. Kilovoltage peak

2. True/False: Every radiographic image must be imprinted with patient identification and date and anatomic side markers.

3. The amount of blackening on a processed radiograph is called:

   A. Density   C. Contrast

   B. Milliamperage seconds   D. Pneumbra

4. Which exposure factor primarily affects radiographic density?

   A. Kilovoltage peak   C. Focal spot size

   B. Milliamperage seconds   D. Source-image distance (SID)

5. True/False: For an underexposed radiograph, the milliamperage seconds must be increased by a factor of four to produce a visible change in radiographic density.

6. **Situation:** A radiograph of the knee reveals that it is overexposed and must be repeated. The original technique used 10 mAs. Which one of the following changes will improve the image during the repeat exposure?

   A. Increase to 15 mAs   C. Increase to 20 mAs

   B. Decrease to 5 mAs   D. Decrease to 7 mAs

7. The primary controlling factor for radiographic contrast is:

   A. Milliamperage seconds   C. Focal spot size

   B. Kilovoltage peak   D. SID

8. **Situation:** A radiographer is asked to produce a radiograph of the chest that will demonstrate long-scale contrast of the anatomy. Which one of the following set of exposure factors will produce this result?

   A. 50 kVp, 20 mAs   C. 110 kVp, 2 mAs

   B. 65 kVp, 15 mAs   D. 90 kVp, 5 mAs

9. Which one of the following set of exposure factors will produce in the highest radiographic contrast?

   A. 60 kVp, 30 mAs   C. 96 kVp, 5 mAs

   B. 80 kVp, 20 mAs   D. 120 kVp, 2 mAs

10. True/False: Kilovoltage peak is also a secondary controlling factor for radiographic density.

11. True/False: A low kilovoltage peak technique (50 kVp) produces a long-scale image.

12. True/False: Recorded detail is optimal with a long object-image distance (OID) and a short SID.

13. Which one of the following factors best controls involuntary cardiac motion?

    A. Careful instructions given to the patient

    B. High kilovoltage peak technique

    C. Practicing with patient when to hold breath

    D. Shortening the exposure time

14. **Situation:** The radiographer is asked to produce a high-quality image of the carpal (wrist) bones. The emergency room physician suspects that the patient has a very small fracture of one of the bones. Which one of following sets of factors will produce an image with the highest degree of radiographic detail?

    A. 1-mm focal spot and 30-inch SID

    B. 2-mm focal spot and 36-inch SID

    C. 0.5 mm focal spot and 40 inch SID

    D. 0.3 mm focal spot and 40-inch SID

15. The misrepresentation of an object's size or shape projected on a radiograph defines:

    A. Magnification   C. Unsharpness

    B. Blurring   D. Distortion

16. Which one of the following sets of factors minimizes radiographic distortion to the greatest degree?

    A. 40-inch SID and 8-inch OID

    B. 44-inch SID and 6-inch OID

    C. 72-inch SID and 3-inch OID

    D. 60-inch SID and 4-inch OID

17. True/False: To best utilize the anode heel effect, the thinner aspect of the anatomic part should be placed under the cathode aspect of the x-ray tube.

SELF-TEST D: Positioning Principles

1. True/False: If a patient is less than 18 years of age, any confidential information obtained during the procedure must be shared with the parent or guardian.

2. True/False: The radiographer must provide a preliminary interpretation of any radiographs if requested by the referring physician.

3. PBL collimators are required for:

    A. All new x-ray equipment manufactured before 1974

    B. All new x-ray equipment manufactured after 1993

    C. All x-ray equipment regardless when it was manufactured

    D. None of the x-ray equipment manufactured after 1994

4. True/False: Measurement of part thickness is not required as part of the positioning routine, if automatic exposure control is utilized.

5. Indicate the minimum number of projections required for the following structures:

_____ 1. Knee   A. Two

_____ 2. Fourth finger   B. Three

_____ 3. Humerus

_____ 4. Sternum

_____ 5. Ankle

_____ 6. Tibia/fibula

_____ 7. Chest

_____ 8. Hand

_____ 9. Hip (proximal femur)

_____ 10. Forearm

6. **Situation:** A patient enters the emergency room with a fractured forearm. The fracture is set, or *reduced.* The orthopedic physician orders a postreduction series. How many projections are required?

A. One   C. Two

B. Three   D. Four

7. A 24 × 30 cm imaging plate is equivalent to a _____ inch imaging plate.

A. 8 × 10   C. 11 × 14

B. 10 × 12   D. 14 × 17

8. A 40-inch SID is equivalent to a(n) _____ -cm SID.

A. 80   C. 100

B. 110   D. 180

9. Which topographical landmark can be palpated to locate the L4-5 vertebral interspace?

A. Iliac crest   C. ASIS

B. Inferior costal margin   D. Xiphoid process

10. Which topographical landmark can be palpated to locate T2-3?

A. Vertebra prominens   C. Sternal angle

B. Jugular notch   D. Inferior costal margin

11. The xiphoid process corresponds to the _____ vertebral level

A. T9-10   B. T4-5   C. L2-3   D. T2-3

12. A "stocky," massive body build describes a/an _____ body habitus.

A. Asthenic   C. Sthenic

B. Hyposthenic   D. Hypersthenic

SELF-TEST E: Digital Imaging

1. True/False: Computed radiography (CR) and digital radiography (DR) both require the use of an image receptor (IR) plate.

2. True/False: Direct capture digital fluoroscopy does not require the use of an image intensifier.

3. Patient information may be recorded on the CR imaging plate by:

   A. Light source   C. X-ray source

   B. Laser   D. Bar code reader

4. The latent image recorded on the CR image plate is read by a:

   A. Laser   C. Photomultiplier tube

   B. Bright light source   D. Ultraviolet light source

5. CR systems permit an underexposure of _____ without having to repeat the exposure when automatic exposure control (AEC) is not used.

   A. 5% to 10%   C. 80%

   B. 100%   D. 500%

6. True/False: Tight or aggressive collimation must be avoided when recording an image on a CR plate.

7. True /False: Grids must not be used with a CR system.

8. True/False: The initial cost for digital mammography systems is much higher as compared with conventional film-screen systems.

9. True/False: Digital chest systems permit postprocessing of the image to correct exposure errors.

10. True/False: PACS is a digital network that permits viewing and storage of digital and chemically produced images.

11. The acronym RIS stands for:

    A. Rapid imaging system

    B. Radiology imaging system

    C. Radiology information system

    D. Reusable imaging system

12. The acronym DICOM refers to:

    A. A set of standards to ensure communication among PACS networks

    B. A new direct digital "flat plate" receptor system

    C. A digital image transmission system

    D. A new-generation CR system

13. A digital transmission system for transferring radiographic images to remote locations by telephone, satellite, or cable is:

    A. PACS   C. HIS

    B. Direct DR   D. Teleradiology

SELF-TEST F: Radiation Protection

1. What is the Internation System (SI) unit of radiation measurement for *absorbed dose?*

   A. Seivert C. Coulombs per kilogram of air

   B. Gray D. Roentgen

2. What traditional unit of measurement describes radiation exposure in air?

   A. Seivert C. Coulombs per kilogram of air

   B. Gray D. Roentgen

3. What is the annual whole body effective dose (ED) for a radiographer?

   A. 10 rem or 100 mSv C. 1 rem or 10 mSv

   B. 0.1 rem or 1 mSv D. 5 rem or 50 mSv

4. What is the cumulative lifetime ED for a 25-year-old radiographer?

   A. 25 rem or 250 mSv C. 50 rem or 500 mSv

   B. 2.5 rem or 25 mSv D. 250 rem or 2500 mSv

5. What is the annual ED limit for an individual less than 18 years of age?

   A. 5 rem or 50 mSv C. 1 rem or 1 mSv

   B. 0.1 rem or 1 mSv D. 10 rem or 100 mSv

6. The federal set limit on exposure rates for intensified fluoroscopy units is:

   A. 3 to 4 R/min C. 1 R/min

   B. 0.5 R/min D. 10 R/min

7. The average intensified fluoroscopy rate for modern equipment is:

   A. 3 to 4 R/min C. 1 R/min

   B. 0.5 R/min D. 10 R/min

8. What is the primary purpose of x-ray tube filtration?

   A. Absorb lower energy x-rays

   B. Harden the x-ray beam

   C. Increase penetrability of the x-ray beam

   D. All of the above

9. Which of the following results in the highest ED for females (assuming no specific area shields are used)?

   A. Anteroposterior (AP) thoracic spine (7×17 collimation)

   B. AP abdomen (14×17 collimation)

   C. AP hip (10×12 collimation)

   D. AP chest (14×17 collimation)

10. The use of a gonadal shield reduces the gonadal dose by _____ if the gonads are within the primary x-ray field.

    A. 20% to 30% C. 50% to 90%

    B. 40% to 50% D. 100%

11. Which type of shield would be ideal when the affected tissue is part of a sterile field?

    A.   Contact shield   C.   Shadow shield

    B.   Lead masking   D.   Gonadal shaped shield

12. True/False: Low kilovoltage peak and high milliamperage seconds techniques greatly reduce patient dose compared with high kilovoltage peak and low milliamperage seconds.

13. True/False: The total ED for females on an AP chest projection is more than double that for a PA chest.

14. True/False: The use of a positive beam limiting (PBL) collimator is no longer required by the FDA for new x-ray equipment manufactured after 1994.

15. True/False: Collimators must be accurate within 5% of the selected SID.

2

Chest

After you have successfully completed **all** the activities of this chapter, you will be able to:

_____ 1. List the parts of the bony thorax.

_____ 2. List specific topographic positioning landmarks of the chest.

_____ 3. Identify the parts and function of specific structures of the respiratory system.

_____ 4. List the four organs of the mediastinum.

_____ 5. Identify specific structures of the chest on line drawings.

_____ 6. Identify specific structures of the chest on posteroanterior (PA) and lateral radiographs.

_____ 7. Identify specific structures of the chest on a computed tomography (CT), transverse image.

_____ 8. Identify the four types of body habitus and their impact on chest positioning.

_____ 9. Describe the methods to ensure proper degree of inspiration during chest radiography.

_____ 10. Describe the importance of employing close collimation, gonadal shielding, and film markers during chest radiography.

_____ 11. Identify the correct exposure factors to be used during chest radiography.

_____ 12. Identify alterations in positioning routine and exposure factors specific to pediatric and geriatric patients.

_____ 13. List three reasons for taking chest radiographs with the patient in the erect position whenever possible.

_____ 14. Describe the three important positioning criteria that must be present on chest radiographs using erect PA and lateral positions.

_____ 15. Describe the advantages of the central ray placement method compared with the traditional method of centering for the PA and lateral chest positions.

_____ 16. Identify advantages and disadvantages in using CT, sonography, nuclear medicine, and magnetic resonance imaging (MRI) to demonstrate specific types of pathologic conditions in the chest.

_____ 17. Match various types of pathologic chest conditions to their correct definition.

_____ 18. For specific forms of pathologic chest conditions, indicate whether manual exposure factors have to be increased, decreased, or remain the same.

_____ 19. List the correct central ray placement, part position, and criteria for specific chest positions.

_____ 20. List the patient dose ranges for skin, midline, thyroid, and breast for specific projections of the chest and upper airway.

_____ 21. Given a hypothetical situation, identify the correct modifications of position, exposure factors, or both to improve the radiographic image.

_____ 22. Given a hypothetical situation, identify the correct position for a radiograph of specific pathologic conditions.

POSITIONING AND FILM CRITIQUE OBJECTIVES

_____ 1. Using a peer, position the patient for PA, anteroposterior (AP), and lateral chest projections.

_____ 2. Using a chest phantom, use routine PA and lateral chest positions to produce satisfactory radiographs (if equipment is available).

_____ 3. Determine whether rotation is present on PA and lateral chest radiographs.

_____ 4. Critique and evaluate chest radiographs based on the four divisions of radiographic criteria: (1) structures shown, (2) position, (3) collimation and central ray, and (4) exposure criteria.

_____ 5. Distinguish between acceptable and unacceptable chest radiographs based on exposure factors, motion, collimation, positioning, or other errors.

Learning Activity Exercises

Complete the following review exercises after reading the associated pages in Chapter 2 of the textbook as indicated by each exercise. Answers to each review exercise are given at the end of the review exercises.

Part I: Radiographic Anatomy

REVIEW EXERCISE A: Radiographic Anatomy of the Chest (see textbook pp. 64-71)

1. The bony thorax consists of (A) the single _____ anteriorly (B), two

    _____ (C), two _____ , (D) twelve pairs of

    _____ , and (E) twelve _____ posteriorly.

2. The two important bony landmarks of the thorax that are used for locating the central ray on a posteroanterior

    (PA) and anteroposterior (AP) chest projection are the (A) _____ and

    (B) _____ , respectively.

3. The four divisions of the respiratory system are:

    A. _____   C. _____

    B. _____   D. _____

4. Identify correct anatomic terms for the following structures:

    A. Adam's apple _____   D. Shoulder blade _____

    B. Voice box _____   E. Collar bone _____

    C. Breastbone _____

5. List the three divisions of the structure located proximally to the larynx that serve as a common passageway for both food and air:

    A. _____   C. _____

    B. _____

6. What is the name of the structure that acts as a lid over the larynx to prevent foreign objects such as food particles

    from entering the respiratory system? _____

7. Circle the correct term. The trachea is located (anteriorly or posteriorly) to the esophagus.

8. The _____ bone is seen in the anterior portion of the neck and is found just below the
    tongue or floor of the mouth.

9. If a person accidentally inhales a food particle, which bronchus is it most likely to enter and why?

    A. The _____ bronchus.

    B. Why? _____

10. A. What is the name of the prominence, or ridge, seen when looking down into the bronchus where it divides into

        the right and left bronchi? _____

    B. This prominence, or ridge, is approximately at the level of the _____ vertebra.

11. What is the term for the small air sacs located at the distal ends of the bronchioles in which oxygen and carbon

    dioxide are exchanged in the blood? _____

12. A. The delicate, double-walled sac, or membrane, containing the lungs is called the _____ .

    B. The outer layer of this membrane adhering to the inner surface of the chest wall and diaphragm is the

        _____ .

    C. The inner layer adhering to the surface of the lungs is the _____ or

        _____ .

    D. The potential space between these two layers (identified in *C* and *D*) is called the

        _____ .

    E. Air or gas that enters the space identified in D results in a condition called _____ .

13. Fill in the correct terms for the following portions of the lungs:

    A. Lower, concave portion: _____

    B. Central area in which bronchi and blood vessels enter the lungs: _____

    C. Upper, rounded portion above the level of the clavicles: _____

    D. Extreme, outermost lower corner of the lungs: _____

14. Explain why the right lung is smaller than the left lung and the right hemidiaphragm is positioned higher than the

    left hemidiaphragm. _____

15. List the four important structures located in the mediastinum:

    A. _____   C. _____

    B. _____   D. _____

16. Identify the following structures in this drawing:

A. _____ gland

B. _____

C. _____

D. _____

E. _____

F. _____ gland

G. _____

H. _____

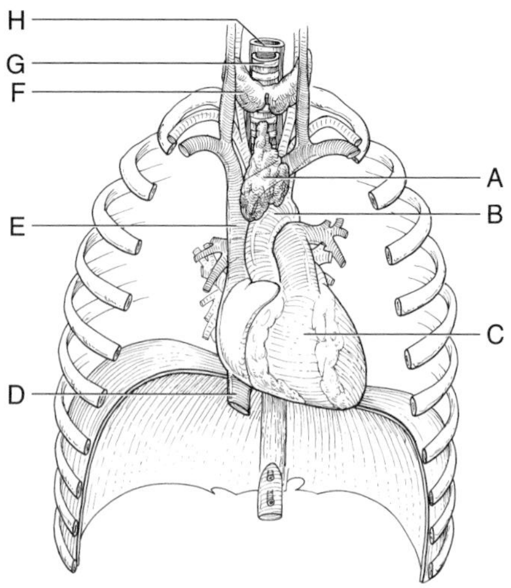

Fig. 2-1 Structures within the mediastinum.

17. The heart is enclosed in a double-walled membrane called the _____ .

18. The three parts of the aorta are the _____ , _____ , and _____ .

19. Identify the following labeled structures as seen on a PA and lateral chest radiograph:

A. _____

B. _____

C. _____

D. _____

E. _____

F. _____

G. _____

H. _____

I. _____

J. _____

K. _____

L. _____

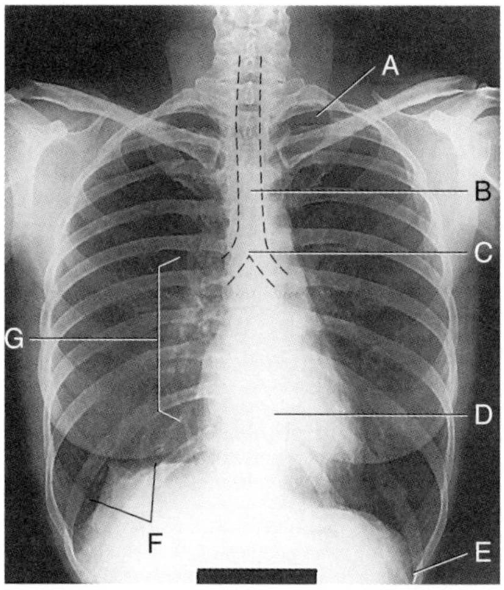

Fig. 2-2 Posteroanterior (PA) chest radiograph.

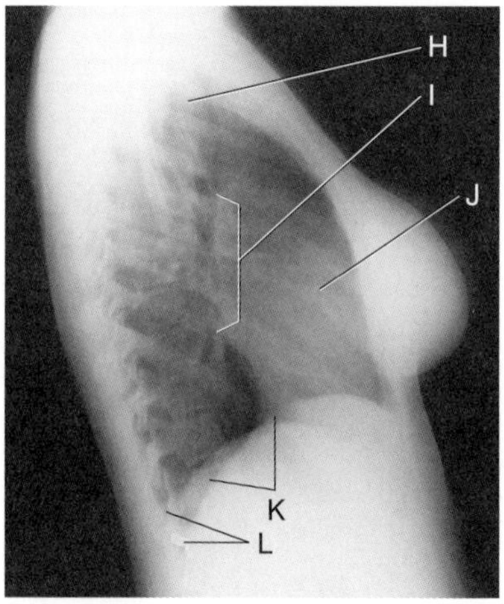

Fig. 2-3 Lateral chest radiograph.

20. Identify the labeled parts on this computed tomography (CT) image of a transverse section of the thorax at the level of T5—the fifth thoracic vertebra, which is also the level of the carina. (HINT: *B*, *G*, and *H* are major blood vessels.)

A. _____

B. _____

C. _____

D. _____

E. _____

F. _____

G. _____

H. _____

I. _____

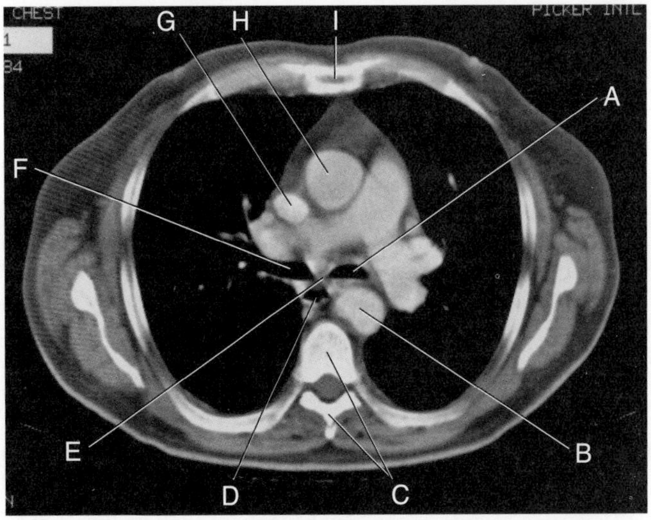

Fig. 2-4 Computed tomography (CT) transverse section of the thorax at the level of T5.

Part II: Radiographic Positioning

REVIEW EXERCISE B: Technical Considerations (see textbook pp. 72-83)

1. Which type of body habitus is associated with a broad and deep thorax? _____

2. Which one of the following types of body habitus may cause the costophrenic angles to be cut off if careful vertical collimation is not used?

   A. Hypersthenic

   B. Hyposthenic

   C. Sthenic

   D. Hyposthenic and asthenic

3. What is the minimum number of ribs that should be demonstrated above the diaphragm on a PA radiograph of the chest with full inspiration? _____

4. Indicate which of the following objects should be removed (or moved) before chest radiography:

   A. Necklace

   B. Bra

   C. Religious medallion around neck

   D. Dentures

   E. Pants

   F. Long-hair fasteners

   G. Oxygen lines

5. True/False: Chest radiography is the most commonly repeated radiographic procedure because of poor positioning or exposure factor selection errors.

6. True/False: Generally, you do not need to use grids for adult patients for PA or lateral chest radiographs.

7. Chest radiography for the adult patient usually employs a kilovoltage peak of _____ to _____ kVp.

8. Optimal technical factor selection ensures proper penetration of the:

   A. Heart

   B. Great vessels

   C. Lung regions

   D. Hilar region

   E. All of the above

9. Describe the way optimum density of the lungs and mediastinal structures can be determined on a PA chest

    radiograph. _____

10. True/False: Because the heart is always located in the left thorax, the use of film markers on a PA chest projection may not be necessary.

11. Which one of the following devices should be used for the PA and lateral chest positions for a young, pediatric patient?

    A. Upright chest device   C. Pigg-O-Stat

    B. Supine table Bucky   D. Plexiglas restraint board

12. Which one of the following set of exposure factors is recommended for a chest examination of a young, pediatric patient?

    A. 60 to 70 kVp, short exposure time   C. 100 to 120 kVp, short exposure time

    B. 90 to 100 kVp, medium exposure time   D. 120 to 150 kVp, long exposure time

13. True/False: Because they have more shallow lung fields, the central ray is often centered higher for geriatric patients.

14. To ensure better lung inspiration during chest radiography, exposure should be made during the _____ inspiration.

15. List four possible pathologic conditions that would suggest the need for both inspiration and expiration PA chest radiographs. (Five were given in the text.):

    A. _____   C. _____

    B. _____   D. _____

16. List and explain briefly the three reasons that chest radiographs should be taken with the patient in the erect position (when the patient's condition permits):

    A. _____   C. _____

    B. _____

17. Explain the primary purpose and benefit of performing chest radiography using a 72-inch source-to-image receptor

    distance (SID). _____

18. Why do the lungs tend to expand more with the patient in an erect position than in a supine position?

    _____

19. Hyperemia refers to:

    A. Fluid in the lungs   C. Free air in the pleural cavity

    B. Hyperinflation of the lungs   D. Excessive blood in a body part caused
                                          by relaxation of small blood vessels

20. Which one of the following anatomic structures is evaluated to determine rotation on a PA chest radiograph?

    A. Appearance of ribs   C. Symmetrical appearance of the sternoclavicular joints

    B. Shape of heart   D. Symmetrical appearance of the costophrenic angles

21. Which positioning tip will help you prevent the patient's chin from being superimposed over the upper airway and apices of the lungs for a PA chest radiograph?

_____

_____

22. Which lateral (right or left) position would you use for patients with the following clinical histories?

    A. Patient with severe pains in left side of chest _____

    B. Patient with no chest pain but recent history of pneumonia in right lung _____

    C. Patient with no chest pain or history of heart trouble _____

23. Why is it important to raise the patients' arms above their head for lateral chest projections?

_____

_____

24. The traditional central ray centering technique for the chest is to place the top of the cassette _____ to _____

    inches (_____ to _____ cm) above the shoulders.

25. A recommended central ray centering technique for a PA chest projection requires the technologist to palpate the

    _____ and measure down from that bony landmark _____ inches (_____ cm) for a male

    and _____ inches (_____ cm) for a female patient.

26. A. How should the cassette be placed for a PA chest projection of a hypersthenic patient: lengthwise or crosswise?

    _____

    B. For a hyposthenic patient? _____

27. True/False: With a digital chest unit, the question of cassette placement into either vertical or crosswise positions is eliminated because of the larger image receptor (IR).

28. Which one of the following bony landmarks is palpated for centering of the AP chest position?

    A. Vertebra prominens   C. Thyroid cartilage

    B. Jugular notch   D. Sternal angle

29. True/False: In general, more collimation should be on the lower film margin than on the top for a PA or lateral chest projection.

30. True/False: For most patients the central ray level for a PA chest projection is near the inferior angle of the scapula.

31. True/False: The height, or vertical dimension, of the average person's chest is greater than the width, or horizontal dimension.

32. True/False: CT has replaced bronchography as the preferred imaging modality to study the bronchial tree

33. True/False: Ultrasound is not an effective modality to detect pleural effusion.

34. True/False: Echocardiography and electrocardiography are basically the same procedure.

35. For the following pathologic indicators, match the following descriptions to the correct term.

    _____ 1. One of the most common inherited diseases   A. Atelectasis

    _____ 2. Condition most frequently associated with   B. Bronchiectasis
             congestive heart failure

    _____ 3. Coughing up blood   C. Bronchitis

    _____ 4. Accumulation of air in the pleural cavity   D. Chronic obstructive pulmonary disease (COPD)

    _____ 5. Accumulation of pus in pleural cavity   E. Hemoptysis

    _____ 6. A form of pneumoconiosis   F. Cystic fibrosis

    _____ 7. A contagious disease caused by an airborne   G. Empyema
             bacterium

    _____ 8. Irreversible dilation of bronchioles   H. Pleurisy

    _____ 9. Most common form is emphysema   I. Pneumothorax

    _____ 10. Acute or chronic irritation of bronchi   J. Pulmonary edema

    _____ 11. Collapse of all or portion of lung   K. Tuberculosis

    _____ 12. Inflammation of pleura   L. Silicosis

36. For the following types of pathologic conditions, indicate whether manual exposure factors would be increased (+), decreased (−), or remain the same (0) as compared with the standard chest exposure factors:

    _____ Atelectasis

    _____ Lung cancer

    _____ Pulmonary edema

    _____ Respiratory distress syndrome (RDS) or adult respiratory distress syndrome (ARDS) hyaline membrane disease (HMD in infants)

    _____ Secondary tuberculosis

    _____ Emphysema

    _____ Pneumothorax

    _____ Pulmonary emboli

    _____ Childhood tuberculosis

    _____ Asbestosis

REVIEW EXERCISE C: Positioning of the Chest (see textbook pp. 84-96)

1. Why is a PA chest preferred to an AP projection? _____

2. The CR is placed at the level of the _____ vertebra for a PA chest projection.

3. The shoulders need to be rolled forward for the PA projection to allow the _____ to move laterally and clear of the lung fields.

4. When using the automatic exposure control system (AEC) for the PA projection, which ionization chambers should be activated?

    A. Left chamber   C. Right chamber

    B. Center chamber   D. Left and right chambers

5. What is the midline dose range for a PA projection of the chest for an average-size female?

    A. 10 to 100 mrad   C. Less than 10 mrad

    B. Greater than 100 mrad   D. 0.5 to 1 rad

6. True/False: The average breast dose and thyroid dose for a PA chest projection are approximately the same.

7. The average female breast dose on an AP chest projection is approximately _____ times that for a PA chest dose.

    A. 1.5   B. 4   C. 10   D. 30

8. How much separation of the posterior ribs on a lateral chest projection indicates excessive rotation from a true lateral position? _____ (Less separation than this is caused by the divergent rays.)

9. To prevent the clavicles from obscuring the apices on an AP projection of the chest, the central ray should be angled

    (A) _____ (caudad or cephalad) so that it is perpendicular to the (B) _____ .

10. What is the name of the condition characterized by fluid entering the pleural cavity? _____

11. Which specific position would be used if a patient were unable to stand but the physician suspected the patient had fluid in the left lung? _____

12. What is the name of the condition characterized by free air entering the pleural cavity?

    _____

13. Which specific position would be used if the patient were unable to stand but the physician suspected the patient had free air in the left pleural cavity? _____

14. What circumstances or clinical indications suggest that an apical lordotic projection should be ordered?

    _____

15. What position/projection would be used for a patient who is too ill or weak to stand for an apical lordotic projection?

    _____

16. A. Which anterior oblique position would best demonstrate the left lung: right anterior oblique (RAO) or left anterior oblique (LAO)? _____

    B. Which posterior oblique position would best demonstrate the left lung: RPO or LPO?

    _____

17. For certain studies of the heart, the _____ (right or left) anterior oblique requires a rotation of _____ °.

18. Which AEC ionization chamber(s) should be activated for an LAO chest projection? _____

19 Where is the central ray placed for a lateral projection of the upper airway? _____

20. Which one of the following tissues receives the greatest dose during an AP projection of upper airway?

A. Thyroid   C. Midline structures   B. Breast   D. Gonads

REVIEW EXERCISE D: Problem Solving for Technical and Positioning Errors (see textbook pp. 72-96)

The following radiographic problems involve technical and positioning errors that lead to substandard images. Other questions involve situations pertaining to different conditions and pathologic findings. As you analyze these problems and situations, use your textbook to help you find solutions to these questions.

1. A radiograph of a PA view of the chest reveals that the sternoclavicular (SC) joints are not the same distance from the spine. The right SC joint is closer to the midline than is the left SC joint. What is the positioning error?

_____

2. A radiograph of a PA view of the chest only shows seven posterior ribs above the diaphragm. What caused this

problem, and how could it be prevented on the repeat exposures?_____

_____

3. A radiograph of a PA and left lateral view of the chest reveals that the mediastinum of the chest is underpenetrated. The technologist used the following for the radiograph: a 72-inch SID, an upright Bucky, a full-inspiration exposure, 75 kVp and 600 mA, and a ¹⁄₆₀-second-exposure time.

A. Which one of these factors is the most likely cause of the problem?_____

B. How can the technologist improve the image when making the repeat exposure?_____

4. A radiograph of a PA view of the chest reveals that the top of the apices are cut off, and a wide collimation border can be seen below the diaphragm. In what way can this be corrected during the repeat radiograph?

_____

5. **Situation:** A patient with a clinical history of advanced emphysema comes to the radiology department for a chest x-ray. AEC will not be used. How should the technologist alter the manual exposure settings for this patient?

A. Do not alter them. Use the standard exposure factors.

B. Decrease the kilovoltage peak moderately (− −).

C. Increase the kilovoltage peak slightly (+).

D. Increase the kilovoltage peak moderately (+ +).

6. **Situation:** A patient with pleural effusion comes to the radiology department for a chest x-ray. AEC will not be used. How should the technologist alter the manual exposure settings for this patient?

A. Do not alter them. Use the standard exposure factors.

B. Decrease the kilovoltage peak moderately (− −).

C. Increase the kilovoltage peak slightly (+).

D. Increase the kilovoltage peak moderately (++).

7. **Situation:** A patient comes to the radiology department for a presurgical chest x-ray. The clinical history indicates a possible situs inversus of the thorax (transposition of structures within the thorax). Which positioning step or action

must be taken to perform a successful chest examination? _____

8. A radiograph of a lateral view of the chest reveals that the posterior ribs and costophrenic angles are separated more than 1/2 inch, or 1 cm, indicating excessive rotation. Describe a possible method of determining the direction of rotation? _____

9. **Situation:** A patient enters the emergency room with a possible hemothorax in the right lung caused by a motor vehicle accident (MVA). The patient is unable to stand or sit erect. Which specific position would best diagnose this condition and why? _____
_____

10. **Situation:** A young child enters the emergency room with a foreign body in one of the bronchi of the lung. The foreign body, a peanut, can't be seen on the PA and lateral views of the chest projection.

    A. Which additional projections could the technologist perform to locate the foreign body?

    _____

    B. Which primary bronchi would most likely contain the peanut? _____

11. **Situation:** A routine chest study indicated a possible mass beneath a patient's right clavicle. The PA and lateral projections were inconclusive. Which additional projection(s) could the technologist take to diagnose this small tumor?

    _____

12. **Situation:** A patient has a possible small pneumothorax. Routine chest projections (PA and lateral) fail to reveal the pneumothorax conclusively. Which additional projections could be taken to rule out this condition?

    _____

13. **Situation:** A patient with a history of pleurisy comes to the radiology department. Which one of the following positioning routines should be used?

    A. Soft tissue lateral of the upper airway   C. Erect PA and lateral

    B. Right and left lateral decubitus   D. CT scan of the chest

REVIEW EXERCISE E: Critique Radiographs of the Chest (see textbook p. 96)

The following questions relate to the radiographs found at the end of Chapter 2 of the textbook. Evaluate these radiographs for the radiographic criteria categories *(1* through *5)* that follow. Describe the corrections needed to improve the overall image. The major, or "repeatable" errors, are specific errors that indicate the need for a repeat exposure, regardless of the nature of the other errors.

A. **PA chest, 43-year-old man (Fig. C2-97)**
   Description of possible error:

   1. Structures shown: _____

   2. Part positioning: _____

   3. Collimation and central ray: _____

   4. Exposure criteria: _____

   5. Markers: _____

   Repeatable error(s): _____

B. PA chest, 74-year-old man (Fig. C2-98)
Description of possible error:

1. Structures shown: _____

2. Part positioning: _____

3. Collimation and central ray: _____

4. Exposure criteria: _____

5. Markers: _____

Repeatable error(s): _____

C. Lateral chest, female (Fig. C2-99)
Description of possible error:

1. Structures shown: _____

2. Part positioning: _____

3. Collimation and central ray: _____

4. Exposure criteria: _____

5. Markers: _____

Repeatable error(s): _____

D. PA chest, 73-year-old female (Fig. C2-100)
Description of possible error:

1. Structures shown: _____

2. Part positioning: _____

3. Collimation and central ray: _____

4. Exposure criteria: _____

5. Markers: _____

Repeatable error(s): _____

E. Lateral chest, female in wheelchair (Fig. C2-101)
Description of possible error:

1. Structures shown: _____

2. Part positioning: _____

3. Collimation and central ray: _____

4. Exposure criteria: _____

5. Markers: _____

Repeatable error(s): _____

Part III: Laboratory Activities (see textbook pp. 84-94)

You must gain experience in chest positioning before performing the following exams on actual patients. You can get experience in positioning and radiographic evaluation of these projections by performing exercises using radiographic phantoms and practicing on other students (although not taking actual exposures).

The following suggested activities assume that your teaching institution has an energized lab and radiographic phantoms. If not, perform Laboratory Exercise B, the physical positioning exercises. (Check off each step and projection as you complete it.)

LABORATORY EXERCISE A: Energized Laboratory

1. Using the chest radiographic phantom, produce radiographs using:

    _____ PA and AP views   _____ A lateral view

2. Evaluate these radiographs, additional radiographs provided by your instructor, or both for:

    _____ Rotation

    _____ Collimation

    _____ Part and central ray centering

    _____ Markers

    _____ Proper exposure factors

    _____ Motion

LABORATORY EXERCISE B: Physical Positioning

1. On another person, simulate taking all basic and special projections of the chest as listed. Follow the suggested positioning steps and sequence as listed in the following section and as described in Chapter 1 of your textbook:

    _____ PA chest

    _____ Anterior and posterior obliques

    _____ Lateral chest

    _____ AP and lateral upper airway

    _____ AP supine or semisupine

    _____ Lateral decubitus

    _____ AP lordotic

For Suggested Positioning Sequence and Routine, see textbook p. 42. For Protocols and Order for General Diagnostic Radiographic Procedures, see textbook p. 40.

Step 1. General Patient Positioning—Protocols #1 through #9, which include:

_____ Select the size and number of cassettes needed.

_____ Prepare the radiographic room. Check that tube is centered to the center of the film holder (or the centerline of the table for Bucky exams).

_____   Correctly identify the patient, and bring the patient into the room.

_____   Explain to the patient what you will be doing.

_____   Assist the patient to the proper place and position for the first radiograph.

Step 2.   Measuring Part Thickness—Protocols #10 and #11 (unless AEC is used):

_____   Measure the body part being radiographed, and set correct exposure factors (technique). (If using an AEC system, select the correct chamber cells on the control panel.)

Step 3.   Part Positioning—Protocol #12:

_____   Align and center the body part to the central ray or vice versa for chest positioning with the chest board. (For Bucky exams on a table, move the patient and table top together as needed [with floating-type table top]). (NOTE: In cases in which the correct central ray position is of primary importance, the central ray icon is included in the textbook on the appropriate positioning page.)

Step 4.   Film Centering:

_____   After the part has been centered to the central ray, the IR (cassette) is also centered to the central ray. (NOTE: This step can be omitted on most chest units where the x-ray tube and IR unit are attached and move together.)

Additional Steps or Actions—Protocols #13 through #18:

_____ 1.   Collimate accurately to include only the area of interest.

_____ 2.   Place the correct marker within the exposure field (so that you do not superimpose pertinent anatomic structures).

_____ 3.   Restrain or provide support for the body part to prevent motion.

_____ 4.   Use contact lead shielding as needed (e.g., gonadal, breast, thyroid).

_____ 5.   Give clear breathing instructions, and make the exposure while watching patient through window.

Answers to Review Exercises

Review Exercise A: Radiographic Anatomy of the Chest

1. A. Sternum
   B. Clavicles
   C. Scapulae
   D. Ribs
   E. Thoracic vertebrae
2. A. Vertebra prominens
   B. Jugular notch
3. A. Pharynx
   B. Trachea
   C. Bronchi
   D. Lungs
4. A. Thyroid cartilage
   B. Larynx
   C. Sternum
   D. Scapula
   E. Clavicle
5. A. Nasopharynx
   B. Oropharynx
   C. Laryngopharynx
6. Epiglottis
7. Anteriorly
8. Hyoid
9. A. Right
   B. It is larger in diameter and more vertical.
10. A. Carina
    B. T5
11. Alveoli
12. A. Pleura
    B. Parietal pleura
    C. Pulmonary or visceral pleura
    D. Pleural cavity
    E. Pneumothorax
13. A. Base
    B. Hilum (hilus)
    C. Apex (apices)
    D. Costophrenic angle
14. Presence of liver on right
15. A. Thymus gland
    B. Heart and great vessels
    C. Trachea
    D. Esophagus
16. A. Thymus gland
    B. Arch of aorta
    C. Heart
    D. Inferior vena cava
    E. Superior vena cava
    F. Thyroid gland
    G. Trachea
    H. Esophagus
17. Pericardial sac
18. Ascending, arch, and descending aorta
19. A. Apex of left lung
    B. Trachea
    C. Carina
    D. Heart
    E. Left costophrenic angle
    F. Right hemidiaphragm (or base)
    G. Hilum
    H. Apex of lungs
    I. Hilum
    J. Heart
    K. Right and left hemidiaphragm
    L. Right and left costophrenic angles
20. A. Left main stem bronchus
    B. Descending aorta
    C. T5 (fifth thoracic vertebra)
    D. Esophagus
    E. Region of carina
    F. Right main stem bronchus
    G. Superior vena cava
    H. Ascending aorta
    I. Sternum

Review Exercise B: Technical Considerations

1. Hypersthenic
2. D. Hyposthenic and asthenic
3. 10 ribs
4. A. Necklace
   B. Bra
   C. Religious medallion around neck
   F. Long-hair fasteners
   G. Oxygen lines
5. True
6. False
7. 110 to 125 kVp
8. E. All of the above
9. To be able to see faint outlines of at least middle and upper vertebrae and ribs through heart and other mediastinal structures
10. False (Situs inversus may be present.)
11. C. Pigg-O-Stat
12. A. 60 to 70 kVp, short exposure time
13. True
14. Second
15. 1. Small pneumothorax
    2. Fixation or lack of normal diaphragm movement
    3. Presence of a foreign body
    4. Distinguish between opacity in rib or lung.
    5. Possible atelectasis (incomplete expansion of the lungs)
16. A. To allow diaphragm to move down farther
    B. To show possible air and fluid levels in the chest
    C. To prevent engorgement and hyperemia of the pulmonary vessels
17. Reduces distortion and magnification of the heart and other chest structures
18. Erect position causes abdominal organs to drop, allowing the diaphragm to move farther down and the lungs to more fully aerate
19. D. Excessive blood in a part caused by relaxation of small blood vessels
20. C. Symmetrical sternoclavicular joints
21. Extend the chin upward.
22. A. Left
    B. Right
    C. Left
23. Prevents upper arm soft tissue from being superimposed over upper chest fields
24. One to two inches (3.8 to 5 cm)
25. Vertebra prominens, 8 inches (20 cm) for male, 7 inches (18 cm) for female
26. A. Crosswise
    B. Lengthwise
27. True
28. B. Jugular notch
29. False (should be equal)
30. True
31. False (greater width)
32. True
33. False
34. False
35. 1. F
    2. J
    3. E
    4. I
    5. G
    6. L
    7. K
    8. B
    9. D
    10. C
    11. A
    12. H
36. + Atelectasis
    + Lung cancer
    + Pulmonary edema
    + RDS or ARDS (HMD in infants)
    + Secondary tuberculosis
    − Emphysema
    − Pneumothorax
    0 Pulmonary emboli
    0 Childhood tuberculosis
    + Asbestosis

Review Exercise C: Positioning of the Chest

1. Places the heart closer to the cassette to reduce magnification of the heart
2. T7
3. Scapulae

4. D. Left and right chambers
5. C. Less than 10 mrad
6. True (Both are about 1 mrad.)
7. B. Four times
8. Greater than 1 cm (½ to ¾ inch)
9. A. Caudad (±5°)
   B. Sternum
10. Pleural effusion
11. Left lateral decubitus
12. Pneumothorax
13. Right lateral decubitus (Affected side should be up.)
14. Rule out calcifications or masses beneath the clavicles
15. AP semiaxial projection, central ray 15° to 20° cephalad
16. A. RAO
    B. LPO
17. Left, 60°
18. Right upper chamber
19. Level of C6-7, midway between thyroid cartilage and jugular notch
20. A. Thyroid

Review Exercise D: Problem-Solving for Technical and Positioning Errors

1. Rotation. The patient is rotated into a slight RAO position (see p. 75).
2. The lungs are underinflated. Explain to the patient the need for a deep inspiration, and take the exposure on the second deep inspiration (see p. 74).
3. A. The 75 kVp is too low. The ideal kilovoltage peak range is 100 to 130.
   B. Increase the kilovoltage peak and reduce the milliamperage seconds for the repeat exposure (see p. 73).
4. Center the central ray higher (to the level of T7, which will be found 7 to 8 inches below the vertebra prominens). Make sure the cassette is centered to the central ray and the top collimation light border is at the vertebra prominens (see p. 77).
5. B. Decrease the kilovoltage peak moderately (− −).
6. C. Increase the kilovoltage peak slightly (+) .
7. Ensure placement of the correct right or left anatomic side marker on the cassette because the heart and other thoracic structures may be transposed from right to left (see Chapter 1).

8. By determining which hemidiaphragm (right or left) is more posterior or more anterior. The left hemidiaphragm can frequently be identified by visualization of the gastric air bubble or the inferior heart shadow, both of which are associated with the left hemidiaphragm (see p. 76).
9. Right lateral decubitus; in a patient with hemothorax (fluid), the side of interest should be down.
10. A. Inspiration and expiration PA projections (see p. 74).
    B. The right bronchus is most likely to contain the foreign body because it is more vertical and larger in diameter (see p. 68).
11. AP apical lordotic (see p. 90).
12. Inspiration and expiration PA projections, and/or a lateral decubitus AP chest with affected side up. (see p. 89)
13. C. Erect PA and lateral

Review Exercise E : Critique Radiographs of the Chest (see textbook, p. 96)

A. PA chest (Fig. C2-97)
   1. Left costophrenic angle cut off*
   2. Slight rotation into an RAO position (hips and lower thorax most rotated, spine shifted to right)
   3. Vertical centering is correct; central ray is centered to T7. Tighter collimation is desirable (to prevent excessive exposure to both neck and abdominal region).
   4. Acceptable
   5. Anatomic side marker present
   Repeatable error(s): criterion 1
B. PA chest (Fig. C2-98)
   1. Additional left anatomic side marker obscuring portion of right lung
   2. Slight rotation into an LAO position
   3. Central ray is centered slightly high (T6-7 interspace) No evident collimation
   4. Acceptable
   5. Anatomic side marker present, but which one is truly correct? This patient may have situs inversus.
   Repeatable error(s): criteria 1 and 5
C. Lateral chest (Fig. C2-99)
   1. All pertinent anatomy is demonstrated (costophrenic angle is nearly cut off).

*NOTE: Cassette should have been placed crosswise,

2. Excessive rotation (±1 inch or 2.5 cm). Right side is anterior. (Right diaphragm is discernible because of association of gastric bubble with the higher [right] diaphragm).
3. Central ray is centered too high (causing excessive exposure of neck and face) No upper collimation as a result of poor central ray centering
4. Acceptable
5. No evident left marker (may be present but is not visible here)
Repeatable error(s): criteria 2 and 5 (if not visible on radiograph)
D. PA chest (Fig. C2-100)
   1. Bra artifact is in lung field. Bra also created increased breast shadow in lung field.
   2. Some rotation into RAO position has occurred. (Right sternoclavicular joint is closer to spine, and spine is shifted to right, indicating entire thorax is somewhat rotated.)
   3. Central ray is centered too high. Collimation is not evident on top because of high central ray centering. Side collimation is excellent.
   4. Acceptable
   5. Left marker is evident.
   Repeatable error(s): criterion 1
E. Lateral chest (Fig. C2-101)
   1. All pertinent anatomy is demonstrated.
   2. Marginal rotation is present. Shoulders are more rotated than hips. (¾ inch or 2 cm measured along the posterior ribs.) The radiograph may or may not have to be repeated for this problem depending on departmental protocol and other factors.
   3. Central ray centering is good (just slightly high). Collimation is excellent.
   4. Motion is present along the diaphragm and lower lung field (more visible on actual radiograph). Shorter exposure time or better instruction is needed.
   5. Left marker is not visible
   Repeatable error(s): criteria 2, 3, and 5

SELF-TEST

My Score = _____%

This self-test should be taken only after completing all of the readings, review exercises, and laboratory activities for a particular section. The purpose of this test is not only to provide a good learning exercise but also to serve as a strong indicator of what your final unit evaluation grade will cover. It is strongly suggested that if you do not get at least a 90% to 95% grade on each self-test, you should review those areas in which you missed questions before going to your instructor for the final unit evaluation exam. (Total 50 blanks, 2 points per blank)

1. Match the following structures with their correct anatomic term:

   _____ A. Breastbone   1. Clavicle

   _____ B. Adam's apple   2. Larynx

   _____ C. Shoulder blade   3. Thyroid cartilage

   _____ D. Voice box   4. Scapula

   _____ E. Collar bone   5. Sternum

2. The correct term for the seventh cervical vertebrae is:

   A. Xiphoid process   C. Axis

   B. Jugular notch   D. Vertebra prominens

3. A notch, or depression, located on the superior portion of the sternum is called the:

   A. Sternal notch   C. Jugular notch

   B. Xiphoid notch   D. Sternal angle

4. The trachea bifurcates and forms the:

   A. Right and left bronchi   C. Costophrenic angles

   B. Right and left hilum   D. Pulmonary arteries

5. A specific prominence, or ridge, found at the point where the internal distal trachea divides into the right and left bronchi is called the:

   A. Hilum   C. Epiglottis

   B. Carina   D. Alveoli

6. The area of each lung where the bronchi and blood vessels enter and leave is called the:

   A. Carina   C. Base

   B. Apex   D. Hilum

7. The structures within the lung where oxygen and carbon dioxide gas exchange occurs are called:

   A. Carina   C. Hila

   B. Alveoli   D. Bronchi

8. Which of the following is *not* an aspect of the pleura?

   A. Parietal pleura   C. Pleural cavity

   B. Hilar pleura   D. Pulmonary pleura

9. The condition in which blood fills the potential space between the layers of pleura is called:

    A. Pneumothorax   B. Atelectasis

    C. Hemothorax   D. Empyema

10. The extreme, outermost lower corner of each lung is called the:

    A. Costophrenic angle   C. Base

    B. Apex   D. Hilar region

11. Which one of the following structures is *not* found in the mediastinum?

    A. Thymus gland   C. Epiglottis

    B. Heart and great vessels D. Trachea

12. A narrow thorax that is shallow from the front to back but very long in the vertical dimension is characteristic of a _____ body habitus.

    A. Hypersthenic   C. Hyposthenic

    B. Sthenic   D. Asthenic

13. Identify the best technique for chest radiography from the following choices:

    A. 85 kVp, 300 mA, $\frac{1}{30}$ second, 40-inch SID

    B. 110 kVp, 100 mA, $\frac{1}{10}$ second, 40-inch SID

    C. 120 kVp, 600 mA, $\frac{1}{60}$ second, 60-inch SID

    D. 130 kVp, 600 mA, $\frac{1}{60}$ second, 72-inch SID

14. Match the correct answer for the structures labeled on this midsagittal section of the pharynx and upper airway:

    _____ A.   1. Laryngopharynx

    _____ B.   2. Uvula

    _____ C.   3. Epiglottis

    _____ D.   4. Esophagus

    _____ E.   5. Spinal cord

    _____ F.   6. Oral cavity

    _____ G.   7. Hyoid bone

    _____ H.   8. Nasopharynx

    _____ I.   9. Thyroid gland

    _____ J.   10. Oropharynx

    _____ K.   11. Larynx

    _____ L.   12. Hard palate

    _____ M.   13. Thyroid cartilage

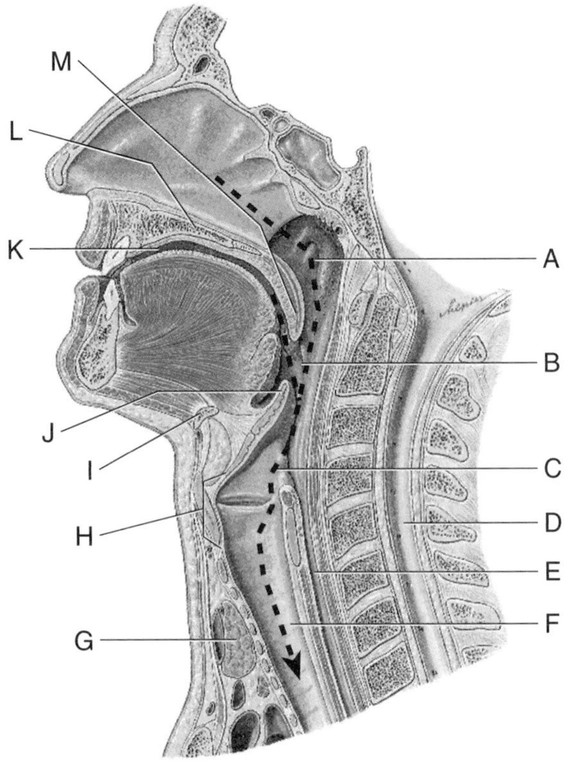

Fig 2-5 Midsaggital section of the pharynx and upper airway.

15. Identify the structures labeled on this computed tomography (CT) axial section of the thorax at the level of T3 (the third thoracic vertebra):

    A. _____

    B. _____

    C. _____

    D. _____

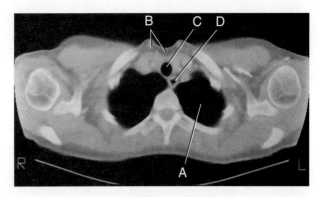

Fig. 2-6 Computed tomography (CT) axial section of the thorax at the level of T3.

16. Identify the structures on this CT axial section of the thorax at the approximate level of T4-5 (1 cm proximal to carina). HINT: B, E, and F are major blood vessels.

    A. _____

    B. _____

    C. _____

    D. _____

    E. _____

    F. _____

    G. _____

    H. _____

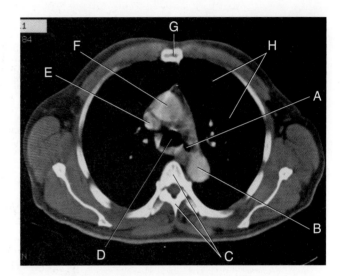

Fig. 2-7 Computed tomography (CT) axial section of the thorax at the approximate level of T4-5.

17. What is the name of the special immobilization device used for pediatric chest studies?

    A. Pigg-O-Stat   C. Chest immobilizer

    B. Restraining chair   D. Franklin unit

18. Which one of the following exposure factors is recommended for a chest study of a young pediatric patient?

    A. 110 kVp, short exposure time   C. 65 kVp, short exposure time

    B. 90 kVp, medium exposure time   D. 60 kVp, long exposure time

19. Which of the following is *not* a valid reason to perform chest projections with the patient in the erect position?

    A. To reduce patient dose

    B. To demonstrate air and fluid levels

    C. To allow the diaphragm to move down further

    D. To prevent hyperemia of pulmonary vessels

20. Why are the shoulders pressed downward for a posteroanterior (PA) projection of the chest?

    A. To remove scapulae from lung fields

    B. To prevent hyperemia of pulmonary vessels

    C. To allow the diaphragm to move down further

    D. To reduce chest rotation

21. Why are the shoulders rolled forward for a PA projection of the chest?

    A. To remove scapulae from lung fields

    B. To prevent hyperemia of pulmonary vessels

    C. To allow the diaphragm to move down further

    D. To reduce chest rotation

22. Where is the central ray placed for an anteroposterior (AP) supine projection of the chest?

    A. 7 to 8 inches (18 to 20 cm) below vertebra prominens

    B. 1 to 2 inches (2.5 to 5 cm) below jugular notch

    C. 3 to 4 inches (8 to 10 cm) below jugular notch

    D. 3 to 4 inches (8 to 10 cm) below thyroid cartilage

23. True/False: CT is replacing bronchography for the study of bronchial tree conditions.

24. A condition in which all or a portion of the lung is collapsed is:

    A. Atelectasis   C. Pneumothorax

    B. Pleural effusion   D. Pneumoconiosis

25. A type of a pleural effusion that involves a milky fluid is:

    A. Empyema   C. Chylothorax

    B. Hemothorax   D. Pneumonia

26. A sudden blockage of an artery in the lung is called:

    A. Pleurisy   C. Adult respiratory distress syndrome (ARDS)

    B. Pulmonary emboli   D. Chronic obstructive pulmonary disease (COPD)

27. Which one of the following is *not* a form of pneumoconiosis?

    A. Asbestosis   C. Anthracosis

    B. Silicosis   D. Tuberculosis

28. The exposure factors for a patient with a large pneumothorax should:

    A. Be reduced   C. Be increased

    B. Remain the same   D. Change from automatic exposure control (AEC) to manual technique

29. A PA chest radiograph reveals that the left sternoclavicular joint is superimposed over the spine (in comparison with the right joint). What specific positioning error is involved?

    A. Poor inspiration

    B. Rotation into a right anterior oblique (RAO) position

    C. Rotation into a left anterior oblique (LAO) position

    D. Tilting of the chest toward the left

30. A PA chest radiograph shows 10 posterior ribs above the diaphragm.

    Is this an acceptable radiograph? _____ Yes _____ No

31. A PA and lateral chest radiographic study has been completed. The PA projection reveals that the right costophrenic angle was collimated off, but both angles are included on the lateral projection.

    Would you repeat the PA projection? _____ Yes _____ No

32. A lateral chest radiograph demonstrates that the soft tissue of the upper limbs is superimposed over the apices of the lungs. How can this situation be prevented?

    A. Deeper inspiration   C. Slight rotation to the patient's left

    B. Extend chin   D. Raise upper limbs higher

33. A lateral chest radiograph reveals that the posterior ribs and costophrenic angles are separated by approximately

    $1/2$ inch (slightly less than 1 cm). Should the technologist repeat this projection? _____ Yes _____ No

34. **Situation:** A radiograph of an apical lordotic projection reveals that the clavicles are projected within the apices. The clinical instructor informs the student radiographer that the study is unacceptable but during the repeat exposure, the patient complains of being too unsteady to lean backward for another projection. What other options are available if the student wants to complete the study?

    A. Perform the PA lordotic projection

    B. Perform an AP semiaxial projection

    C. Perform both lateral decubitus projections

    D. Perform inspiration and expiration PA projections

35. **Situation:** An ambulatory patient with a clinical history of advanced emphysema enters the emergency room. The patient is having difficulty breathing and is receiving oxygen. The physician has ordered a PA and lateral chest study. Should the technologist alter the normal exposure factors for this patient?

    A. No. Use the standard exposure factors

    B. Yes. Increase the exposure factors

    C. Yes. Decrease the exposure factors

    D. No. Increase the SID instead of changing the exposure factors

36. **Situation:** A patient enters the ER with an injury to the chest. The ER physician suspects a pneumothorax may be present in the right lung. The patient is unable to stand or sit erect. Which specific position can be performed to confirm the presence of the pneumothorax?

    A. Left lateral decubitus   C. Right lateral decubitus

    B. Inspiration and expiration PA   D. AP lordotic

37. **Situation:** A PA and lateral chest study reveals a suspicious mass located near the heart in the right lung. The radiologist would like a radiograph of the patient in an anterior oblique position to delineate the mass from the heart. Which position should the technologist use to accomplish this objective?

    A. 45° LAO   B. 60° LAO   C. 45° RAO   D. AP lordotic

38. **Situation:** A patient with a history of pulmonary edema comes to the radiology department and is unable to stand. The physician suspects fluid in the left lung. Which specific position should be used to confirm this diagnosis?

    A. Right lateral decubitus   C. AP lordotic

    B. AP semiaxial   D. Left lateral decubitus

39. For the following critique questions, refer to textbook, p. 96 (Fig. C2-97) (PA chest)

   A. Which positioning errors are visible on this radiograph? More than one answer may be selected.

      (a) All essential anatomic structures are not demonstrated.

      (b) Central ray is incorrectly centered.

      (c) Collimation not evident.

      (d) Exposure factors are incorrect.

      (e) No anatomic marker is visible.

      (f) Rotation into the RAO position is evident. (The spine is shifted to the right.)

      (g) Rotation into the LAO position is evident. (The spine is shifted to the left.)

      (h) The chin is not elevated.

   B. Which of the above criteria errors on this radiograph is/are considered "repeatable errors"?

   C. Which of the following modifications must be made during the repeat exposure? More than one answer may be selected.

      (a) Increase closer collimation

      (b) Center CR correctly to T7

      (c) Decrease exposure factors

      (d) Increase exposure factors

      (e) Place anatomic marker on IR prior to exposure

      (f) Correct for rotation of shoulders and hips

      (g) Place image receptor crosswise

      (h) Elevate chin higher

40. For the following critique questions, refer to Fig. C2-99 (Lateral Chest)

   A. What are the positioning error(s) seen on this radiograph? More than one answer may be selected.

      (a) All essential anatomy is not demonstrated on the radiograph

      (b) Incorrect CR centering

      (c) Collimation not evident

      (d) Exposure factors are incorrect

      (e) No anatomic marker seen on radiograph

      (f) Excessive rotation of the chest

   B. Which of the previous error(s) on this radiograph is/are considered "repeatable errors?"

   C. Which of the following modifications must be made during the repeat exposure? More than one answer may be selected.

      (a) Center the central ray correctly—to T7.

      (b) Decrease the exposure factors.

      (c) Increase the exposure factors.

      (d) Place an anatomic marker correctly on the image receptor (IR) before exposure.

      (e) Ensure that the shoulders and hips are superimposed to eliminate rotation.

      (f) Raise the upper limbs higher.

Abdomen

After you have successfully completed **all** the activities in this chapter, you will be able to:

_____ 1. List the location of the three muscles of the abdomen that are important in abdominal radiography.

_____ 2. List the major organs and structures of the digestive, biliary, and urinary systems.

_____ 3. Using drawings and radiographs, identify the principle structures of the digestive system, biliary system, urinary system, and accessory organs involved in digestion.

_____ 4. Identify whether select organs of the abdomen are intraperitoneal, retroperitoneal, or infraperitoneal.

_____ 5. Identify the correct quadrant or region of the abdomen where specific organs are located.

_____ 6. Identify specific bony topographic landmarks used for positioning of the abdomen.

_____ 7. Using drawings, radiographs, and computed tomography (CT) images, identify the major bony and soft tissue structures of the abdomen.

_____ 8. List specific types of pathologic findings that are clinical indications for an acute abdominal series.

_____ 9. List specific methods for controlling involuntary and voluntary motion during abdominal radiography.

_____ 10. Describe the factors that affect collimation and the use of gonadal shielding during abdominal radiography.

_____ 11. Identify the correct exposure factors to be employed during abdominal radiography.

_____ 12. Identify alterations in positioning routine and exposure factors for pediatric and geriatric patients.

_____ 13. Identify the pathologic conditions and diseases of the abdomen that are best demonstrated with CT, sonography, nuclear medicine, and magnetic resonance imaging (MRI).

_____ 14. Match various types of abdominal pathologic findings to their correct definition.

_____ 15. Match specific types of abdominal pathologic findings to their correct radiographic appearance.

_____ 16. Describe variations in cassette and central ray placement that can be used to accommodate differences in body habitus.

_____ 17. List the dose ranges for skin, midline, and gonadal doses for the various projections of the abdomen on an average-size patient.

_____ 18. Identify the reason for the difference in female ovarian doses on an anteroposterior (AP) versus a posteroanterior (PA) abdomen projection with the same exposure factors.

_____ 19. List the correct central ray placement, part position, and radiographic criteria for specific abdomen positions.

_____ 20. List the pathologic indications for the acute abdominal series.

_____ 21. List the projections taken for the acute abdominal series and variations of it that can be used to accommodate patient conditions.

_____ 22. Given various hypothetical situations, identify the correct modification of position, exposure factors, or both to improve the radiographic image.

_____ 23. Given various hypothetical situations, identify the correct position for a specific pathologic feature or condition.

POSITIONING AND FILM CRITIQUE OBJECTIVES

_____ 1. Use another student as a model to practice putting a patient in supine, erect, and lateral decubitus abdominal positions.

_____ 2. Using an abdomen phantom, produce an AP projection of the abdomen that results in a satisfactory radiograph (if equipment is available).

_____ 3. Determine whether rotation, tilt, or both are present on a radiograph of an AP projection of the abdomen.

_____ 4. Critique and evaluate abdomen radiographs based on the four divisions of radiographic criteria: (1) structures shown, (2) position, (3) collimation and central ray, and (4) exposure criteria.

_____ 5. Distinguish between acceptable and unacceptable abdomen radiographs based on exposure factors, motion, collimation, positioning, or other errors.

_____ 6. Identify specific bony and soft tissue structures seen radiographically.

_____ 7. Discriminate among radiographs taken in supine, erect, or lateral decubitus positions.

Learning Exercises

Complete the following review exercises after reading the associated pages in Chapter 3 of the textbook as indicated by each exercise. Answers to each review exercise are given at the end of the review exercises.

Part I: Radiographic Anatomy

REVIEW EXERCISE A: Abdominopelvic Anatomy (see textbook pp. 98-105)

1. What is the name of the two large muscles that are found in the posterior abdomen adjacent to the lumbar vertebra and are usually visible on an anteroposterior (AP) radiograph? _____

2. The medical prefix for stomach is _____

3. List the three parts of the small intestine:

   A. _____ B. _____ C. _____

4. Which portion of the small intestine is considered to be the longest? _____

5. The large intestine begins in the _____ quadrant with a saclike area called the

   _____ .

6. The sigmoid colon is located between the _____ and _____ of the large intestine.

7. List the three accessory digestive organs:

   A. _____ B. _____ C. _____

8. Circle the correct term. The pancreas is located **anteriorly or posteriorly** to the stomach.

9. Which one of the following organs is _not_ directly associated with the digestive system?

   A. Gallbladder   C. Jejunum

   B. Spleen   D. Pancreas

10. Which one of the following organs is considered to be part of the lymphatic system?

    A. Liver   C. Pancreas

    B. Spleen   D. Gallbladder

11. Why is the right kidney found in a more inferior position than the left kidney?

    _____

12. Which endocrine glands are superomedial to each kidney?

    _____

13. True/False: The correct term for the radiographic study of the urinary system is intravenous pyelogram (IVP).

14. The double-walled membrane lining the abdominopelvic cavity is called the _____ .

15. The organs located posteriorly to, or behind, the serous membrane lining of the abdominopelvic cavity are referred

    to as _____ .

16. Which one of the following structures helps stabilize and support the small intestine?

    A. Omentum   C. Viscera

    B. Peritoneum   D. Mesentery

17. Which one of the following structures is a double fold of peritoneum that connects the transverse colon to the greater curvature of the stomach?

    A. Mesocolon   C. Greater omentum

    B. Lesser omentum   D. Mesentery

18. Match the following structures to the correct portion of the peritoneum:

    _____ 1. Liver   A. Intraperitoneum

    _____ 2. Urinary bladder   B. Retroperitoneum

    _____ 3. Kidneys   C. Infraperitoneum

    _____ 4. Spleen

    _____ 5. Ovaries

    _____ 6. Duodenum

    _____ 7. Transverse colon

    _____ 8. Testes

    _____ 9. Adrenal glands

    _____ 10. Stomach

    _____ 11. Pancreas

    _____ 12. Ascending and descending colon

19. List the correct abdominal quadrant where the following organs would be found (left upper quadrant [LUQ], left lower quadrant [LLQ], right lower quadrant [RLQ], or right upper quadrant [RUQ]):

    A. Liver _____

    B. Spleen _____

    C. Sigmoid colon _____

    D. Left colic flexure _____

    E. Stomach _____

    F. Appendix _____

    G. Two thirds of jejunum _____

20. What is the correct name for the abdominal region found directly in the middle of the abdomen?
    A. Epigastric   C. Umbilical
    B. Inguinal   D. Pubic

21. Which one of the following abdominal regions contains the rectum?
    A. Pubic   D. Epigastric
    B. Inguinal   E. Hypochondriac
    C. Umbilical   F. Lumbar

22. Identify the bony landmarks in Fig. 3-1:

    A. _____

    B. _____

    C. _____

    D. _____

    E. _____

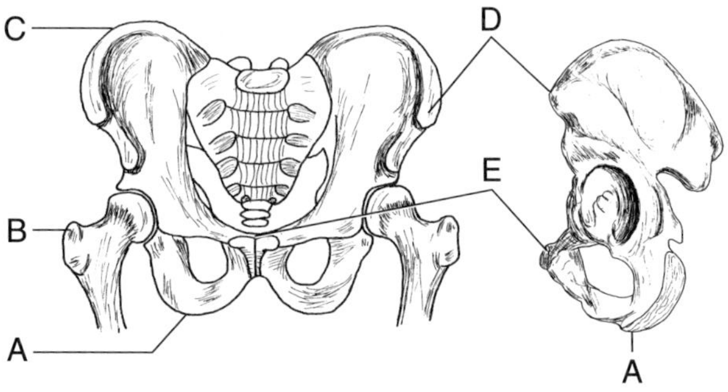

Fig. 3-1 Osteology of the pelvis.

23. The superior margin of the greater trochanter is about _____ inches (_____ cm) _____

    (superior or inferior) to the level of the symphysis pubis, and the ischial tuberosity is about _____ inches (_____ cm)

    _____ (superior or inferior) to the superior aspect of the symphysis pubis.

24. Which topographic landmark corresponds with the inferior margin of the abdomen and is formed by the anterior

    junction of the two pelvic bones? _____

25. Which topographic landmark is found at the level of L2-3? _____

26. The iliac crest is at the level of the _____ vertebra.

27. Identify the labeled parts of the digestive system (Fig. 3-2):

    A. _____

    B. _____

    C. _____

    D. _____ valve

    E. _____

    F. _____

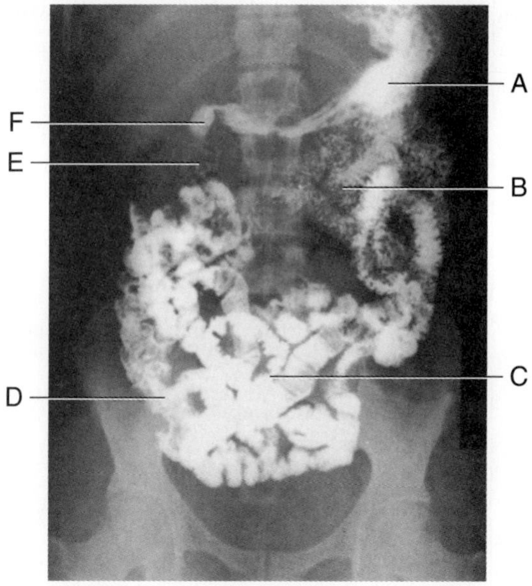

Fig. 3-2 Radiograph of the digestive tract.

28. Identify the labeled structures present on the computed tomography (CT) image (Fig. 3-3).

    A. _____

    B. _____

    C. _____

    D. _____

    E. _____

    F. _____

    G. _____

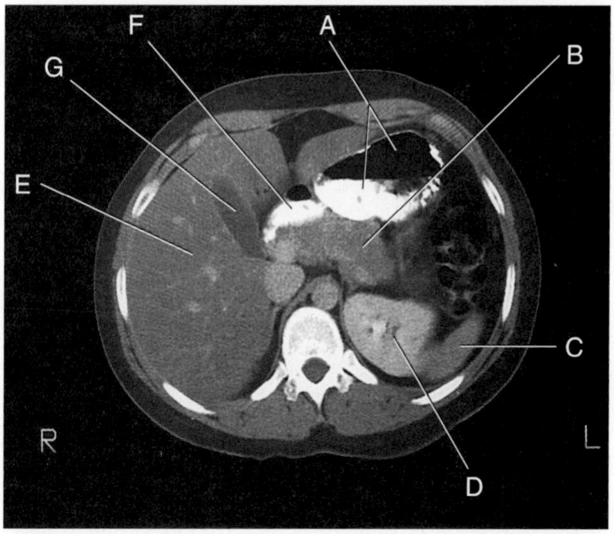

Fig. 3-3 Computed tomography (CT) cross-sectional image of abdomen at the level of L1 or L2.

Part II: Radiographic Positioning and Other Patient Considerations

REVIEW EXERCISE B: Shielding, Patient Dose, Pathology, Exposure Factors, and Positioning (see textbook pp. 106-115)

1. What are the two causes of voluntary motion?

    A. _____   B. _____

2. Voluntary motion can best be prevented by _____ to the patient.

3. What is the primary cause for involuntary motion in the abdomen?

    _____

4. What is the best mechanism to control involuntary motion?

_____

5. True/False: Because the liver margin is visible in the right upper quadrant of the abdomen, it is not necessary to place a right or left film marker on the cassette before exposure.

6. Gonadal shielding should *not* be used during abdomen radiography if:

   A. It obscures essential anatomy   C. The technologist does not elect to use it

   B. The patient requests that it not be used   D. The patient is 40 years or older

7. True/False: For an adult abdomen, a collimation margin must be visible on all four sides of the radiograph.

8. Gonadal shielding for _____ may be impossible for studies of the lower abdominopelvic region.

   A. Males   C. Both males and females

   B. Females   D. Small children

9. Gonadal shielding for females involves placing the top of the shield at or slightly above the level of the

   _____ , with the bottom at the _____ .

10. Which one of the following exposure factors would be most ideal for an AP abdomen of a small- to average-size adult?

    A. 110 kV, 200 mA, ¼ second, grid, 40-inch SID

    B. 85 kV, 300 mA, ⅕ second, grid, 40-inch SID

    C. 75 kV, 600 mA, ⅟₃₀ second, grid, 40-inch SID

    D. 60 kV, 400 mA, ⅟₁₅ second, grid, 40-inch SID

11. Which of the following technical factors is essential when performing abdomen studies on a young pediatric patient?

    A. Short exposure times   C. High milliamperage

    B. High speed screens and film   D. All of the above

12. True/False: A radiolucent pad should be placed underneath geriatric patients for added comfort.

13. With the use of iodinated contrast media, _____ is able to distinguish between a simple cyst or tumor of the liver:

    A. Ultrasound   C. Computed tomography (CT)

    B. Nuclear medicine   D. Magnetic resonance imaging (MRI)

14. _____ is being used to evaluate patients with acute appendicitis:

    A. Ultrasound   C. CT

    B. Nuclear medicine D. MRI

15. The preferred imaging modality for examining the gallbladder quickly is:

    A. Ultrasound   C. Barium enema study

    B. Nuclear medicine   D. MRI

16. Match the following definitions to the correct pathologic indicator:

_____ 1. Free air or gas in the peritoneal cavity   A.   Volvulus

_____ 2. Inflammatory condition of the colon   B.   Paralytic ileus

_____ 3. Telescoping of a section of bowel into another loop of bowel   C.   Ascites

_____ 4. Abnormal accumulation of fluid in the peritoneal cavity   D.   Ulcerative colitis

_____ 5. Bowel obstruction caused by a lack of intestinal peristalsis   E.   Pneumoperitoneum

_____ 6. A twisting of a loop of bowel creating an obstruction   F.   Intussusception

_____ 7. Chronic inflammation of the intestinal wall that may result   G.   Crohn's disease
             in bowel obstruction

17. Match the following radiographic appearances of the abdomen to the correct type of pathologic condition:

_____ 1. Distended loops of air-filled small intestine   A.   Ascites

_____ 2. Air-filled "coiled spring" appearance   B.   Volvulus

_____ 3. General abdominal haziness   C.   Pneumoperitoneum

_____ 4. Thin crest-shaped radiolucency underneath diaphragm   D.   Ulcerative colitis

_____ 5. Deep air-filled mucosal protrusions of colon wall   E.   Intussusception

_____ 6. A large amount of air trapped in sigmoid colon with a   F.   Crohn's disease
             tapered narrowing at the site of obstruction

18. The central ray is centered to the level of the _____ for a supine AP projection of the abdomen.

19. Exposure for an AP projection of the abdomen should be taken on _____ (inspiration or
     expiration).

20. Rotation can be determined on a KUB radiograph by the loss of symmetrical appearance of:

     A. _____   C. _____

     B. _____   D. _____

21. Which type of body habitus may require two lengthwise films if the entire abdomen is to be included?

     _____

22. True/False: A tall, asthenic patient may require two, 14 × 17 inch (35 × 43 cm) cassettes placed lengthwise if the
     entire abdomen is to be included.

23. Which of the following generates the largest gonadal dose?

     A. Female AP abdomen   C. Female posteroanterior (PA) abdomen

     B. Male lateral decubitus abdomen   D. Male erect AP abdomen

24. What is the gonadal dose range for an average-size female patient with an AP projection of the abdomen?

     A. 1 to 5 mrad   C. 35 to 75 mrad

     B. 5 to 10 mrad   D. 200 to 300 mrad

25. Which one of the following abdominal structures is not visible on a well-exposed KUB?

    A. Kidneys   C. Pancreas

    B. Margin of liver processes   D. Lumbar transverse

26. Why may the PA projection of a KUB generally be less desirable than the AP projection?

    _____

27. Which decubitus position of the abdomen best demonstrates intraperitoneal air in the abdomen?

    _____

28. Why should a patient be placed in the decubitus position for a minimum of 5 minutes before exposure?

    _____

29. Which decubitus position best demonstrates possible aneurysms, calcifications of the aorta, or umbilical hernias?

    _____

30. Which position best demonstrates a possible aortic aneurysm in the prevertebral region of the abdomen?

    _____

31. List the projections commonly performed for an acute abdominal series or three-way abdomen series:

    A. _____   B. _____   C. _____

32. Which position of the three-way acute abdominal series best demonstrates free air under the diaphragm?

    _____

33. Which positioning routine should be used for an acute abdominal series if the patient is too ill to stand?

    _____

34. To ensure that the diaphragm is included on an erect abdomen projection, the central ray should be at the level of

    _____ , which places the top of the 14 × 17 inch (35 × 43 cm) cassette at the level of the

    _____ .

35. Which one of the following projections involves a kilovoltage peak setting of 110 to 120?

    A. Erect abdomen for ascites

    B. Supine abdomen for intraabdominal mass

    C. PA, erect chest for free air under diaphragm

    D. Dorsal decubitus abdomen for calcified aorta

36. When using automatic exposure control (AEC) systems, which ionization chamber(s) should be activated for an average- to large-size patient when performing an AP projection of the abdomen?

    _____

37. True/False: A larger patient receives a greater amount of skin dose and midline dose as compared with a smaller patient during an AP projection of the abdomen.

REVIEW EXERCISE C: Problem Solving for Technical and Positioning Errors

The following radiographic problems involve technical and positioning errors that may lead to substandard images. As you analyze these problems, review your textbook to find solutions to these questions.

Other questions involve situations pertaining to different patient conditions and pathologic findings. If you need more information about a particular pathologic condition, review your textbook or a medical dictionary to learn more about it.

1. A radiograph of a KUB reveals that the symphysis pubis is cut off along the bottom of the film. Is this an acceptable image? If it is not, how can this problem be prevented on the repeat exposure?

   _____

   _____

2. A radiograph of an AP projection of an average-size adult abdomen was produced using the following exposure factors: 90 kVp, 400 mA, $^1/_{10}$ second, grid, 40-inch SID. The overall density of the radiograph was acceptable, but the soft tissue structures such as the psoas muscles and kidneys were not visible. Which adjustment to the technical factors will enhance the visibility of these structures on the repeat exposure?

   _____

   _____

3. A radiograph image of an AP projection of the abdomen is blurry. The following exposure factors were selected: 78 kV, 200 mA, $^2/_{10}$ second, grid, 40-inch SID. The technologist is sure that the patient didn't breathe or move during the exposure. What may have caused this blurriness? What can be done to correct this problem on the repeat exposure?

   _____

   _____

4. A radiograph of an AP abdomen reveals that the left iliac wing is more narrowed than the right. What specific positioning error caused this?

   _____

   _____

5. **Situation:** A patient with a possible **ileus** enters the emergency room. The patient is able to stand. The physician has ordered an acute abdominal series. What specific positioning routine should be used?

   _____

   _____

6. **Situation:** A patient with a possible perforated duodenal ulcer enters the emergency room. The emergency room physician is concerned about the presence of free air in the abdomen. The patient is in severe pain and **cannot** stand. What positioning routine should be used to diagnose this condition?

   _____

   _____

7. **Situation:** The emergency room physician suspects a patient has a kidney stone. The patient is sent to the radiology department to confirm the diagnosis. What specific positioning routine would be performed to rule out the presence of a kidney stone?

   _____

   _____

8. **Situation:** A patient in intensive care may have developed intraabdominal bleeding. The patient is in critical condition and cannot go to the radiology department. The physician has ordered a portable study of the abdomen. Which specific position or projection can be used to determine the extent of the bleeding?

   _____

   _____

9. **Situation:** A patient with a history of ascites comes to the radiology department. Which one of the following positions best demonstrates this condition?

   A. Erect AP abdomen   B. Erect PA chest   C. Supine KUB   D. Prone KUB

10. **Situation:** A radiograph of a KUB reveals that the gonadal shielding is superior to the upper margin of the symphysis pubis. The female patient has a history of kidney stones. What is the next step the technologist should take?

    A. Accept the radiograph because the kidneys were not obscured by the shielding.

    B. Repeat the exposure without using gonadal shielding.

    C. Repeat the exposure only if the patient complains of pain in the lower abdomen.

    D. Repeat the exposure with gonadal shielding, but position it below the symphysis pubis.

11. **Situation:** A hypersthenic patient comes to the radiology department for a KUB. The radiograph reveals that the symphysis pubis is included on the image, but the upper abdomen, including the kidneys, are cut off. What is the next step the technologist should take?

    A. Accept the radiograph.

    B. Repeat the exposure, but expose during inspiration to force the kidneys lower into the abdomen

    C. Ask the radiologist if the upper abdomen really needs to be seen. Repeat only if requested.

    D. Repeat the exposure. Use two, 14 × 17 inch (35 × 43 cm) cassettes crosswise to include the entire abdomen.

12. **Situation:** A patient comes from the emergency room with a largely, distended abdomen caused by an ileus. The physician suspects that the distention is caused by a large amount of bowel gas that is trapped in the small intestine. The standard technique for a KUB on an adult is 76 kVp, 30 mAs. Should the technologist change any of these exposure factors for this patient? (AEC is not being used.)

    A. No. Use the standard exposure settings.

    B. Yes. Decrease the milliamperage seconds.

    C. Yes. Increase the milliamperage seconds.

    D. Yes. Increase the kilovoltage peak.

REVIEW EXERCISE D: Critique Radiographs of the Abdomen (see textbook p.116)

The following questions relate to the radiographs found at the end of Chapter 3 of the textbook. Evaluate these radiographs for the radiographic criteria categories (*1* through *5*) that follow. Describe the corrections needed to improve the overall image. The major, or "repeatable" errors, are specific errors that indicate the need for a repeat exposure, regardless of the nature of the other errors.

A. Abdomen (left lateral decubitus) (Fig. C3-48)
   Description of possible error:

   1. Structures shown: _____

   2. Part positioning: _____

3. Collimation and central ray: _____

4. Exposure criteria: _____

5. Markers: _____

Repeatable error(s): _____

B. AP supine abdomen (KUB) (Fig. C3-49)
Description of possible error:

1. Structures shown: _____

2. Part positioning: _____

3. Collimation and central ray: _____

4. Exposure criteria: _____

5. Markers: _____

Repeatable error(s): _____

C. AP supine abdomen (KUB) (Fig. C3-50)
Description of possible error:

1. Structures shown: _____

2. Part positioning: _____

3. Collimation and central ray: _____

4. Exposure criteria: _____

5. Markers: _____

Repeatable error(s): _____

D. AP supine abdomen (KUB) (Fig. C3-51)
Description of possible error:

1. Structures shown: _____

2. Part positioning: _____

3. Collimation and central ray: _____

4. Exposure criteria: _____

5. Markers: _____

Repeatable error(s): _____

Part III: Laboratory Exercises (see textbook pp. 106-115)

You must gain experience in chest positioning before performing the following exams on actual patients. You can get experience in positioning and radiographic evaluation of these projections by performing exercises using radiographic phantoms and practicing on other students (although you will not be taking actual exposures).

The following suggested activities assume that your teaching institution has an energized lab and radiographic phantoms. If not, perform Laboratory Exercise B, the physical positioning exercises. (Check off each step and projection as you complete it.)

LABORATORY EXERCISE A: Energized Laboratory

1. Using the abdominal radiographic phantom, produce a radiograph of:

   _____ KUB

2. Evaluate the KUB radiograph, additional radiographs provided by your instructor, or both for:

   _____ Rotation   _____ Part and central ray centering

   _____ Proper exposure factors   _____ Motion

   _____ Collimation   _____ Markers

LABORATORY EXERCISE B: Physical Positioning

1. On another person, simulate taking all basic and special projections of the chest as listed. Follow the suggested positioning steps and sequence as listed in the following section and as described in Chapter 1 of your textbook:

   _____ KUB of the abdomen   _____ Dorsal decubitus

   _____ Left lateral decubitus   _____ Acute abdominal series to include: AP supine, AP erect, PA chest

For Suggested Positioning Sequence and Routine, see textbook p. 42. For Protocols for General Diagnostic Radiographic Procedures, see textbook p. 40.

Step 1. General Patient Positioning–Protocols #1 to #9, which include:

_____ Select the size and number of cassettes needed.

_____ Prepare the radiographic room. Check that tube is centered to the center of the film holder (or the centerline of the table for Bucky exams).

_____ Correctly identify the patient, and bring the patient into the room.

_____ Explain to the patient what you will be doing.

_____ Assist the patient to the proper place and position for the first radiograph.

Step 2. Measuring Part Thickness—Protocols #10 and #11 (unless AEC is used):

_____ Measure the body part being radiographed, and set correct exposure factors (technique). (If using an AEC system, select the correct chamber cells on the control panel.)

Step 3. Part Positioning—Protocol #12:

_____ Align and center the body part to the central ray or vice versa. For Bucky exams on a table, move the patient and table top together as needed (with floating-type table top). (NOTE: In cases in which the correct central ray position is of primary importance, the central ray icon is included in the textbook on the appropriate positioning page.)

Step 4. Film Centering:

_____ After the part has been centered to the central ray, the IR (cassette) is also centered to the central ray.

Additional Steps or Actions—Protocols #13 through #18:

_____ 1. Collimate accurately to include only the area of interest.

_____ 2. Place the correct marker within the exposure field (so that you do not superimpose pertinent anatomic structures).

_____ 3. Restrain or provide support for the body part to prevent motion.

_____ 4. Use contact lead shielding as needed.

_____ 5. Give clear breathing instructions, and make the exposure while watching the patient through the window.

Answers to Review Exercises

Review Exercise A: Abdominopelvic Anatomy

1. Psoas muscles
2. Gastro-
3. A. Duodenum
   B. Jejunum
   C. Ileum
4. Ileum
5. Right Lower, cecum
6. Descending colon, rectum
7. A. Pancreas
   B. Liver
   C. Gallbladder
8. Posteriorly
9. B. Spleen
10. B. Spleen
11. Presence of liver on right
12. Suprarenals (adrenal)
13. False (intravenous urogram [IVU])
14. Peritoneum
15. Retroperitoneal
16. D. Mesentery
17. C. Greater omentum
18. 1. A
    2. C
    3. B
    4. A
    5. C
    6. B
    7. A
    8. C
    9. B
    10. A
    11. B
    12. B
19. A. RUQ
    B. LUQ
    C. LLQ
    D. LUQ
    E. LUQ
    F. RLQ
    G. LUQ
20. C. Umbilical
21. A. Pubic
22. A. Ischial tuberosity
    B. Greater trochanter
    C. Iliac crest or crest of ilium
    D. Anterior superior iliac spine (ASIS)
    E. Symphysis pubis
23. 1.5 inches (3 to 4 cm) superior
    1.5 inches (3 to 4 cm) inferior
24. Symphysis pubis
25. Inferior costal margin
26. Interspace between L4-5
27. A. Stomach
    B. Jejunum
    C. Ileum
    D. Region of ileocecal valve
    E. Duodenum
    F. Duodenal bulb

28. A. Stomach
    B. Pancreas
    C. Spleen
    D. Kidney (left)
    E. Liver
    F. Duodenum
    G. Gallbladder

Review Exercise B: Shielding, Patient Dose, Pathology, Exposure Factors, and Positioning

1. A. Patient breathing
   B. Patient movement during exposure
2. Careful breathing instructions
3. Peristaltic action of the bowel
4. Use the shortest exposure time possible.
5. False
6. A. It obscures essential anatomy
7. False
8. B. Female
9. ASISs
   Symphysis pubis
10. C (70 to 80 kVp range)
11. D. All of the above
12. True
13. C. Computed tomography (CT)
14. A. Ultrasound
15. A. Ultrasound
16. 1. E
    2. D
    3. F
    4. C
    5. B
    6. A
    7. G
17. 1. F
    2. E
    3. A
    4. C
    5. D
    6. B
18. Iliac crest
19. Expiration
20. A. Iliac wings
    B. Obturator foramina (if visible)
    C. Ischial spines
    D. Outer rib margins
21. Tall, hyposthenic or asthenic
22. True
23. A. (female AP abdomen)
24. C. (35 to 75 mrad)
25. C. Pancreas
26. Increased object-image distance (OID) of kidneys on PA
27. Left lateral decubitus (free air best visualized in upper right abdomen in area of liver)
28. To allow intraabdominal air to rise or abnormal fluids to accumulate

29. Dorsal decubitus (p. 113)
30. Lateral position
31. A. AP supine
    B. AP erect or lateral decubitus abdomen
    C. PA erect chest
32. PA chest
33. Two-way abdomen; AP supine abdomen, and left lateral decubitus
34. A. 2 inches (5 cm) above crest
    B. Axilla
35. C. (chest technique)
36. Center and upper left chambers
37. True (p. 109)

Review Exercise C: Problem-Solving for Technical and Positioning Errors

1. No. A KUB must include the symphysis pubis on the radiograph to ensure that the bladder is seen. The positioning error involves centering of the central ray to the iliac crest. The technologist should also palpate the symphysis pubis or greater trochanter to ensure that it is above the bottom of the cassette.
2. The selected kilovoltage peak (90 kVp) was too high. The technologist needs to lower the kilovoltage peak to between 70 and 80 kVp. The milliamperage and exposure time can be altered to maintain the density.
3. The blurriness may be caused by involuntary motion. To control this motion, the technologist needs to increase the milliamperage and decrease the exposure time (e.g., 400 mA at $1/10$ second).
4. Patient was rotated into a slight right posterior oblique (RPO) position. (The downside will appear wider.)
5. The three-way acute abdominal series, including the anteroposterior (AP) supine and erect abdomen, and posteroanterior (PA) erect chest projections.
6. The two-way acute abdomen series: AP supine abdomen, and left lateral decubitus
7. A KUB would be performed with the correct exposure factors to visualize the possible stone.
8. A bedside portable left lateral decubitus projection could be performed to demonstrate any fluid levels in the abdomen.
9. A. The erect AP abdomen position best demonstrates air/fluid levels. Ascites produces free fluid in the intraperitoneal cavity

10. B. Because the patient may have renal calculi in the distal ureters and urinary bladder, gonadal shielding cannot be used.
11. D. Repeat the exposure using two 14 × 17 inch cassettes placed crosswise. The hypersthenic patient often requires this type of film placement for abdomen studies
12. B. Decrease the milliamperage seconds. Because trapped air is easier to penetrate than soft tissue with x-rays, reducing the milliamperage seconds will prevent overexposing the radiograph

Review Exercise D: Critique Radiographs of the Abdomen

A. Left lateral decubitus abdomen (Fig. C3-48)
   1. Diaphragm cut off
   2. Slight rotation of pelvis evident by asymmetric appearance of pelvis
   3. Central ray centered too low (right upper quadrant cut off)
      Collimation not evident
   4. Exposure factors acceptable
   5. Anatomic side marker missing
      Repeatable error(s): criteria 1 and 3 (central ray centering)
B. AP supine abdomen (Fig. C3-49)
   1. Top of kidneys cut off
   2. Slight rotation toward right (RPO). (NOTE: Left obturator foramen is wider than right, and patient is slightly off center to the right.)
   3. Central ray centered correctly to the iliac crest, but image receptor (IR) not centered to central ray—too low
      Unequal collimation because of centering error; too close side collimation
   4. Exposure factors acceptable
   5. Anatomic side marker present
      Repeatable error(s): criteria 1 and 3 (central ray to image receptor [CR-to-IR] centering)
C. AP supine abdomen (Fig. C3-50)
   1. Upper abdomen cut off because central ray and IR centered too low
   2. No rotation evident; upper abdomen slightly off center toward left because of body tilt
   3. Central ray and IR centered too low

Only lower collimation visible because of poor CR-to-IR centering
   4. Motion present; must use shorter exposure time or give more complete breathing instructions
   5. Anatomic side marker evident (over femur)
      Repeatable error(s): criteria 1 (upper abdomen cut off), 3 (central ray centered too low), and 4 (motion present, general blurring of gas pattern margins—maybe difficult to discern on this printed radiograph)
D. AP supine abdomen (Fig. C3-51)
   1. Region of bladder cut off
   2. No rotation
   3. Central ray and IR centered too high
      Excellent side-to-side collimation
   4. Exposure factors acceptable
   5. Anatomic side marker present (but difficult to see)
      Repeatable error(s): criteria 1 and 3

SELF-TEST

My Score = _____%

This self-test should be taken only after completing all of the readings, review exercises, and laboratory activities for a particular section. The purpose of this test is not only to provide a good learning exercise but also to serve as a strong indicator of what your final unit evaluation grade will cover. It is strongly suggested that if you do not get at least a 90% to 95% grade on each self-test, you should review those areas in which you missed questions before going to your instructor for the final unit evaluation exam.

1. The double-walled membrane lining the abdominal cavity is called the:

    A. Greater omentum   C.   Lesser omentum

    B. Mesentery   D.   Peritioneum

2. Which one of the following soft-tissue structures are seen on a well-exposed KUB?

    A. Spleen   C.   Psoas muscles

    B. Pancreas   D.   Stomach

3. The first portion of the small intestine is called the:

    A. Duodenum   C.   Jejunum

    D. Ileum   D.   Pylorus

4. At the junction of the small and large intestine is the:

    A. Sigmoid colon   C.   Ileocecal valve

    B. Rectum   D.   Ascending colon

5. Match the correct answer to the structures labeled on Fig. 3-4:

    _____ 1.   A. Sigmoid colon

    _____ 2.   B. Liver

    _____ 3.   C. Jejunum

    _____ 4.   D. Oral cavity

    _____ 5.   E. Spleen

    _____ 6.   F. Stomach

    _____ 7.   G. Esophagus

    _____ 8.   H. Oropharynx

    _____ 9.   I. Pancreas

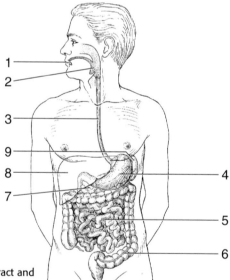

Fig. 3-4 Digestive tract and surrounding structures.

6. Which one of the following is not an accessory organ of digestion?

    A. Liver   C.   Pancreas

    B. Spleen   D.   Kidney

7. The kidneys are connected to the bladder by way of the:

    A. Urethra   B. Renal artery   C. Ureter   D. Renal vein

8. Which structure stores and releases bile?

    A. Liver   B. Spleen   C. Pancreas   D. Gallbladder

9. Which one of the following structures connects the small intestine to the posterior abdominal wall?

    A. Greater omentum   C. Lesser omentum

    B. Peritoneum   D. Mesentery

10. List the correct quadrant(s) where the following organs would be found on an average sthenic patient (right upper quadrant [RUQ], right lower quadrant [RLQ], left upper quadrant [LUQ], left lower quadrant [LLQ]):

    A. Cecum _____

    B. Liver _____

    C. Spleen _____

    D. Stomach _____

    E. Right colic flexure _____

    F. Sigmoid colon _____

    G. Appendix _____

    H. Pancreas _____

    I. Gallbladder _____

11. Which region of the abdomen would contain the T12 vertebra?

    A. Epigastric   C. Hypochondriac

    B. Umbilical   D. Pubic

12. Match the following structures to the correct aspect of the peritoneum:

    _____   1. Cecum   A. Intraperitoneum

    _____   2. Jejunum   B. Retroperitoneum

    _____   3. Ascending colon   C. Infraperitoneum

    _____   4. Liver

    _____   5. Adrenal glands

    _____   6. Gallbladder

    _____   7. Ovaries

    _____   8. Duodenum

    _____   9. Urinary bladder

    _____ 10. Pancreas

13. The xiphoid process corresponds with the vertebral level:

    A. T9-10   C. L2-3

    B. L4-5   D. T4-5

14. Identify the topographical positioning landmarks as labeled on Figs. 3-5 and 3-6:

    _____ 1. Iliac crest

    _____ 2. Ischial tuberosity

    _____ 3. Xiphoid process

    _____ 4. Symphysis pubis

    _____ 5. Greater trochanter

    _____ 6. Lower costal margin

    _____ 7. Anterior superior iliac spine (ASIS)

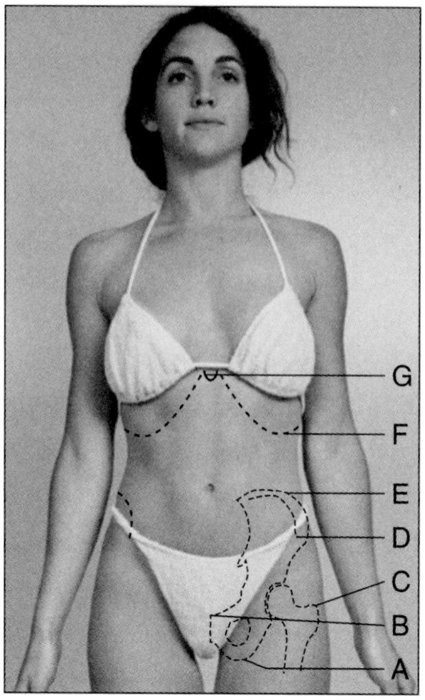

Fig. 3-5 Anterior surface landmarks. 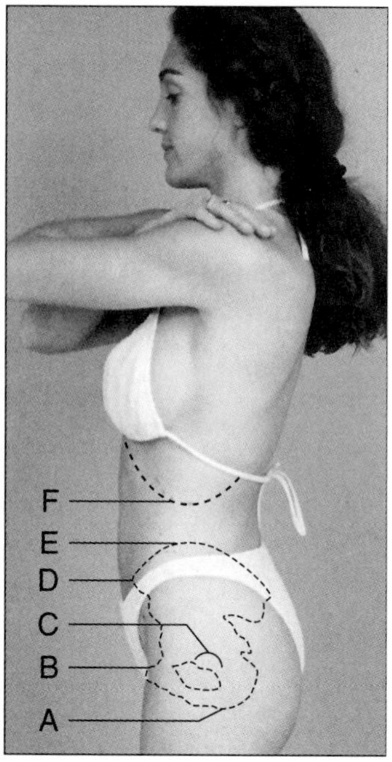   **Fig. 3-6** Lateral surface landmarks.

15. To identify the **inferior margin** of the abdomen, the technologist can palpate the symphysis pubis or:

    A. Iliac crest   C. ASIS

    B. Greater trochanter   D. Ischial tuberosity

16. The most important anatomic landmark that is commonly used to locate the center of the abdomen is the:

    A. Iliac crest   C. ASIS

    B. Greater trochanter   D. Ischial tuberosity

17. Which one of the following factors best controls the involuntary motion of a pediatric patient during abdominal radiography?

    A. Short exposure time

    B. High kilovoltage peak (100 to 125)

    C. Clear, concise breathing instructions

    D. Use of compression band across abdomen

18. An abnormal accumulation of fluid in the abdominal cavity is called:

    A. Ileus   C. Volvulus

    B. Ulcerative colitis   D. Ascites

19. The general term describing a nonmechanical bowel obstruction is:

    A. Pneumoperitoneum   C. Ascites

    B. Ileus   D. Intussusception

20. The telescoping of a section of bowel into another loop is called:

　　A. Intussusception　　　C. Volvulus

　　B. Ascites　　　　　　　D. Ulcerative colitis

21. A chronic disease involving inflammation of the colon is:

　　A. Ascites　　　　　C. Crohn's disease

　　B. Volvulus　　　　D. Ulcerative colitis

22. Free air or gas in the peritoneal cavity is:

　　A. Pneumothorax　　　C. Pneumoperitoneum

　　B. Ileus　　　　　　　D. Volvulus

23. Free air in the intraabdominal cavity rises to the level of the _____ in a patient who is in the erect position:

　　A. Greater omentum　　　C. Intraperitoneal cavity

　　B. Diaphragm　　　　　　D. Liver

24. Which one of the following conditions is demonstrated radiographically as general abdominal haziness?

　　A. Pneumoperitoneum　　　C. Ileus

　　B. Ascites　　　　　　　　D. Volvulus

25. Which one of the following conditions is demonstrated radiographically as distended, air-filled loops of small bowel?

　　A. Ascites　　　　　　　C. Pneumoperitoneum

　　B. Ulcerative colitis　　D. Ileus

26. Identify the structures labeled on this anteroposterior (AP) KUB radiograph (Fig. 3-7):

　　A. _____

　　B. _____

　　C. _____

　　D. _____

　　E. _____

　　F. _____

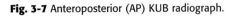

Fig. 3-7 Anteroposterior (AP) KUB radiograph.

27.   Identify the organs or structures labeled on this computed tomography (CT) scan (Fig. 3-8) at the level of L1 or L2.

A.   _____

B.   _____

C.   _____

D.   _____

E.   _____

F.   _____

G.   _____

H.   _____

Major blood vessels:

I.   _____

J.   _____

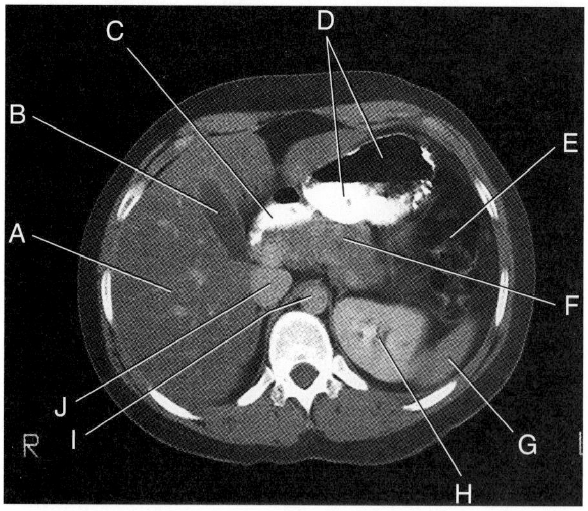

Fig. 3-8 Computed tomography (CT) cross-sectional image at the level of L1 or L2.

28.   Which one of the following exposure factors would be the best for abdominal radiography (for an average-size adult)?

A.   110 kVp, 400 mA, $^1\!/_{20}$ second, grid, 40-inch source-image distance (SID)

B.   78 kVp, 600 mA, $^1\!/_{30}$ second, grid, 40-inch SID

C.   78 kVp, 200 mA, $^1\!/_{10}$ second, grid, 40-inch SID

D.   65 kVp , 600 mA, $^1\!/_{15}$ second, grid, 40-inch SID

29.   A radiograph of an AP projection of the abdomen reveals that the right iliac wing is wider than the left. What type of positioning error was involved?

A.   Rotation toward the left   C.   Rotation toward the right

B.   Tilt to the left   D.   Tilt to the right

30.   Most abdominal projections are taken during:

A.   Expiration   C.   Inspiration

B.   Shallow breathing   D.   Deep breathing

31.   A radiograph of a KUB on a large, hypersthenic patient reveals that the entire abdomen is not included on the 35 × 43 cm (14 × 17 inch) image receptor (IR). What can be done to correct this on the repeat radiograph?

A.   Use two cassettes placed lengthwise.

B.   Use two cassettes placed crosswise.

C.   Expose during deep inspiration.

D.   Perform KUB with patient in erect position.

32.   What is the **minimum** amount of time a patient should be upright before taking a projection to demonstrating intraabdominal free air?

A.   20 minutes   C.   2 minutes

B.   30 minutes   D.   5 minutes

33. If the posteroanterior (PA) chest projection is *not* performed for the acute abdominal series, centering for the erect abdomen projection **must** include the:

    A. Inferior liver margin   C. Entire kidneys

    B. Diaphragm   D. Bladder

34. Which specific decubitus position of the abdomen should be used in an acute abdomen series if the patient cannot stand?

    A. Left lateral decubitus   C. Right lateral decubitus

    B. Dorsal decubitus   D. Ventral decubitus

35. **Situation:** A patient with a possible ileus enters the emergency room. The physician orders an acute abdominal series. The patient can stand. Which specific position best demonstrates air/fluid levels in the abdomen?

    A. AP supine abdomen   C. Dorsal decubitus

    B. Right lateral decubitus   D. AP erect abdomen

36. **Situation:** A patient with a possible perforated bowel caused by trauma enters the emergency room. The patient is unable to stand. Which projection(s) should be performed to confirm the diagnosis?

    A. Dorsal decubitus   C. AP supine abdomen

    B. Left lateral decubitus   D. Right lateral decubitus

37. **Situation:** A patient with a clinical history of a possible umbilical hernia comes to the radiology department. The KUB is inconclusive Which additional projection can be taken to help confirm the diagnosis?

    A. AP erect abdomen   C. Dorsal decubitus

    B. Left lateral decubitus   D. Ventral decubitus

38. True/False: The following statements concern average-size patient doses for abdominal radiographs:

    _____ A. The female ovarian dose on a PA abdomen is close the midline dose ($\pm10\%$).

    _____ B. The skin dose for an average-size AP or PA abdomen is in the 75- to 150-mrad range.

    _____ C. The female ovarian dose for an AP abdomen is about double that for a PA projection.

    _____ D. The male testes dose is less than $^1/_{10}$ that of the female ovarian dose with proper collimation.

39. For the following critique questions, refer to the textbook, p. 116 (Fig. C3-49) (AP supine abdomen):

    A. Which positioning errors are visible on this radiograph? More than one answer may be selected.

       (a) All essential anatomic structures are not demonstrated.

       (b) CR-to-IR centering is incorrect.

       (c) CR-to-anatomy centering incorrect.

       (d) Collimation is not evident.

       (e) Exposure factors are incorrect.

       (f) No marker is seen on the radiograph.

       (g) Rotation is toward the right.

       (h) Rotation is toward the left.

    B. Which of the previous criteria errors on this radiograph is/are considered "repeatable errors?"

    _____

C. Which of the following modifications must be made during the repeat exposure? More than one answer may be selected.

   (a) Open up collimation.

   (b) Center CR-to-IR correctly.

   (c) Center CR-to-anatomy correctly.

   (d) Decrease exposure factors.

   (e) Increase exposure factors.

   (f) Place marker on IR before exposure.

   (g) Ensure ASISs are equal distance from table top to eliminate rotation.

40. For the following critique questions, refer to Fig. C3-51 (AP supine abdomen) on p. 116 in your textbook.

   A. What are the positioning error(s) seen on this radiograph? More than one answer may be selected.

      (a) All essential anatomic structures are not demonstrated.

      (b) CR-to-IR centering is incorrect.

      (c) Collimation is not evident.

      (d) Exposure factors are incorrect.

      (e) No marker is seen on the radiograph.

      (f) Rotation is toward the right.

      (g) Rotation is toward the left.

   B. Which of the previous criteria errors on this radiograph is/are considered "repeatable errors?"

   C. Which of the following modifications must be made during the repeat exposure? More than one answer may be selected.

      (a) Open up collimation.

      (b) Center CR-to-IR correctly.

      (c) Decrease exposure factors.

      (d) Increase exposure factors.

      (e) Place marker on IR before exposure.

      (f) Ensure ASISs are equal distance from table top to eliminate rotation.

Upper Limb

CHAPTER OBJECTIVES

After you have successfully completed **all** the activities in this chapter, you will be able to:

_____ 1. List the total number of bones of the hand and wrist.

_____ 2. Identify specific aspects of the phalanges, metacarpals, and carpal bones.

_____ 3. On drawings and radiographs, identify specific anatomic structures of the hand and wrist.

_____ 4. List and describe the location, size, and shape of each carpal bone of the wrist.

_____ 5. Match specific joints of the hand and wrist according to classification and movement type.

_____ 6. List four specific ligaments of the wrist.

_____ 7. On drawings and radiographs, identify specific fat pads and stripes of the upper limb.

_____ 8. Distinguish between ulnar and radial deviation wrist movements.

_____ 9. Identify specific parts of the forearm, elbow, and distal humerus.

_____ 10. On drawings and radiographs, identify specific anatomic structures of the forearm, elbow, and distal humerus.

_____ 11. List the technical factors commonly used for upper limb radiography.

_____ 12. Match specific pathologic features of the upper limb to their correct definition.

_____ 13. Match specific pathologic features of the upper limb to their correct radiographic appearance.

_____ 14. For select pathologic conditions of the upper limb, indicate whether manual exposure factors should be increased or decreased or remain the same.

_____ 15. Identify the correct central ray placement, part position, and radiographic criteria for specific positions of the fingers, thumb, hand, wrist, forearm, and elbow.

_____ 16. Identify which structures are best seen with each basic and special projection of the upper limb.

_____ 17. Based on clinical situations, describe the preferred positioning routine to assist the physician with the diagnosis of a specific condition or disease process.

_____ 18. Identify and apply the exposure conversion chart for various sizes of plaster and fiberglass casts.

_____ 19. List the three radiographic criteria for a true lateral elbow position.

_____ 20. List the skin and midline dose ranges and the relative differences among these doses for each body part of the upper limb.

_____ 21. Given various hypothetical situations, identify the correct modification of a position, exposure factors, or both to improve the radiographic image.

_____ 22. Given various hypothetical situations, identify the correct position for a specific condition or pathologic feature.

_____ 23. Given radiographs of specific upper limb positions, identify specific positioning and exposure factors errors.

POSITIONING AND FILM CRITIQUE

_____   1. Using another student as a model, practice basic and special projections of the upper limb.

_____   2. Using a hand and elbow radiographic phantom, produce satisfactory radiographs of the hand, thumb, wrist, and elbow (if equipment is available).

_____   3. Critique and evaluate upper limb radiographs based on the four divisions of radiographic criteria: (1) structures shown, (2) position, (3) collimation and central ray, and (4) exposure criteria.

_____   4. Distinguish between acceptable and unacceptable upper limb radiographs based on exposure factors, motion, collimation, positioning, or other errors.

Learning Exercises

Complete the following review exercises after reading the associated pages in the textbook as indicated by each exercise. Answers to each review exercise are given at the end of the review exercises.

PART I: Radiographic Anatomy

REVIEW EXERCISE A: Anatomy of the Hand and Wrist (see textbook pp. 118-124)

1. Fill in the number of bones in the following:

    A. Phalanges (fingers and thumb) _____   C. Carpals (wrist) _____

    B. Metacarpals (palm) _____   D. Total _____

2. The two portions of the thumb (first digit) are the:

    A. _____   B. _____

3. The three portions of each finger (second through fifth digits) are the:

    A. _____

    B. _____

    C. _____

4. The three parts of each phalanx, starting distally, are the:

    A. _____   B. _____   C. _____

5. List the three parts of each metacarpal, starting proximally:

    A. _____   B. _____   C. _____

6. The name of the joint between the proximal and distal phalanges of the first digit is the _____.

7. The joints between metacarpals and phalanges are the _____.

8. Fill in the names and parts of the following bones
    and joints of the right hand shown in Fig. 4-1. In-
    clude abbreviations for joints if applicable:

    A. _____

    B. _____

    C. _____

    D. _____

    E. _____

    F. _____

    G. _____

    H. _____

    I. _____

    J. _____

    K. _____

    L. _____

    M. _____

    N. _____

    O. _____

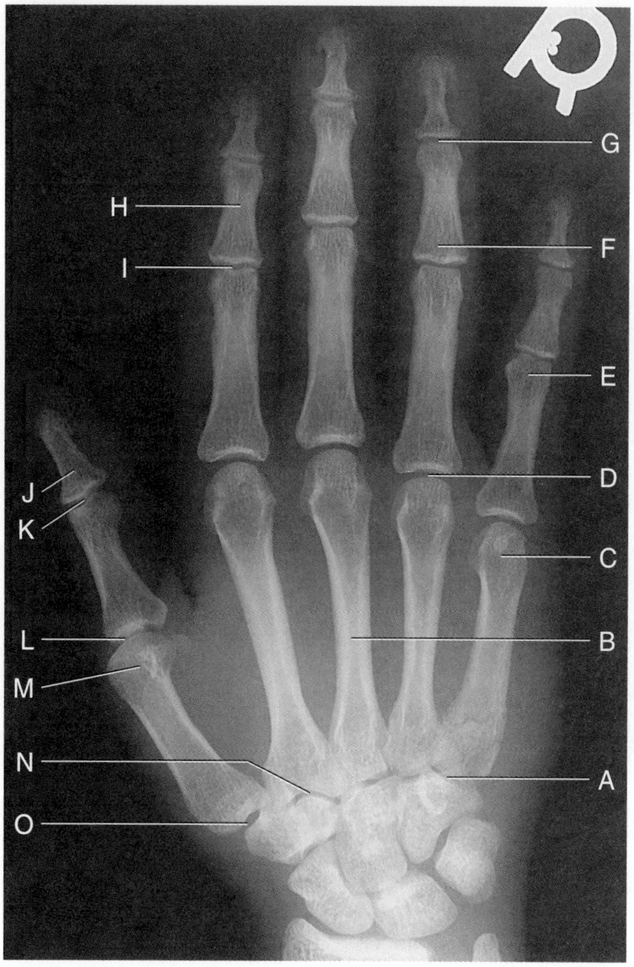

Fig. 4-1 Posteroanterior (PA) right hand.

9. Match each of the following carpal bones shown in Figs. 4-2 and 4-3:

    _____ A.   1. Lunate

    _____ B.   2. Hamate

    _____ C.   3. Trapezium

    _____ D.   4. Pisiform

    _____ E.   5. Triquetrum

    _____ F.   6. Trapezoid

    _____ G   7. Capitate

    _____ H.   8. Scaphoid

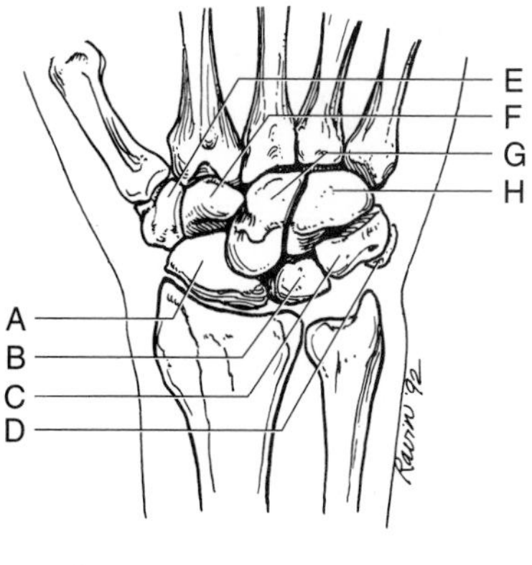

Fig. 4-2 Posterior view of wrist.

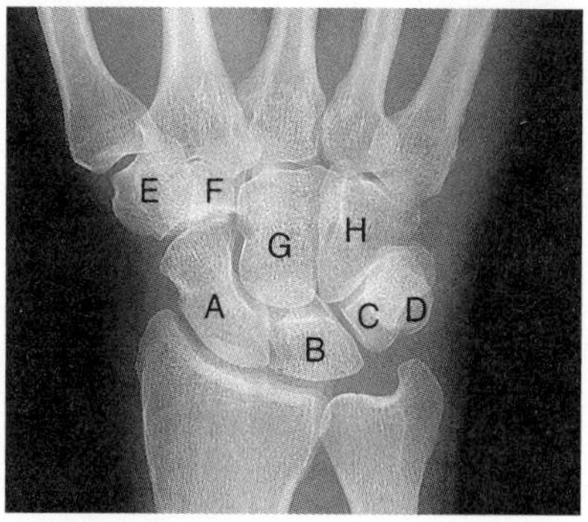

Fig. 4-3 Posteroanterior (PA) wrist.

10. Which is the largest of the carpal bones? _____

11. What is the name of the hooklike process extending anteriorly from the hamate? _____

12. Which is the most commonly fractured carpal bone? _____

13. List one of the mnemonics given in the textbook that uses the first letter of the preferred terms of the eight carpal

    bones. _____

    _____

14. Match the structures labeled *A-I* on Figs. 4-4 and 4-5 with the
    correct bones listed *1-9*:

    _____ A.   1. Capitate

    _____ B.   2. Scaphoid

    _____ C.   3. Base of first metacarpal

    _____ D.   4. Pisiform

    _____ E.   5. Trapezoid

    _____ F.   6. Hamulus (hamular process)

    _____ G.   7. Triquetrum

    _____ H.   8. Hamate

    _____ I.   9. Trapezium

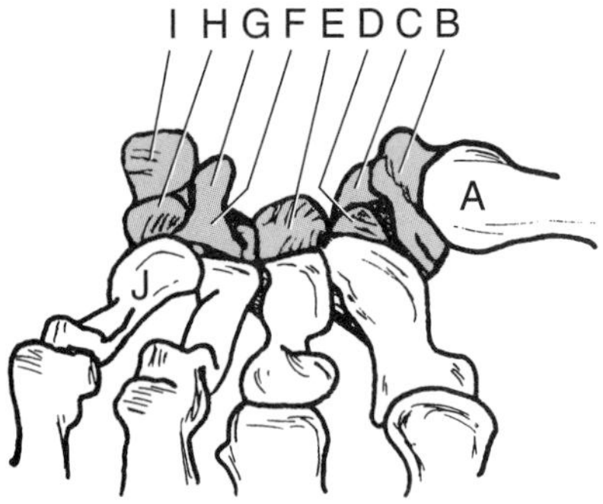

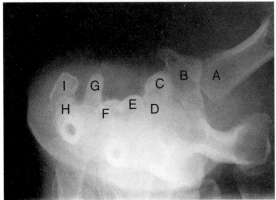

Fig. 4-4 Carpal tunnel view.

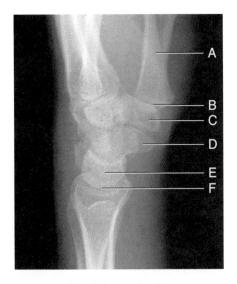

Fig. 4-5 Carpal canal, inferosuperior projection.

15. Identify the carpals and other structures labeled on Fig. 4-6:

    A. _____

    B. _____

    C. _____

    D. _____

    E. _____

    F. _____

Fig. 4-6 Lateral wrist.

REVIEW EXERCISE B: Anatomy of the Forearm, Elbow, and Distal Humerus (see textbook pp. 122-127)

1. In the anatomic position, identify which of the bones of the forearm is located on the lateral (thumb) side (A)

   _____ and which is on the medial side (B) _____ .

2. Indicate whether the following structures are part of the radius (R), ulna (U), or distal humerus (H) by listing the appropriate letter next to the structure:

   _____ A. Trochlear notch   _____ E. Coronoid tubercle

   _____ B. Radial notch   _____ F. Coronoid process

   _____ C. Olecranon fossa   _____ G. Olecranon process

   _____ D. Trochlea   _____ H. Coronoid fossa

3. Which two joints of the forearm allow for rotation of the forearm during pronation?

   _____

4. A. The articular portion of the medial aspect of the distal humerus is called the _____ .

   B. The similar structure found on the lateral aspect of the distal humerus is called the _____ .

5. The deep depression located on the posterior aspect of the distal humerus is the _____ .

6. The criteria for evaluating a true lateral position of the elbow is the appearance of three concentric arcs (Fig. 4-7). These arcs include:

   A. The first and smallest of the arcs: _____

   B. The intermediate double arc, consisting of the outer ridges of:

   The smaller arc: _____

   The larger arc: _____

   C. The third arc, which is part of the ulna: _____

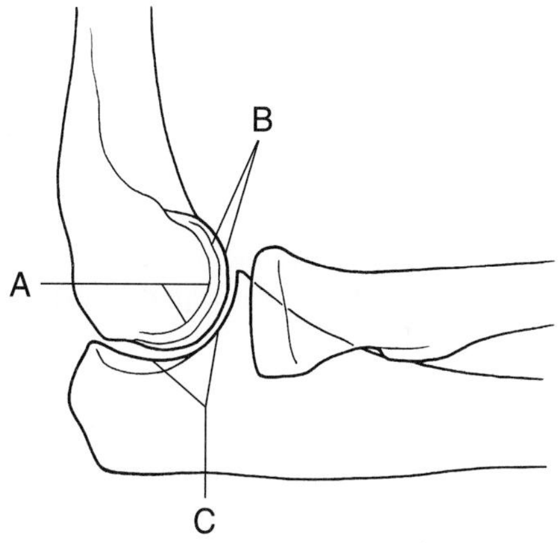

Fig. 4-7 True lateral elbow. Three concentric circles

7. Match the following articulations with the correct joint movement types:

   _____ A. Interphalangeal   1. Ginglymus (hinge)

   _____ B. Carpometacarpal of first digit   2. Ellipsoidal (condyloid)

   _____ C. Elbow joint (humeroulnar and humeroradial)   3. Trochoidal (pivot)

   _____ D. Metacarpophalangeal of second to fifth digits   4. Plane (gliding)

   _____ E. Radiocarpal   5. Sellar (saddle)

   _____ F. Intercarpal

   _____ G. Elbow joint (proximal radioulnar)

   _____ H. Proximal and distal radioulnar joint

8. Ellipsoidal or condyloid joints are classified as freely movable or _____ and allow movement

   in _____ directions.

9. List the four ligaments of the wrist:

   A. _____   C. _____

   B. _____   D. _____

10. Which one of the ligaments of the wrist extends from the styloid process of the radius to the lateral aspect of the

    scaphoid and trapezium bones? _____

11. What is the name of the two special turning or bending positions of the hand and wrist that demonstrate medial and
    lateral aspects of the carpal region?

    A. _____   B. _____

12. Of the two positions listed in the previous question, which one is most commonly performed to detect a fracture of

    the scaphoid bone? _____

13. How does the forearm appear radiographically if pronated for a posteroanterior (PA) projection?

    _____

14. The two important fat stripes around the wrist joint are the:

    A. _____   B. _____

15. The fat pads around the elbow joint are valuable diagnostic indicators if the following three technical/positioning re-
    quirements are met with the lateral position:

    A. _____   C. _____

    B. _____

16. True/False: If the posterior fat pad of the elbow is not visible radiographically, it suggests that a nonobvious radial
    head or neck fracture is present.

17. True/False: If the elbow is flexed correctly at 90°, the posterior fat pad is visible if pathologic elbow trauma is
    present.

18. True/False: Trauma or infection makes the anterior fat pad more difficult to see on a lateral elbow radiograph.

19. Which projections best demonstrate the scaphoid fat pad? _____

20. Which projection best demonstrates the pronator fat stripe? _____

21. Identify the parts labeled on Fig. 4-8 and Fig. 4-9:

A. _____   I. _____

B. _____   J. _____

C. _____   K. _____

D. _____   L. _____

E. _____   M. _____

F. _____   N.* _____

G. _____   O.* _____

H. _____   P.* _____

*HINT: These are concentric arcs as evidence of a true lateral position.

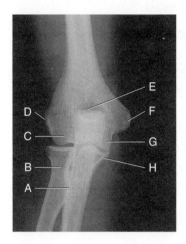

Fig. 4-8 Anteroposterior (AP) elbow.   **Fig. 4-9** Lateral elbow.

22. Identify the parts labeled on Figs. 4-10 and 4-11:

A. _____

B. _____

C. _____

D. _____

E. _____

F. _____

G. _____

H. _____

I. _____

J. _____

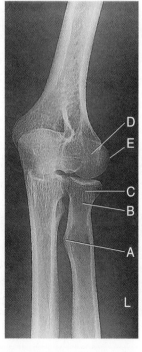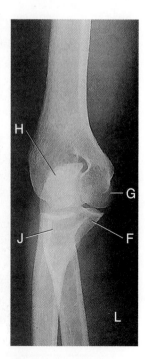

Fig. 4-10 Lateral (external) rotation of the elbow.   **Fig. 4-11** Medial (internal) rotation of the elbow.

PART II: Radiographic Positioning

REVIEW EXERCISE C: Positioning of the Fingers, Thumb, Hand, and Wrist (see textbook pp. 128-151)

1. List the following technical factors most commonly used for upper limb radiography:

    A. Kilovoltage peak (kVp) range: _____

    B. Long or short exposure time? _____

    C. Large or small focal spot? _____

    D. Most common minimum source-image distance (SID): _____

    E. Grids are used if the body part measures more than _____ cm.

    F. Type of intensification screens most commonly used: _____

    G. Small to medium dry plaster casts: Increase _____ kilovoltage peak

    H. Large or wet plaster casts: Increase _____ kilovoltage peak

        or _____ milliamperage seconds

    I. Fiberglass casts: Increase _____ kilovoltage peak

        or _____ milliamperage seconds

    J. Correctly exposed radiographs: Visualize _____ margins as well as

        _____ markings of all bones

2. The general rule for collimation for upper limb radiography states: _____

    _____

3. Circle all pertinent factors that help control distortion during upper limb radiography:

    A. Kilovoltage peak

    B. 40 to 44 inches (100 to 110 cm) SID

    C. Milliamperage seconds

    D. Minimal object-image distance (OID)

    E. Correct central ray placement

    F. Use of small focal spot

4. Gonadal shielding is especially important for upper limbs on all persons who are _____ .

5. True/False: Guardians of young pediatric patients who are having upper limb studies can be asked to hold their child during the radiographic study.

6. _____ is a radiographic procedure that utilizes contrast media to visualize soft tissue pathology of the wrist, elbow, and shoulder joints.

7. What is the basic positioning routine for the second through fifth digits of the hand? _____

    _____

8. How much of the metacarpals should be included for PA projection of the digits? _____

_____

9. List the two radiographic criteria used to determine whether rotation is present on the PA projection of the digits?

    A. _____

    B. _____

10. Which positioning modifications may be used for a study of the second digit to improve definition for the:

    A. PA oblique projection _____

    B. Lateral position _____

11. Where is the central ray centered for a PA oblique projection of the second digit? _____

12. Why is it important to keep the affected digit parallel to the image receptor (IR) for the PA oblique and lateral projections?

    A. To prevent distortion of the phalanx   C. To demonstrate small, nondisplaced fractures near the joint

    B. To prevent distortion of the joints   D. All of the above

13. Why is the anteroposterior (AP) position of the thumb recommended instead of the PA? _____

_____

14. Which projection of the thumb is achieved naturally by placing the palmar surface of the hand in contact with the

    cassette? _____

15. Which IR size should be used for a thumb routine? _____

16. A sesamoid bone is frequently found adjacent to the _____ joint of the thumb.

17. True/False: The entire metacarpal and trapezium must be demonstrated on all projections of the thumb.

18. Where is the central ray centered for an AP projection of the thumb?

    A. First interphalangeal (IP) joint   C. First metacarpophalangeal (MP) joint

    B. Mid aspect of proximal phalanx   D. First proximal interphalangeal (PIP) joint

19. A Bennett's fracture involves:

    A. Base of first metacarpal   C. Scaphoid bone

    B. Trapezium bone   D. Fracture extending through first IP joint

20. A. Which special positioning method can be performed to demonstrate a Bennett's fracture? _____

_____

    B. Which type of central ray angulation is required for this projection? _____

21. Where is the central ray centered for a PA projection of the hand?

    A. Third MP joint   C. Second MP joint

    B. Mid aspect of third metacarpal   D. Third PIP joint

22. A minimum of _____ inch(es) (_____ cm) of the forearm should be included radiographically for a PA projection of the hand.

23. True/False: Some superimposition of the distal third, fourth, and fifth metacarpals is expected with a well-positioned PA oblique projection of the hand.

24. Which preferred lateral position of the hand best demonstrates the phalanges without excessive superimposition?

_____

25. Which lateral projection of the hand best demonstrates a possible foreign body in the palm of the hand?

_____

26. What is the proper name for the position referred to as the "ball-catcher's position?" _____

27. The "ball-catcher's position" is commonly used to evaluate for early signs of:

A. Osteoporosis   C. Osteopetrosis

B. Gout   D. Rheumatoid arthritis

28. The elbow generally should be flexed _____° for the basic positions of the wrist.

29. How much rotation is required for an oblique projection of the wrist? _____

30. Which alternative projection to the routine PA wrist best demonstrates the intercarpal joint spaces and wrist joint?

_____

31. Which positioning error is involved if significant aspects of the third, fourth, and fifth metacarpals are superimposed

in an oblique wrist projections? _____

32. Which one of the following fractures is not demonstrated in a wrist routine?

A. Barton's   C. Smith's

B. Pott's   D. Colles'

33. During the PA scaphoid projection with central ray angle and ulnar flexion, the central ray must be

angled _____° _____ (distally or proximally).

34. How much is the hand and wrist elevated from the IR for the modified Stecher method?

A. None   C. 20°

B. 10°   D. 15°

35. How much central ray angle to the long axis of the hand is required for the carpal canal (tunnel) projection?

_____

36. Which special projection of the wrist best demonstrates the interspaces on the ulnar side of the wrist between the

lunate, triquetrum, pisiform, and hamate bones? _____

37. Which special projection of the wrist helps rule out abnormal calcifications in the carpal sulcus?

_____

38. How much central ray angle from the long axis of the forearm is required for the carpal bridge projection?

   _____

39. What is the approximate difference in mrad between skin and midline doses for the hand and wrist?

   _____

REVIEW EXERCISE D: Pathologic Features of the Fingers, Thumb, Hand, and Wrist (see textbook pp. 132-151)

1. List the correct pathology term for the following definitions:

   A. _____ Fracture and dislocation of the posterior lip of the distal radius

   B. _____ Hereditary form of arthritis

   C. _____ Reduction in the quantity of bone or atrophy of skeletal tissue

   D. _____ Accumulated fluid in the joint cavity

   E. _____ An abnormality of the cartilage affecting long bones

   F. _____ Transverse fracture extending through the distal aspect of the fifth metacarpal

   G. _____ Hereditary condition marked by abnormally dense bone

   H. _____ Transverse fracture of the distal radius with posterior displacement of the distal
      fragment

2. Match the pathologic condition or disease to its radiographic appearance:

   _____ A. Narrowing of joint space with periosteal growths   A. Achondroplasia
              on the joint margins
                                                                            B. Bursitis
   _____ B. Fluid-filled joint space with possible calcification
                                                                            C. Carpal tunnel syndrome
   _____ C. Possible calcification in the carpal sulcus
                                                                            D. Osteoarthritis
   _____ D. Underdeveloped arms with trumpeting of the shafts of the
              long bones   E. Osteopetrosis

   _____ E. Chalky white or opaque appearance with a lack of distinction
              between the bony cortex and trabeculation

3. For the following types of pathologic conditions, indicate whether the manual exposure factors should be increased
   (+), decreased (−), or remain the same (0) as compared with the standard exposure factors.

   _____ Gout   _____ Osteoporosis

   _____ Joint effusion   _____ Osteopetrosis

   _____ Rheumatoid arthritis   _____ Bursitis

REVIEW EXERCISE E: Positioning of the Forearm, Elbow, and Humerus (see textbook pp. 152-164)

1. Which basic projections are required for a study of the forearm? _____

2. True/False: The technologist only needs to include the joint closest to the site of the injury for a forearm study.

3. To properly position the patient for an AP projection of the elbow, the epicondyles must be _____ to the film.

4. If the patient cannot fully extend the elbow for the AP projection, what alternative projection(s) should be performed?

   _____

5. Which basic projection of the elbow best demonstrates the radial head, neck, and tuberosity without any super-

   imposition? _____

6. True/False: Gonadal shielding is not required for upper limb radiographs if the patient can sit upright for these exams.

7. Which projection of the elbow best demonstrates the coronoid process? _____

8. The best position to evaluate the posterior fat pads of the elbow joint is: _____

9. Which special projection(s) of the elbow should be performed instead of the basic AP if the patient's elbow is

   tightly flexed and cannot be extended? _____

10. The basic positioning routine for a nontraumatic study of the middle or distal humerus is: _____

    _____

11. How should the epicondyles be aligned for a lateral projection of the humerus? _____

    _____

12. How much and in which direction should the central ray be angled for the Coyle method involving the radial head?

    _____

13. Which type of central ray angle must be used for the Coyle method involving the coronoid process?

    _____

14. What is the only difference among the four radial head lateral projections of the elbow?

    _____

15. Match the nearest skin dose for:

    _____ A. PA finger   1. 5 mrad

    _____ B. AP forearm   2. 10 mrad

    _____ C. Lateral humerus   3. 15 mrad

    _____ D. Lateral hand   4. 20 mrad

    _____ E. Carpal canal wrist   5. 25 mrad

    _____ F. PA hand   6. 30 mrad

REVIEW EXERCISE F: Problem Solving for Technical and Positioning Errors (see textbook pp. 132-165)

The following radiographic problems involve technical and positioning errors that may lead to substandard images. As you analyze these problems, review your textbook to find solutions to these questions.

   Other questions involve situations pertaining to different patient conditions and pathologic findings. If you need more information about a particular pathologic condition, review your textbook or a medical dictionary to learn more about it.

1. A three-projection study of the hand was taken using the following exposure factors: 64 kVp, 1000 mA, $^1/_{100}$ second, large focal spot, 36-inch (91-cm) SID, and high-speed screens. Which of these factors should be changed on future hand studies to produce more optimal images?

_____

2. A radiograph of a PA projection of the second digit reveals that the phalanges are not symmetric on both sides of the bony shafts. Which specific positioning error is involved?

_____

3. A radiograph of an oblique position of the hand reveals that the midshafts of the fourth and fifth metacarpals are superimposed. Which specific positioning error is involved?

_____

4. In a radiographic study of the forearm, the proximal radius crossed over the ulna in the frontal projection. Which specific positioning error led to this radiographic outcome?

_____

5. A PA scaphoid projection of the wrist using a central ray angle of 15° distally and ulnar flexion was performed. The resulting radiograph reveals that the scaphoid bone is foreshortened. How must this projection be modified to produce a more diagnostic image of the scaphoid ?

_____

6. A radiograph of an AP elbow reveals that considerable superimposition between the proximal radius and ulna. Which specific positioning error is involved?

_____

7. A routine radiograph of an AP oblique elbow with lateral rotation reveals that the radial tuberosity is partially superimposed on the ulna. In what way must this position be modified during the repeat exposure?

_____

8. A radiograph of a lateral projection of the elbow reveals that the humeral epicondyles are not superimposed and the trochlear notch is not clearly demonstrated. Which specific type of positioning error is involved?

_____

9. **Situation:** A patient with a possible fracture of the radial head enters the emergency room. When the technologist attempts to place the arm in the AP oblique-lateral rotation position, the patient is unable to extend or rotate the elbow laterally. Which other positions can be used to demonstrate the radial head and neck without superimposition on the proximal ulna? _____

10. **Situation:** A patient with a metallic foreign body in the palm of the hand enters the emergency room. Which specific positions should be used to locate the foreign body? _____

_____

11. **Situation:** A patient with a trauma injury enters the emergency room with an evident Colles' fracture. Which positioning routine should be used to determine the extent of the injury?

_____

12. **Situation:** A patient with a dislocated elbow enters the emergency room. The patient has it tightly flexed and is careful not to move it. Which specific positioning routine can be used to determine the extent of the injury?

_____

13. **Situation:** A patient with a possible Bennett's fracture enters the emergency room. The routine projections do not clearly demonstrate a possible fracture. Which other special projection can be taken? _____

_____

14. **Situation:** A patient with a history of carpal tunnel syndrome comes to the radiology department. The orthopedic physician suspects that bony changes in the carpal sulcus may be causing compression of the median nerve. Which special projection best demonstrates this region of the wrist? _____

_____

15. **Situation:** A patient comes to the radiology department for a hand series to evaluate early evidence of rheumatoid arthritis. Which special position can be used in addition to the basic hand projections to evaluate this patient?

_____

REVIEW EXERCISE G: Critique Radiographs of the Upper Limb (see textbook pp. 128-165)

The following questions relate to the radiographs found at the end of Chapter 4 of the textbook. Evaluate these radiographs for the radiographic criteria categories *(A through F)* that follow. Describe the corrections needed to improve the overall image. The major, or "repeatable," errors are specific errors that indicate the need for a repeat exposure, regardless of the nature of the other errors.

A. **PA hand (Fig. C4-171)**
   Description of possible error:

   1. Structures shown: _____

   2. Part positioning: _____

   3. Collimation and central ray: _____

   4. Exposure criteria: _____

   5. Markers: _____

   Repeatable error(s): _____

B. **Lateral hand (Fig. C4-172)**
   Description of possible error:

   1. Structures shown: _____

   2. Part positioning: _____

3. Collimation and central ray: _____

4. Exposure criteria: _____

5. Markers: _____

Repeatable error(s): _____

C. **AP elbow (Fig. C4-173)**
   Description of possible error:

   1. Structures shown: _____

   2. Part positioning: _____

   3. Collimation and central ray: _____

   4. Exposure criteria: _____

   5. Markers: _____

   Repeatable error(s): _____

D. **PA wrist (Fig. C4-174)**
   Which special wrist projection is demonstrated on this radiograph?
   Description of possible error:

   1. Structures shown: _____

   2. Part positioning: _____

   3. Collimation and central ray: _____

   4. Exposure criteria: _____

   5. Markers: _____

   Repeatable error(s): _____

E. **PA oblique hand (Fig. C4-175)**
   Description of possible error:

   1. Structures shown: _____

   2. Part positioning: _____

   3. Collimation and central ray: _____

   4. Exposure criteria: _____

   5. Markers: _____

   Repeatable error(s): _____

F. **Lateral elbow (Fig. C4-176)**
Description of possible error:

1. Structures shown: _____

2. Part positioning: _____

3. Collimation and central ray: _____

4. Exposure criteria: _____

5. Markers: _____

Repeatable error(s): _____

PART III: Laboratory Exercises (see textbook pp. 128-164)

You must gain experience in upper limb positioning before performing the following exams on actual patients. You can get experience in positioning and radiographic evaluation of these projections by performing exercises using radiographic phantoms and practicing on other students (although you will not be taking actual exposures).

The following suggested activities assume that your teaching institution has an energized lab and radiographic phantoms. If not, perform Laboratory Exercises B and C, the radiographic evaluation, and the physical positioning exercises. (Check off each step and projection as you complete it.)

LABORATORY EXERCISE A: Energized Laboratory

1. Using the hand radiographic phantom, produce radiographs of the following basic routines:

   _____ Hand (PA, oblique, lateral)   _____ Thumb (AP, oblique, lateral)

   _____ Wrist (PA, oblique, lateral)

2. Using the elbow radiographic phantom, produce radiographs of the following basic routines:

   _____ AP   _____ AP oblique, medial rotationg

   _____ Lateral elbow   _____ AP oblique, lateral rotation

LABORATORY EXERCISE B: Radiographic Evaluation

1. Evaluate and critique the radiographs produced during the previous experiments, additional radiographs provided by your instructor, or both. Evaluate each radiograph for the following points. (Check off when completed.):

   _____ Evaluate the completeness of the study. (Are all of the pertinent anatomic structures included on the radiograph?)

   _____ Evaluate for positioning or centering errors (e.g., rotation, off centering).

   _____ Evaluate for correct exposure factors and possible motion. (Are the density and contrast of the images acceptable?)

   _____ Determine whether markers and an acceptable degree of collimation and/or area shielding are seen on the images.

LABORATORY EXERCISE C: Physical Positioning

1. On another person, simulate performing all basic and special projections of the upper limb as follows. (Check off each when completed satisfactorily.) Include the following six steps as described in the textbook.

Step 1. Appropriate size and type of film holder with correct markers
Step 2. Correct central ray placement and centering of part to central ray and/or film
Step 3. Accurate collimation
Step 4. Area shielding of patient where advisable
Step 5. Use of proper immobilizing devices when needed
Step 6. Approximate correct exposure factors, breathing instructions where applicable, and "making" exposure

Projections	Step 1	Step 2	Step 3	Step 4	Step 5	Step 6
• Second to fifth digit routines (PA, oblique, lateral)	___	___	___	___	___	___
• Thumb routine (AP, oblique, lateral)	___	___	___	___	___	___
• Hand (PA, oblique, lateral)	___	___	___	___	___	___
• Wrist basic routine (PA, oblique, lateral)	___	___	___	___	___	___
• Scaphoid, carpal canal, and carpal bridge projections	___	___	___	___	___	___
• Elbow routine (AP, oblique, lateral)	___	___	___	___	___	___
• Partial flexion APs	___	___	___	___	___	___
• Acute flexion (Jones)	___	___	___	___	___	___
• Trauma axial laterals (Coyle)	___	___	___	___	___	___
• Radial head projections	___	___	___	___	___	___
• Forearm routine (AP, lateral)	___	___	___	___	___	___
• AP and rotational lateral projections of midhumerus and distal humerus	___	___	___	___	___	___

Answers to Review Exercises

Review Exercise A: Anatomy of Hand and Wrist

1. A. 14
   B. 5
   C. 8
   D. 27
2. A. Proximal phalanx
   B. Distal phalanx
3. A. Proximal phalanx
   B. Middle phalanx
   C. Distal phalanx
4. A. Head
   B. Body (shaft)
   C. Base
5. A. Base
   B. Body (shaft)
   C. Head
6. Interphalangeal joint
7. Metacarpophalangeal joints
8. A. Fifth carpometacarpal (CM) joint
   B. Body of third metacarpal
   C. Head of fifth metacarpal
   D. Fourth metacarpophalangeal (MP) joint
   E. Head of proximal phalanx of fifth digit
   F. Base of middle phalanx of fourth digit
   G. Distal interphalangeal (DIP) joint of fourth digit
   H. Body of middle phalanx of second digit
   I. Proximal interphalangeal (PIP) joint of second digit
   J. (Body of) distal phalanx of first digit
   K. Interphalangeal (IP) joint of first digit
   L. Metacarpophalangeal (MP) joint of first digit
   M. Head of first metacarpal
   N. Second carpometacarpal (CM) joint
   O. First carpometacarpal (CM) joint
9. A. 8. Scaphoid
   B. 1. Lunate
   C. 5. Triquetrum
   D. 4. Pisiform
   E. 3. Trapezium
   F. 6. Trapezoid
   G. 7. Capitate
   H. 2. Hamate
10. Capitate
11. Hamulus or hamular process
12. Scaphoid
13. (1) **S**end **L**etter **T**o **P**eter **T**o **T**ell'im (to) **C**ome **H**ome

(2) **S**teve **L**eft **T**he **P**arty **T**o **T**ake **C**arol **H**ome

14. A. 3. Base of first metacarpal (thumb)
    B. 9. Trapezium
    C. 2. Scaphoid
    D. 5. Trapezoid
    E. 1. Capitate
    F. 8. Hamate
    G. 6. Hamulus (hamular process)
    H. 7. Triquetrum
    I. 4. Pisiform
15. A. Body of first metacarpal (thumb)
    B. Carpometacarpal joint of first digit
    C. Trapezium
    D. Scaphoid
    E. Lunate
    F. Radiocarpal (wrist) joint (between radius and carpals)

Review Exercise B: Anatomy of the Forearm, Elbow, and Distal Humerus

1. A. Radius
   B. Ulna
2. A. U
   B. U
   C. H
   D. H
   E. U
   F. U
   G. U
   H. H
3. Proximal and distal radioulnar joints
4. A. Trochlea
   B. Capitulum
5. Olecranon fossa
6. A. Trochlear sulcus (groove)
   B. Capitulum, trochlea
   C. Trochlear notch
7. A. 1
   B. 5
   C. 1
   D. 2
   E. 2
   F. 4
   G. 3
   H. 3
8. Diarthrodial, 4 (four)
9. A. Ulnar collateral
   B. Radial collateral
   C. Dorsal radiocarpal
   D. Palmar radiocarpal
10. Radial collateral ligament
11. A. Ulnar deviation
    B. Radial deviation

12. Ulnar deviation
13. The proximal radius crosses over the ulna
14. A. Scaphoid fat stripe
    B. Pronator fat stripe
15. A. Elbow flexed 90°
    B. Optimal exposure techniques are used.
    C. In a true lateral position
16. False A nonvisible fat pad suggests a negative exam.
17. True
18. False
19. Posteroanterior (PA) and oblique wrist
20. Lateral wrist
21. A. Radial tuberosity
    B. Radial neck
    C. Capitulum
    D. Lateral epicondyle
    E. Olecranon fossa
    F. Medial epicondyle
    G. Trochlea
    H. Coronoid tubercle
    I. Olecranon process
    J. Superimposed epicondyles
    K. Radial head
    L. Radial neck
    M. Radial tuberosity
    N. Outer ridges of trochlea and capitulum
    O. Trochlear sulcus (groove)
    P. Trochlear notch
22. A. Radial tubercle
    B. Radial neck
    C. Radial head
    D. Capitulum
    E. Lateral epicondyle
    F. Coronoid process
    G. Trochlea
    H. Olecranon process
    I. Trochlear notch
    J. Radial head

Review Exercise C: Positioning of the Fingers, Thumb, Hand, and Wrist

1. A. Low to medium
   B. Short exposure
   C. Small focal spot
   D. 40 inches (100 cm)
   E. 10 cm
   F. Detail screens
   G. 5 to 7
   H. 8 to 10, 100%
   I. 3 to 4; 25% to 30%
   J. Soft tissue, trabecular markings

2. Collimation borders should be visible on all four sides if the image receptor (IR) is large enough to allow this without cutting off essential anatomy
3. B, D, E, F
4. Child-bearing age or younger
5. True
6. Arthrography
7. PA, PA oblique and lateral
8. Distal metacarpals
9. A. Symmetric appearance of both sides of the shafts of phalanges and distal metacarpals
   B. Equal amounts of tissue on each side of the phalanges
10. A. Perform the medial oblique rather than lateral oblique to decrease object-image distance (OID).
    B. Perform a thumb down lateral (mediolateral projection) to decrease OID.
11. Proximal interphalangeal (PIP) joint
12. D
13. The AP position produces a decrease in OID and increased definition.
14. PA oblique
15. 8 × 10 inch (18 × 24 cm)
16. Metacarpophalangeal
17. True
18. C
19. A
20. A. Modified Robert's method
    B. 15° proximal
21. A
22. 1 inch (2.5 cm)
23. True
24. Fan lateral
25. Lateral in extension
26. Norgaard method
27. D
28. 90
29. 45°
30. Anteroposterior (AP) projection (with the hand slightly arched)
31. Excessive lateral rotation from PA
32. B
33. 10 to 15, proximally
34. C
35. 25° to 30°
36. PA projection with radial deviation
37. Carpal canal or Gaynor-Hart projection
38. 45°
39. No difference

Review Exercise D: Radiographic Positioning of the Fingers, Thumb, Hand, and Wrist

1. A. Barton's fracture
   B. Gout
   C. Osteoporosis
   D. Joint effusion
   E. Achondroplasia
   F. Boxer's fracture
   G. Osteopetrosis
   H. Colles' fracture
2. A. D
   B. B
   C. C
   D. A
   E. E
3. A. Gout (−)
   B. Joint effusion (0)
   C. Rheumatoid arthritis (−)
   D. Osteoporosis (−)
   E. Osteopetrosis (+)
   F. Bursitis (0)

Review Exercise E: Positioning of the Forearm, Elbow, and Humerus

1. AP and lateral
2. False
3. Parallel
4. Two AP projections, one with humerus parallel to IR and one with forearm parallel to IR
5. AP oblique with 45° lateral rotation
6. False (because of scatter, divergent rays, or both reaching gonads)
7. AP oblique with 45° medial rotation
8. Lateral, flexed 90°
9. Two projections, central ray perpendicular to humerus and central perpendicular to forearm (Jones method)
10. AP and lateral projections
11. Perpendicular to IR
12. 45° toward shoulder
13. 45° away from shoulder
14. The rotational position of hand and wrist
15. A. PA finger: (1) 5 mrad
    B. AP forearm: (5) 25 mrad
    C. Lateral humerus: (6) 30 mrad
    D. Lateral hand: (3) 15 mrad
    E. Carpal canal wrist: (4) 20 mrad
    F. PA hand: (2) 10 mrad

Review Exercise F: Problem-Solving for Technical and Positioning Errors

1. Use a small focal spot, minimum 40-inch (102-cm) source-image distance (SID), and detail speed screens to produce a higher quality study.
2. Rotation
3. Excessive lateral rotation
4. PA forearm projection was performed rather than AP.
5. The central ray needs to be angled 15° proximally, toward the elbow.
6. The elbow is rotated medially.
7. Increase lateral rotation of the elbow to separate the radius from the ulna.
8. The forearm and humerus are not on the same horizontal plane.
9. Coyle method for radial head (lateral elbow, central ray 45° toward shoulder)
10. PA and lateral-in-extension hand
11. AP and lateral forearm projections to include the wrist
12. Two AP projections with acute flexion (Jones method) and a lateral projection
13. Modified Robert's method
14. Carpal canal position
15. Norgaard method—ball catcher's position

Review Exercise G: Critique Radiographs of the Upper Limb

A. PA hand (Fig. C4-171)
   1. All pertinent anatomic structures included
   2. Some lateral rotation evident; asymmetric appearance of distal third, fourth, and fifth metacarpals and slight overlap of distal ulna and radius at distal radioulnar joint
   3. No collimation evident on this printed radiograph; centering satisfactory for hand
   4. Selected exposure factors acceptable, but streaking artifacts visible on the radiograph (but they may be printing artifacts)
   5. Good placement of anatomic markers
      Repeatable error(s): criteria 4 (streaking artifacts) and 2

B. Lateral hand (Fig. C4-172)
   1. All pertinent anatomic structures included
   2. Hand rotated medially; radius and ulna not directly superimposed; metacarpals not all superimposed
   3. No collimation evident on this printed radiograph; centering slightly off; central ray centered to the midmetacarpals rather than the second metacarpophalangeal joint; includes too much forearm
   4. Acceptable selected exposure factors
   5. No anatomic marker evident on this projection
      Repeatable error(s): criteria 2 and 5 (unless marker is visible elsewhere on radiograph)
C. AP external (lateral) oblique elbow (Fig. C4-173)
   1. All essential anatomic structures included
   2. Arm insufficiently rotated; radial tuberosity partially superimposed; capitulum insufficiently elongated and not in total profile
   3. No collimation borders evident; central ray centering excellent for elbow

   4. Excellent selected exposure factors
   5. No anatomic marker evident on this projection
      Repeatable error(s): 2 and 5 (unless markers are visible elsewhere on radiograph)
D. PA wrist (Fig. C4-174)
   NOTE: This demonstrates a radial deviation for the ulnar side carpals (the opposite of the ulnar deviation for scaphoid).
   1. Part of pisiform cut off laterally
   2. Excellent part positioning with good radial deviation
   3. Central ray centering error—central ray centered over scaphoid and medial carpals; would have excellent collimation if central ray were centered correctly
   4. Excellent exposure factors
   5. Evidence of satisfactory anatomic marker
      Repeatable error(s): criteria 1 and 3
E. PA oblique hand (Fig. C4-175)
   1. All pertinent anatomic structures included
   2. Excellent part positioning (no overlap of midshafts of third, fourth, and fifth metacarpals)
   3. No collimation evident on this printed radiograph; acceptable

central ray centering, but it is centered to middle of third metatarsal rather than to third metacarpophalangeal joint
   4. Hand underexposed (soft tissue too evident, trabecular marking of bones not visible)
   5. No evident anatomic side marker
      Repeatable error(s): criteria 4 and 5 (unless marker is visible elsewhere on radiograph)
F. Lateral elbow (Fig. C4-176)
   1. All pertinent anatomic structures demonstrated
   2. Elbow overflexed (beyond 90°) and not true lateral; too much distance between parts of concentric circles 1 and 2; trochlear notch space not open
   3. Satisfactory collimation (that is, collimation that is evident); central ray centering slightly off center to the elbow joint
   4. Acceptable exposure factors
   5. Anatomic marker partially off radiograph and is unacceptable (unless it is demonstrated on the actual radiograph).
      Repeatable error(s): criteria 2 and 5 (unless marker is more visible on actual radiograph)

SELF-TEST

My Score = _____%

This self-test should be taken only after completing all of the readings, review exercises, and laboratory activities for a particular section. The self-test is divided into six sections. The purpose of this test is not only to provide a good learning exercise but also to serve as a strong indicator of what your final unit evaluation grade will cover. It is strongly suggested that if you do not get at least a 90% to 95% grade on each self-test, you should review those areas in which you missed questions before going to your instructor for the final unit evaluation exam.

1. A. How many bones make up the phalanges of the hand?

    A. 14   C. 5

    B. 8   D. 16

    B. How many bones make up the carpal region?

    A. 14   C. 5

    B. 8   D. 7

    C. What is the total number of bones that make up the hand and wrist?

    A. 21   C. 26

    B. 27   D. 32

2. Match the correct term for the following joints:

    _____ A. Between the two phalanges of the first digit (thumb)   1. Radiocarpal

    _____ B. Between the first metacarpal and the proximal phalanx of the thumb   2. Fourth DIP

    _____ C. Between the middle and distal phalanges of the fourth digit   3. Fourth PIP

    _____ D. Between the carpals and the first metacarpal   4. First MP

    _____ E. Between the forearm and the carpals   5. First CM

    _____ F. Between the distal radius and ulna   6. Distal radioulnar

                                                                             7. IP

3. Match the structures labeled *A-R* on Fig. 4-12 to the correct term as listed *1-18:*

    ____ A.   1. Distal phalanx of fourth digit

    ____ B.   2. Head of fifth metacarpal

    ____ C.   3. Base of fourth metacarpal

    ____ D.   4. Scaphoid

    ____ E.   5. Base of first metacarpal

    ____ F.   6. Pisiform

    ____ G.   7. Trapezoid

    ____ H.   8. Body of proximal phalanx of fifth digit

    ____ I.   9. Fifth carpometacarpal joint

    ____ J.   10. Triquetrum

    ____ K.   11. Radius

    ____ L.   12. Proximal phalanx of first digit

    ____ M.   13. Radiocarpal joint

    ____ N.   14. Hamate

    ____ O.   15. Capitate

    ____ P.   16. Distal interphalangeal joint of fifth digit

    ____ Q.   17. Trapezium

    ____ R.   18. First metacarpophalangeal joint

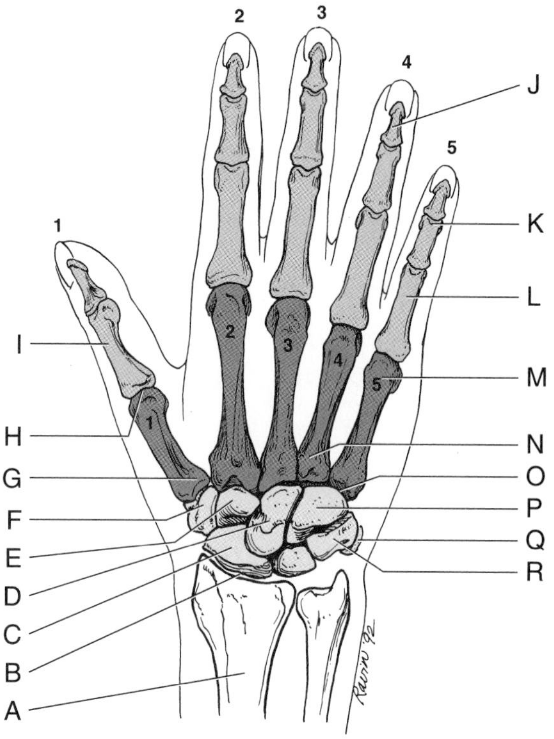

Fig. 4-12 Osteology of the hand and wrist.

4. Which carpal contains a "hooklike" process?

    A. Scaphoid   C. Hamate

    B. Trapezium   D. Pisiform

5. Which carpal articulates with the thumb?

    A. Scaphoid   C. Trapezoid

    B. Lunate   D. Trapezium

6. Which carpal is most commonly fractured?

    A. Scaphoid   C. Trapezium

    B. Capitate   D. Triquetrum

7. Which two carpal bones are located most **anteriorly** as seen on a lateral wrist radiograph? (HINT: They are on the radial side of the wrist.)

    A. Hamate and pisiform   C. Capitate and lunate

    B. Trapezium and trapezoid   D. Scaphoid and trapezium

8. Identify the structures of the wrist labeled on Figs. 4-13, 4-14, and 4-15.

_____ A.   1. Pisiform

_____ B.   2. Trapezoid

_____ C.   3. Scaphoid

_____ D.   4. Triquetrum

_____ E.   5. Base of first metacarpal

_____ F.   6. Radius

_____ G.   7. Lunate

_____ H.   8. Trapezium

_____ I.   9. Hamate

_____ J.   10. Ulna

_____ K.   11. Capitate

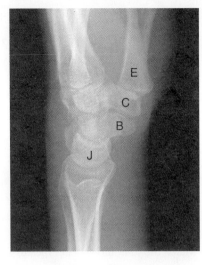

Fig. 4-13 Lateral wrist.

9. Which wrist projection does Fig. 4-14 represent?

    A. PA wrist   C. PA—radial deviation

    B. PA—ulnar deviation   D. Carpal canal

10. Which one of the following carpals is *not* well seen in the Fig. 4-14 projection?

    A. Pisiform   C. Scaphoid

    B. Lunate   D. Triquetrum

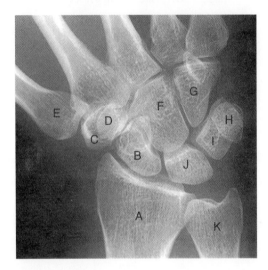

Fig. 4-14 Anteroposterior (AP) wrist with radial deviation.

11. Which projection does Fig. 4-15 represent?

    A. PA—ulnar deviation   C. PA—radial deviation

    B. Carpal canal   D. Modified Stecher method

12. Which one of the following carpal bones is best demonstrated in the Fig. 4-15 projection?

    A. Trapezium   C. Trapezoid

    B. Scaphoid   D. Hamate

13. Which bone of the upper limb contains the coronoid process?

    A. Humerus   C. Radius

    B. First metacarpal   D. Ulna

14. Where are the coronoid and radial fossae located?

    A. Anterior aspect of distal humerus

    B. Posterior aspect of distal humerus

    C. Proximal radius and ulna

    D. Distal end of radius

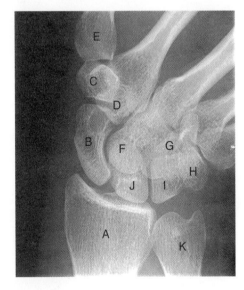

Fig. 4-15 Anteroposterior (AP) wrist with ulnar deviation.

15. Which two bony landmarks are palpated to assist with positioning of the upper limb?

    A. Coronoid and olecranon processes

    B. Pisiform and hamate

    C. Lateral and medial epicondyle

    D. Radial and ulnar styloid processes

16. Where is the coronoid tubercle located?

    A. Medial aspect of coronoid process

    B. Anterior aspect of distal humerus

    C. Lateral aspect of proximal radius

    D. Posterior aspect of distal humerus

17. In an erect anatomic position, which one of the following structures is considered to be most inferior or distal?

    A. Head of ulna

    B. Olecranon process

    C. Radial tuberosity

    D. Head of radius

18. Match the joint movement types to the following articulations. (Each answer may be used more than once.):

    _____ A. Intercarpal joints

    _____ B. Radiocarpal joint

    _____ C. Elbow joint

    _____ D. First carpometacarpal joint

    _____ E. Third carpometacarpal joint

    1. Sellar

    2. Ginglymus

    3. Ellipsoidal

    4. Plane

19. The following four radiographs represent
    the most common routine or basic projections
    for the elbow. Match each of these projections
    to the correct figure number:

    _____ A. Fig. 4-16   1. AP projection

    _____ B. Fig. 4-17   2. Lateral position

    _____ C. Fig. 4-18   3. AP oblique—
                                   lateral rotation

    _____ D. Fig. 4-19   4. AP oblique—
                                   Medial rotation

Identify the soft tissue and bony structures
labeled on Figs. 4-16, 4-17, 4-18, and 4-19).
(Each answers may be used more than once.):

    _____ E.   1. Trochlea

    _____ F.   2. Olecranon process

    _____ G.   3. Coronoid process

    _____ H.   4. Medial epicondyle

    _____ I.   5. Supinator fat pad

    _____ J.   6. Capitulum

    _____ K.   7. Anterior fat pad

    _____ L.   8. Radial head and neck

    _____ M.   9. Region of posterior
                     fat pad

    _____ N.   10. Coronoid tubercle

    _____ O.

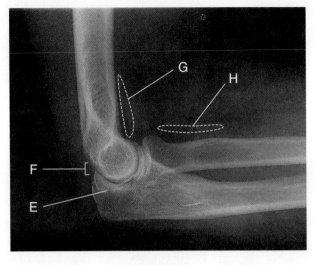

Fig. 4-16

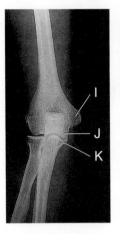

Fig. 4-17

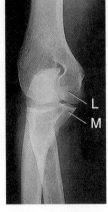

Fig. 4-18

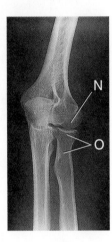

Fig. 4-19

20. Identify the structures labeled *A-K* on Figs. 4-20 and 4-21:

    ____ A.   1. Coronoid fossa

    ____ B.   2. Medial epicondyle

    ____ C.   3. Head of radius

    ____ D.   4. Trochlea

    ____ E.*   5. Radial tuberosity

    ____ F.*   6. Coronoid process

    ____ G.   7. Lateral epicondyle

    ____ H.   8. Capitulum

    ____ I.   9. Trochlear sulcus

    ____ J.   10. Coronoid tubercle

    ____ K.   11. Radial fossa

(Notice difference between structures *J* and *L*.)
*Not visible on radiograph.

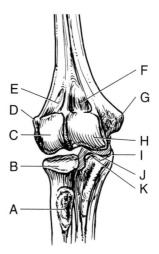

Fig. 4-20 Anterior view of the elbow.

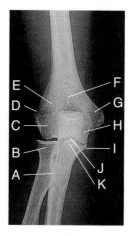

Fig. 4-21 Elbow. Anteroposterior (AP) extended.

21. True/False: To visualize fat pads surrounding the elbow, exposure factors must be adjusted to see both bony and soft tissue structures.

22. True/False: Fat pads of the elbow are normally seen on correctly positioned and correctly exposed anteroposterior (AP) elbow projections.

23. Why should a forearm never be taken as an PA projection?

A. Too painful for the patient

B. Causes the proximal radius to cross over the ulna

C. Causes the distal radius to cross over the ulna

D. Increases the object-image distance (OID) of the distal radius

24. In what position should the hand be for an AP elbow projection?

A. Supinated   C. Rotated 20° from supinated position

B. Pronated   D. True lateral position

25. In what position should the hand be for an AP medial rotation oblique elbow position?

A. Supinated   C. Rotated 20° from supinated position

B. Pronated   D. True lateral position

26. Match the projection of the elbow that best demonstrates the following structures:

_____ A. Coronoid process in profile   1. Lateral elbow

_____ B. Radial head and tuberosity without superimposition   2. AP elbow

_____ C. Olecranon process in profile   3. AP, medial rotation oblique

_____ D. Coronoid tubercle   4. AP, lateral rotation oblique

_____ E. Trochlear notch in profile

_____ F. Capitulum and lateral epicondyle in profile

_____ G. Olecranon process seated in olecranon fossa

27. True/False: Lead masking is not required when placing multiple images on the same digital image receptor (IR) plate.

28. The long axis of the anatomic part being imaged should be placed:

A. Perpendicular to the long axis of the IR

B. Parallel to long axis of the IR

C. 30° angle to the long axis of the IR

D. Any way that will accommodate multiple images being placed on a single IR

29. *Arthrography* is a radiographic study of:

A. Fat pads and stripes

B. Epiphyses of long bones

C. Medullary aspect of long bones

D. Soft tissues structures within certain synovial joints

30. Match the following pathologic term to the correct definition:

_____ 1. Accumulated fluid within the joint cavity   A. Achondroplasia

_____ 2. A reduction in the quantity of bone or atrophy of skeletal tissue   B. Bursitis

_____ 3. Local or generalized infection of bone or bone marrow   C. Carpal tunnel syndrome

_____ 4. Reverse of a Colles' fracture   D. Bennett's fracture

_____ 5. Inflammation of the fluid-filled sacs enclosing the joints   E. Smith's fracture

_____ 6. Fracture of the base of the first metacarpal   F. Joint effusion

_____ 7. Abnormality of the cartilage of long bones   G. Osteomyelitis

_____ 8. Painful disorder of hand and wrist resulting   H. Osteoporosis
            from compression of the median nerve

31. Which one of the following pathologic indications requires a decrease in manual exposure factors?

A. Achondroplasia   C. Gout

B. Osteopetrosis   D. Joint effusion

32. Where is the central ray centered for a PA projection of the second digit?

    A. Affected PIP joint   C. Affected MP joint

    B. Affected middle phalanx   D. Affected CM joint

33. Why is it important to keep the long axis of the digit parallel to the IR?

    A. To reduce distortion of the phalanges   C. To demonstrate small fractures

    B. To preparedly visualize joints   D. All of the above

34. Where is the central ray placed for a PA projection of the hand?

    A. Second MP joint   C. Middle phalanx of third digit

    B. Third MP joint   D. Third PIP

35. What is the major disadvantage of performing a PA projection of the thumb rather than an AP?

    A. Increased OID   C. More painful for patient

    B. Increase in patient dose   D. Awkward position for patient

36. What type of fracture is best demonstrated with a modified Robert's method?

    A. Barton's fracture   C. Bennett's fracture

    B. Colles' fracture   D. Smith's fracture

37. True/False: Both hands are examined with one single exposure when using the Norgaard method.

38. True/False: The hand(s) is/are placed in a true PA position when using the Norgaard method.

39. Choose the **best** set of exposure factors for upper limb radiography:

    A. 75 kVp, 200 mA, $\frac{1}{20}$ second, small focal spot, 40-inch (102-cm) SID, high-speed screens

    B. 75 kVp, 600 mA, $\frac{1}{60}$ second, large focal spot, 40-inch (102-cm) SID, detail-speed screens

    C. 64 kVp, 100 mA, $\frac{1}{10}$ second, small focal spot, 40-inch (102-cm) SID, high-speed screens

    D. 64 kVp, 200 mA, $\frac{1}{20}$ second, small focal spot, 40-inch (102-cm) SID, detail-speed screens

40. True/False: The midline dose for a lateral forearm is greater than the skin dose for a PA finger.

41. A radiograph of a PA oblique of the hand reveals that the mid aspect of the third, fourth, and fifth metacarpals are slightly superimposed. What must be done to correct this positioning problem on the repeat exposure?

    A. Increase obliquity of hand.   C. Decrease obliquity of hand.

    B. Spread fingers out further.   D. Form a tight fist with fingers.

42. A radiograph of an AP elbow projection demonstrates total separation between the proximal radius and ulna. What must be done to correct this positioning error on the repeat exposure?

    A. Rotate upper limb medially.   C. Angle central ray 5° to 10° caudad.

    B. Rotate upper limb laterally   D. Fully extend elbow.

43. A radiograph of the carpal canal (inferosuperior) projection reveals that the pisiform and hamulus are superimposed. What can be done to correct this problem on the repeat exposure?

    A. Flex wrist slightly.   C. Rotate wrist laterally 5° to 10°

    B. Extend wrist slightly.   D. Rotate wrist medially 5° to 10°

44. A radiograph of an AP oblique-medial rotation reveals that the coronoid process is not in profile and the radial head is only partially superimposed over the ulna. What specific positioning error was involved?

    A. Insufficient medial rotation   C. Excessive extension of elbow

    B. Excessive medial rotation   D. Excessive flexion of elbow

45. A radiograph of a lateral projection of the elbow reveals that the epicondyles are not superimposed and the trochlear notch is not clearly seen. What must be done to correct this positioning error during the repeat exposure?

    A. Angle central ray 45° toward shoulder   C. Angle central ray 45° away from shoulder

    B. Place humerus/forearm in same horizontal plane   D. Extend elbow to form an 80° horizontal plane angle

46. **Situation:** A patient with a possible Barton's fracture enters the emergency room. Which positioning routine should be performed to confirm the diagnosis?

    A. Elbow   C. Hand

    B. Wrist   D. Thumb

47. **Situation:** A patient with a possible Smith's fracture enters the emergency room. Which positioning routine should be performed to confirm this diagnosis?

    A. Hand   C. Wrist/forearm

    B. Thumb   D. Elbow

48. **Situation:** A patient has a Colles' fracture reduced, and a large plaster cast is placed on the upper limb. The orthopedic surgeon orders a postreduction study. The original technique, used before the cast placement, involved 60 kVp and 5 mAs. What new technique measurements should be used with a wet plaster cast?

    A. Same measurements   C. 65 kVp and 5 mAs

    B. 75 to 78 kVp and 10 mAs   D. 68 to 70 kVp or 10 mAs

49. **Situation:** A pediatric patient with a possible radial head fracture enters the emergency room. It is too painful for the patient to extend the elbow beyond 90° or rotate the hand. What type of special (i.e., optional) projection could be performed on this patient to confirm the diagnosis without causing further discomfort?

    A. Coyle method   C. Norgaard method

    B. Modified Robert's method   D. Modified Stecher method

50. For the following critique questions, refer to the AP oblique elbow radiograph shown in F C4-173 in your textbook, p. 165.

    1. Which rotation is represented?   A. Lateral rotation
                                            B. Medial rotation

    A. Which positioning errors is/are visible on this radiograph? More than one answer may be selected.

        (a)All essential anatomic structures are not demonstrated.

      (b) Central ray is centered incorrectly.

      (c) Collimation is not evident.

      (d) Exposure factors are incorrect.

      (e) No anatomic marker is visible.

      (f) Excessive rotation in the lateral direction is evident.

      (g) Insufficient rotation in the lateral direction is evident.

      (h) Excessive flexion of the joint is evident.

B. Which of the previous criteria errors are considered "repeatable errors?" _____

NOTE: Insufficient lateral rotation itself may only be considered a marginal repeatable error but if no anatomic marker is visible, it is a repeatable error.

C. Which of the following modifications must be made during the repeat exposure? More than one answer may be selected.

   (a) Increase collimation.

   (b) Center central ray correctly.

   (c) Decrease exposure factors.

   (d) Increase exposure factors.

   (e) Place anatomic marker on IR before exposure.

   (f) Rotate elbow slightly more in the medial direction.

   (g) Rotate elbow slightly more in the lateral direction.

   (h) Extend elbow completely.

51. For the following critique questions, refer to the position of the wrist (shown in Fig. C4-174 in the texbook, p. 165)

   1. Which special wrist projection does this represent?   A. Ulnar deviation
                                                              B. Radial deviation

A. What are the positioning error(s) seen on this radiograph? More than one answer may be selected.

   (a) All essential anatomic structures are not demonstrated.

   (b) Central ray is centered incorrectly

   (c) Exposure factors are incorrect.

   (d) No anatomic marker is visible.

   (e) Excessive rotation in the lateral direction is evident.

   (f) Excessive rotation in the medial direction is evident.

   (g) Excessive deviation of the joint is evident.

B. Which of the previous criteria errors are considered as "repeatable errors?" _____

C. Which of the following modifications must be made during the repeat exposure? More than one answer may be selected.

   (a) Open up collimation to include all soft tissue and bony structures.

   (b) Center central ray correctly to midcarpal region.

   (c) Decrease exposure factors.

   (d) Increase exposure factors.

   (e) Place marker on IR before exposure.

   (f) Pronate hand toward IR.

   (g) Supinate hand away from IR.

   (h) Extend wrist.

   (i) Increase deviation movement.

   (j) Decrease deviation movement.

CHAPTER 5

Proximal Humerus and Shoulder Girdle

CHAPTER OBJECTIVES

After you have successfully completed **all** the activities in this chapter, you will be able to:

_____ 1. Identify the bones and specific features of the proximal humerus and shoulder girdle.

_____ 2. On drawings and radiographs, identify specific anatomic structures of the proximal humerus and the shoulder girdle.

_____ 3. Match specific joints of the shoulder girdle to their structural classification and movement type.

_____ 4. Describe anatomic relationships of prominent structures of the proximal humerus and the shoulder girdle.

_____ 5. On radiographic images, identify rotational positions of the proximal humerus.

_____ 6. List the technical and shielding considerations commonly used for proximal humerus and shoulder girdle radiography.

_____ 7. Match specific pathologic indications of the shoulder girdle to the correct definition.

_____ 8. Match specific pathologic indications of the shoulder girdle to the correct radiographic appearance.

_____ 9. For select forms of pathologic conditions of the shoulder girdle, indicate whether manual exposure factors should be increased or decreased or remain the same.

_____ 10. List basic and special projections of the proximal humerus and shoulder, including the type and size of film holder, the central ray location with correct angles, and the structures best demonstrated.

_____ 11. List the various patient dose ranges for select projections of the proximal humerus and shoulder.

_____ 12. Given various hypothetical situations, identify the correct modification of a position and/or exposure factors to improve the radiographic image.

_____ 13. Given various hypothetical situations, identify the correct position for a specific pathologic feature or condition.

_____ 14. Given radiographs of specific shoulder girdle projections, identify specific positioning and exposure factors errors.

POSITIONING AND FILM CRITIQUE

_____ 1. Using a peer, position for basic and special projections of the proximal humerus and shoulder girdle

_____ 2. Using a shoulder radiographic phantom, produce satisfactory radiographs of the shoulder girdle (if equipment is available).

_____ 3. Critique and evaluate shoulder girdle radiographs based on the four divisions of radiographic criteria: (1) structures shown, (2) position, (3) collimation and central ray, and (4) exposure criteria.

_____ 4. Distinguish between acceptable and unacceptable shoulder girdle radiographs based on exposure factors, motion, collimation, positioning, or other errors.

Learning Exercises

Complete the following review exercises after reading the associated pages in the textbook as indicated by each exercise. Answers to each review exercise are given at the end of the review exercises.

PART I: Radiographic Anatomy

REVIEW EXERCISE A: Radiographic Anatomy of the Proximal Humerus and Shoulder Girdle (see textbook pp. 168-172)

1. The shoulder girdle consists of (A) _____ , (B) _____ , and (C)

   _____ .

2. Identify the following parts on Figs. 5-1 and 5-2. Include secondary terms where indicated.

   A. _____ (_____)

   B. _____ (_____)

   C. _____

   D. _____

   E. _____ (_____)

   F. _____

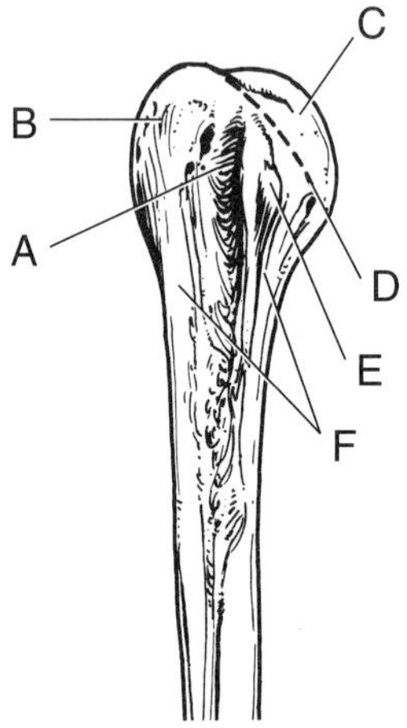

Fig. 5-1. Frontal view, proximal humerus.

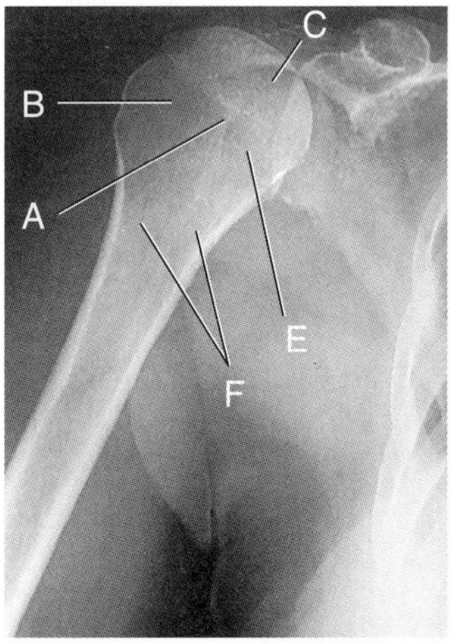

Fig. 5-2. Radiograph, proximal humerus.

   G. Which projection of the proximal humerus is represented by this drawing and radiograph (internal, external, or

   neutral rotation)? _____

3. The three aspects of the clavicle are the (A) _____ , (B) _____ ,

   and (C) _____ .

4. The _____ (male or female) clavicle tends to be thicker and more curved in shape.

5. The three angles of the scapula include the (A) _____ , (B) _____ ,

   and (C) _____ .

6. The anterior surface of the scapula is referred to as the _____ surface.

7. What is the anatomic name for the armpit? _____

8. What are the names of the two fossae located on the posterior scapula? (Use the newer terms.)

   A. _____ B. _____

9. All of the joints of the shoulder girdle are classified as being _____ .

10. List the movement types for the following joints:

    A. Scapulohumeral _____

    B. Sternoclavicular _____

    C. Acromioclavicular _____

11. Match the following anatomic structures with the correct answer:

    _____ 1. Greater tubercle   A. Scapula

    _____ 2. Coracoid process   B. Clavicle

    _____ 3. Crest of spine   C. Proximal humerus

    _____ 4. Coronoid process   D. Not part of the shoulder girdle

    _____ 5. Acromial extremity

    _____ 6. Intertubercular groove

    _____ 7. Condylar process

    _____ 8. Surgical neck

12. Identify the following structures labeled on Figs. 5-3 and 5-4. Include secondary terms where indicated.

    A. _____

    B. _____ (_____)

    C. _____

    D. _____

    E. _____

    F. _____

    G. _____ (_____) border

    H. _____ (_____) border

    I. _____ (_____) surface

    J. _____ surface

    K. _____

    L. _____

    M. _____

    N. _____ (_____)

    O. _____

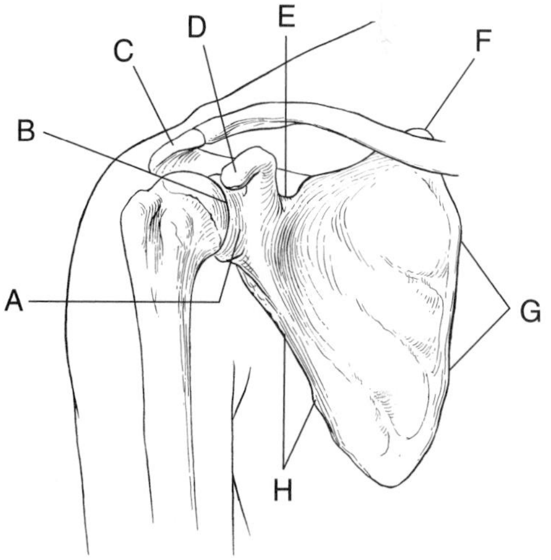

Fig. 5-3. Frontal view, scapula.

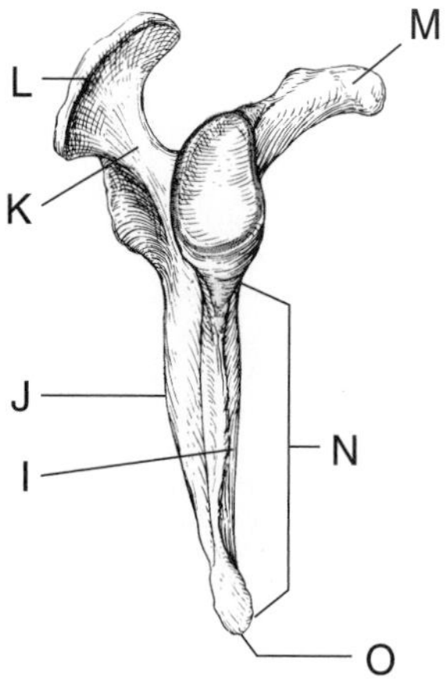

Fig. 5-4. Lateral view, scapula.

13. Identify the structures labeled on Figs. 5-5 and 5-6:

A. _____

B. _____ (joint)

C. _____

D. _____

E. _____

F. _____

G. Is this an **internal** or **external** rotation AP proximal humerus and shoulder?

   _____

H. Does Fig. 5-5 represent an **AP** or a **lateral** projection of the proximal humerus?

   _____

I. Are the epicondyles of the distal humerus **parallel** or **perpendicular** to the IR on this projection?

   _____

J. _____

K. _____

L. _____

M. _____

N. What is the correct term to describe the projection shown in Fig. 5-6?

   _____

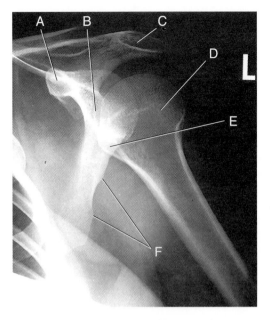

Fig. 5-5. Anteroposterior shoulder, neutral rotation

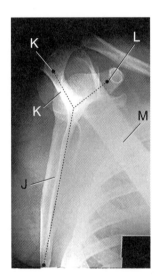

Fig. 5-6. Radiograph.

14. Identify the structures labeled on Fig. 5-7.

A. _____

B. _____

C. _____

D. _____

E. What is the name of the projection shown in Fig. 5-7?

   _____

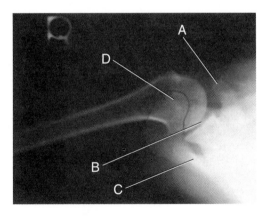

Fig. 5-7. Radiograph.

F. How much is the affected arm abducted from the body for this projection? _____

PART II: Radiographic Positioning

REVIEW EXERCISE B: Positioning of the Proximal Humerus and Shoulder Girdle (see textbook pp. 173-193)

1. Identify the correct proximal humerus rotation for the following:

    _____ 1. Greater tubercle profiled laterally   A. External rotation

    _____ 2. Humeral epicondyles angled 45° to image receptor (IR)   B. Internal rotation

    _____ 3. Epicondyles perpendicular to IR   C. Neutral rotation

    _____ 4. Supination of hand

    _____ 5. Palm of hand against thigh

    _____ 6. Epicondyles parallel to IR

    _____ 7. Lesser tubercle profiled medially

    _____ 8. Proximal humerus in a lateral position

    _____ 9. Proximal humerus in position for an anteroposterior (AP) projection

2. Identify the proximal humerus rotation represented on the following radiographs (Figs. 5-8 to 5-10):

    A. Fig. 5-8 represents _____ rotation

    B. Fig. 5-9 represents _____ rotation

    C. Fig. 5-10 represents _____ rotation

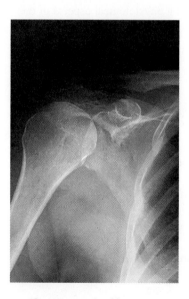

Fig. 5-8. Proximal humerus.

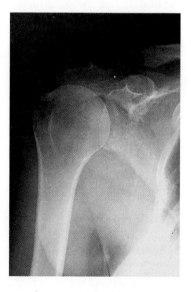

Fig. 5-9. Proximal humerus.

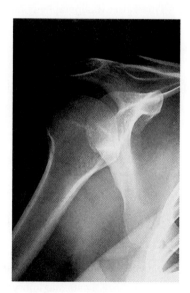

Fig. 5-10. Proximal humerus.

3. Indicate which of the following positioning and technical considerations are true or false for the shoulder girdle:

   A. True/False: The use of grids is not required for shoulders that measure less than 10 cm.

   B. True/False: The kilovoltage peak range for adult shoulder projections is between 80 and 90 kVp.

   C. True/False: Low milliamperage with short exposure times should be used for adult shoulder studies.

   D. True/False: Large focal spot setting should be selected for most adult shoulder studies.

   E. True/False: A high-speed screen-film system is recommended for shoulder studies when using a grid.

   F. True/False: A 72-inch (180-cm) source-image distance (SID) is recommended for most shoulder girdle studies.

   G. True/False: The gonadal dose for most shoulder projections is 0.1 mrad or less.

   H. True/False: The use of contact shields over the breast, lung, and thyroid regions is recommended for most shoulder projections

4. Which one of the following kilovoltage peak ranges should be used for a shoulder series on an average adult?

   A. 70 to 80   C. 80 to 90

   B. 55 to 60   D. 65 to 75

5. If physical immobilization is required, which individual should be asked to restrain a child for a shoulder series?

   A. Parent or guardian   C. Radiography student

   B. Radiologic technologist   D. Nurse aide

6. True/False: Arthrography of the shoulder joint requires the use of iodinated contrast media injected into the joint space.

7. True/False: Magnetic resonance imaging (MRI) is an excellent modality for demonstrating nondisplaced fractures of the shoulder girdle.

8. True/False: Nuclear medicine bone scans can demonstrate signs of osteomyelitis and cellulitis.

9. True/False: Radiography is more sensitive than nuclear medicine for demonstrating physiological aspects of the shoulder girdle.

10. True/False: Ultrasound can provide a functional (dynamic) evaluation of joint movement that MRI cannot.

11. Match the following pathologic indications to the correct definition:

   _____ 1. Encroachment of the supraspinous muscle on the anterior acromion   A. Acromioclavicular joint dislocation

   _____ 2. Lesion of the anteroinferior glenoid rim   B. Bankart lesion

   _____ 3. Inflammatory condition of the tendon   C. Hill-Sachs defect

   _____ 4. Displacement of the distal clavicle superiorly   D. Impingement syndrome

   _____ 5. Compression fracture of the humeral head   E. Osteoporosis

   _____ 6. Traumatic injury to one or more muscles of the shoulder   F. Rotator cuff tear

   _____ 7. Atrophy of skeletal tissue   G. Tendonitis

12. Match the following radiographic appearances to the correct pathologic indication:

    _____ 1. Subacromial spurs   A. Rheumatoid arthritis

    _____ 2. Fluid-filled joint space   B. Bankart lesion

    _____ 3. Thin bony cortex   C. Hill-Sachs defect

    _____ 4. Widening of acromioclavicular joint space   D. Osteoarthritis

    _____ 5. Calcified tendons   E. Bursitis

    _____ 6. Lesion on the glenoid rim   F. Osteoporosis

    _____ 7. Narrowing of joint space   G. Impingement syndrome

    _____ 8. Closed joint space   H. Acromioclavicular joint dislocation

    _____ 9. Compression fracture of humeral head   I. Tendinitis

13. Which one of the following pathologic indications requires a decrease in manual exposure factors?

    A. Impingement syndrome   C. Bankart lesion

    B. Bursitis   D. Osteoporosis

14. Which two basic shoulder projections are routinely taken for a shoulder (with no traumatic injury) and proximal humerus?

    A. _____   B. _____

15. Specifically, where is the central ray placed for an AP projection of the shoulder? _____

    _____

16. Which two special projections of the shoulder best demonstrate a possible Hill-Sachs defect (as described in the textbook in the "Structure Best Shown" section).

    A. _____   B. _____

17. To best demonstrate a possible Hill-Sachs defect, which additional positioning technique should be used with the projections listed in the previous question?

    A. Angle central ray 10° to 15° caudad   C. Angle central ray 3° to 5°caudad

    B. Rotate affected arm externally approximately 45°   D. Place humeral epicondyles parallel to IR

18. What type of central ray angulation is required for the inferosuperior axial projection—Lawrence method?

    A. 25° to 30° medially   C. 25° anterior and 25° medially

    B. 35° to 45° medially   D. Central ray perpendicular to IR

19. Which projection of the shoulder produces an image of the glenoid process in profile (A)

    _____ ? This projection is also referred to as the (B) _____

    method.

20. Which one of the following projections produces a tangential projection of the intertubercular groove?

    A. Fisk method   C. Westpoint method

    B. Grashey method   D. Lawrence method

21. The supine version of the tangential projection for the intertubercular groove requires that the central ray be angled

    _____ posteriorly from the horizontal plane.

22. Which one of the following projections would be best for demonstrating a possible dislocation of the proximal humerus?

    A. Grashey method   C. Inferosuperior axiolateral

    B. Fisk method   D. Scapular Y

23. Which special projection of the shoulder best demonstrates the acromiohumeral space for possible subacromial

    spurs that create shoulder impingement symptoms (A) _____ ? This projection is also re-

    ferred to as the (B) _____ method.

24. True/False: The transthoracic lateral projection is performed for possible fractures or dislocations of the proximal humerus.

25. True/False: The use of a breathing technique is recommended for the transthoracic lateral projection.

26. True/False: The affected arm must be placed into external rotation for the transthoracic lateral projection.

27. True/False: A central ray angle of 10° to 15° caudad may be used for the transthoracic lateral projections if the patient is unable to elevate the uninjured arm and shoulder sufficiently.

28. True/False: The scapular Y lateral position requires the body to be rotated 45° to 60° anteriorly toward the affected side.

29. Which one of the following shoulder projections delivers the greatest skin dose to the patient?

    A. AP axial clavicle   C. Transthoracic lateral

    B. AP projection, neutral position D. Tangential projection for intertubercular groove

30. Which of the following requires the smallest thyroid dose?

    A. AP neutral rotation shoulder   C. AP clavicle

    B. Transthoracic lateral   D. Scapular Y lateral

31. Which of the answers (*A* through *D*) in the previous questions would result in the highest thyroid dose?_____

32. Which special projection of the shoulder requires that the affected side be rotated 45° toward the cassette and a 45°

    caudad central ray angle? _____

33. A posterior dislocation of the humerus projects the humeral head _____ (superior or inferior) to the glenoid cavity with the special projection described in the previous question.

34. A thin-shouldered patient requires _____ (**more** or **less**) angle for an AP axial clavicle projection than a large-shouldered patient.

35. What must be ruled out before performing the weight-bearing study for acromioclavicular joints?

    _____

36. Match the following projections with their correct proper name method. Choices may be used more than once:

    _____ 1. Inferosuperior axiolateral   A. Neer method

    _____ 2. AP oblique for glenoid cavity   B. Grashey method

    _____ 3. Tangential for intertubercular (bicipital) groove   C. Lawrence method

    _____ 4. Supraspinatus outlet tangential   D. Fisk method

    _____ 5. Transthoracic lateral   E. Garth method

    _____ 6. AP apical oblique

REVIEW EXERCISE C: Problem Solving for Technical and Positioning Errors

1. The following factors were used to produce a radiograph of an AP projection of the shoulder: 85 kVp, 20 mAs, high-speed screens, 40-inch (102-cm) SID, grid, and suspended respiration. The resultant radiograph demonstrated poor radiographic contrast between bony and soft tissue structures. Which of these factors can be altered during the repeat exposure to improve radiographic quality?

    ———————————————————————————————————

2. A radiograph of an AP axial clavicle projection reveals that the clavicle is projected below the superior border of the scapula. What can the technologist do to correct this problem during the repeat exposure?

    ———————————————————————————————————

3. A radiograph of an AP scapula reveals that the scapula is within the lung field and difficult to see. Which two things can the technologist do to improve the visibility of the scapula during the repeat exposure?

    ———————————————————————————————————

4. A radiograph of an AP projection (with external rotation) of a shoulder (with no traumatic injury) reveals that neither the greater nor lesser tubercles are profiled. What must be done to correct this during the repeat exposure?

    ———————————————————————————————————

5. A radiograph of a lateral scapula position reveals that it is not a true lateral projection. (Considerable separation exists between the axillary and vertebral borders.) The projection was taken using the following factors: erect position, 40-inch (102-cm) SID, 45° rotation toward cassette from posteroanterior (PA), central ray centered to midscapula, and no central ray angulation. Based on these factors, how can the this position be improved during the repeat exposure?

    ———————————————————————————————————

6. A radiograph of the AP oblique (Grashey) taken as a 35° oblique projection reveals that the borders of the glenoid cavity are not superimposed. The patient had large, rounded shoulders. What must be done to get better superimposition of the cavity during the repeat exposure?

    ———————————————————————————————————

7. **Situation:** A patient with a possible right shoulder dislocation enters emergency room. The technologist attempts to perform a erect transthoracic lateral projection, but the patient is unable to raise the left arm and shoulder high enough. The resultant radiograph reveals that the shoulders are superimposed, and the right shoulder and humeral head are not well visualized. What can be done to improve this image during the repeat exposure?

    ———————————————————————————————————

8. **Situation:** A patient with a possible fracture of the right proximal humerus from an automobile accident enters the emergency room. The patient has other injuries and is unable to stand or sit erect. Which positioning routine should

   be used to determine the extent of the injury? _____

9. **Situation:** A patient with a clinical history of chronic shoulder dislocation comes to the radiology department. The orthopedic physician suspects that a Hill-Sachs defect may be present. Which specific position(s) may be used to

   best demonstrate this pathologic feature? _____

10. **Situation:** A patient with a possible Bankart lesion comes to the radiology department. Which position of the

    shoulder girdle would best demonstrate this? _____

11. **Situation:** A patient with a possible rotator cuff tear comes to the radiology department. Which one of the following imaging modalities would best demonstrate this injury?

    A. Arthrography   C. Nuclear medicine

    B. MRI   D. Radiography

12. **Situation:** A patient with a clinical history of tendon injury in the shoulder region comes to the radiology department. The orthopedic physician needs a *functional* study of the shoulder joint performed to determine the extent of the tendon injury. Which of the following modalities would best demonstrate this injury?

    A. Arthrography   C. Ultrasound

    B. MRI   D. Nuclear medicine

REVIEW EXERCISE D: Critique Radiographs of the Proximal Humerus and Shoulder Girdle (see textbook p. 194)

The following questions relate to the radiographs found at the end of Chapter 5 of the textbook. Evaluate these radiographs for the radiographic criteria categories *(1 through 5)* that follow. Describe the corrections needed to improve the overall image. The major, or "repeatable," errors are specific errors that indicate the need for a repeat exposure, regardless of the nature of the other errors.

A. **AP clavicle (Fig. C5-85)**
    Description of possible error:

    1. Structures shown: _____

    2. Part positioning: _____

    3. Collimation and central ray: _____

    4. Exposure criteria: _____

    5. Markers: _____

    Repeatable error(s): _____

B. **AP apical oblique axial shoulder (Fig. C5-86)**
    Description of possible error:

    1. Structures shown: _____

    2. Part positioning: _____

    3. Collimation and central ray: _____

4. Exposure criteria: _____

5. Markers: _____

Repeatable error(s): _____

C. **AP scapula (Fig. C5-87)**
Description of possible error:

1. Structures shown: _____

2. Part positioning: _____

3. Collimation and central ray: _____

4. Exposure criteria: _____

5. Markers: _____

Repeatable error(s): _____

D. **AP shoulder and proximal humerus (Fig. C5-88)**
Description of possible error:

1. Structures shown: _____

2. Part positioning: _____

3. Collimation and central ray: _____

4. Exposure criteria: _____

5. Markers: _____

Repeatable error(s): _____

Which projection (AP, lateral, or oblique) and which rotation of the proximal humerus are evident (internal, external, or

neutral)? _____

PART III: Laboratory Exercises (see textbook pp. 173-193)

You must gain experience in positioning each part of the proximal humerus and shoulder girdle before performing the following exams on actual patients. You can get experience in positioning and radiographic evaluation of these projections by performing exercises using radiographic phantoms and practicing on other students (although you will not be taking actual exposures).

The following suggested activities assume that your teaching institution has an energized lab and radiographic phantoms. If not, perform Laboratory Exercises B and C, the radiographic evaluation and the physical positioning exercises. (Check off each step and projection as you complete it.)

LABORATORY EXERCISE A: Energized Laboratory

1. Using the thorax radiographic phantom, produce radiographs of the following basic routines:

_____ AP shoulder   _____ AP oblique (Grashey)

_____ AP and AP axial clavicle   _____ AP and lateral scapula

LABORATORY EXERCISE B: Radiographic Evaluation

1. Evaluate and critique the radiographs produced during the previous experiments, additional radiographs provided by your instructor, or both. Evaluate each radiograph for the following points. (Check off when completed.):

    _____   Evaluate the completeness of the study. (Are all of the pertinent anatomic structures included on the radiograph?)

    _____   Evaluate for positioning or centering errors (e.g., rotation, off centering).

    _____   Evaluate for correct exposure factors and possible motion. (Are the density and contrast of the images acceptable?)

    _____   Determine whether markers and an acceptable degree of collimation and/or area shielding are seen on the images.

LABORATORY EXERCISE C: Physical Positioning

On another person, simulate performing all basic and special projections of the proximal humerus and shoulder girdle as follows. (Check off each when completed satisfactorily.) Include the following six steps as described in the textbook.

Step 1. Appropriate size and type of film holder with correct markers
Step 2. Correct central ray placement and centering of part to central ray and/or film
Step 3. Accurate collimation
Step 4. Area shielding of patient where advisable
Step 5. Use of proper immobilizing devices when needed
Step 6. Approximate correct exposure factors, breathing instructions where applicable, and "making" exposure

Projections	Step 1	Step 2	Step 3	Step 4	Step 5	Step 6
• Shoulder series (nontrauma)	____	____	____	____	____	____
(AP internal and external rotation)	____	____	____	____	____	____
• Inferosuperior axiolateral (Lawrence)	____	____	____	____	____	____
• AP oblique (Grashey)	____	____	____	____	____	____
• Tangential (Fisk) for intertubercular groove	____	____	____	____	____	____
• Scapular Y	____	____	____	____	____	____
• Transthoracic lateral	____	____	____	____	____	____
• AP apical oblique (Garth)	____	____	____	____	____	____
• AP and AP axial clavicle	____	____	____	____	____	____
• AP and lateral scapula	____	____	____	____	____	____
• Acromioclavicular joints (with and without weights)	____	____	____	____	____	____

ANSWERS TO REVIEW EXERCISES

Review Exercise A: Anatomy of Proximal Humerus and Shoulder Girdle

1. A. Proximal humerus
   B. Scapula
   C. Clavicle
2. A. Intertubercular groove (bicipital groove)
   B. Greater tubercle (tuberosity)
   C. Head of humerus
   D. Anatomic neck
   E. Lesser tubercle (tuberosity)
   F. Surgical neck
   G. Neutral (Neither the greater nor lesser tubercle are in profile.)
3. A. Sternal extremity
   B. Body (shaft)
   C. Acromial extremity
4. Male
5. A. Lateral angle
   B. Superior angle
   C. Inferior angle
6. Costal
7. Axilla
8. A. Infraspinous fossa
   B. Supraspinous fossa
9. Synovial (diarthroidal)
10. A. Spheroidal or ball and socket
    B. Plane or gliding
    C. Plane or gliding
11. 1. C
    2. A
    3. A
    4. D
    5. B
    6. C
    7. D
    8. C
12. A. Neck of scapula
    B. Scapulohumeral joint (glenohumeral joint)
    C. Acromion
    D. Coracoid process
    E. Scapular notch
    F. Superior angle
    G. Medial (vertebral) border
    H. Lateral (axillary) border
    I. Ventral (costal) surface
    J. Dorsal surface
    K. Spine of scapula
    L. Acromion
    M. Coracoid process
    N. Body (blade, wing, or ala)
    O. Inferior angle
13. A. Coracoid process
    B. Scapulohumeral joint
    C. Acromion
    D. Greater tubercle
    E. Lesser tubercle
    F. Lateral (axillary) border
    G. Internal (Lesser tubercle is in profile medially.)
    H. Lateral
    I. Perpendicular
    J. Body of scapula
    K. Spine of scapula and acromion
    L. Coracoid process
    M. Body (shaft) of humerus
    N. Scapular Y lateral
14. A. Coracoid process
    B. Glenoid process
    C. Spine of scapula
    D. Acromion
    E. Inferosuperior axial projection
    F. 90°

Review Exercise B: Positioning of Proximal Humerus and Shoulder Girdle

1. 1. A
   2. C
   3. B
   4. A
   5. C
   6. A
   7. B
   8. B
   9. A
2. A. Neutral
   B. External
   C. Internal
3. A. True
   B. False
   C. False
   D. False
   E. True
   F. False
   G. True
   H. True
4. D. 65 to 75 kVp
5. A. Parent or guardian
6. True
7. False
8. True
9. False
10. True
11. 1. D
    2. B
    3. G
    4. A
    5. C
    6. F
    7. E
12. 1. G
    2. E
    3. F
    4. H
    5. I

6. B
7. D
8. A
9. C
13. D. Osteoporosis
14. A. AP, external rotation
    B. AP, internal rotation
15. To midscapulohumeral joint, ³/₄ inch (2 cm) inferior and lateral to coracoid process
16. A. Inferosuperior axial projection—Lawrence method
    B. Inferosuperior axial projection—Westpoint method
17. B. Rotate affected arm externally approximately 45°.
18. A. 25° to 30° medially
19. A. AP oblique
    B. Grashey
20. A. Fisk method
21. 10° to 15°
22. D. Scapular Y
23. A. Supraspinatus outlet tangential projection
    B. Neer
24. True
25. True
26. False
27. False
28. True
29. C. Transthoracic lateral
30. D. Scapular Y lateral
31. B. Transthoracic lateral
32. AP apical oblique
33. Superior
34. More
35. Fracture of clavicle
36. 1. C
    2. B
    3. D
    4. A
    5. C
    6. E

Review Exercise C: Problem-Solving for Technical and Positioning Errors

1. Lower kilovoltage peak to 75 kVp and double milliamperage seconds (to 40 mAs), which increases radiographic contrast.
2. Increase central ray cephalad angle.
3. Ensure that the affected arm is abducted 90°, and use a breathing technique.
4. Supinate the hand and ensure that the epicondyles are parallel to the IR for a true AP.

5. Palpate the scapular borders to ensure true lateral and increase body obliquity if needed to between 50° and 60° from a posteroanterior (PA) position.

6. Increase rotation of affected shoulder toward film to closer to 45°.

7. Angle the central ray 10° to 15° cephalad to separate the shoulders.

8. Anteroposterior (AP) of right shoulder and humerus without rotation (neutral rotation); and a supine, horizontal beam, right transthoracic shoulder

   NOTE: In those cases in which the opposite arm cannot be elevated or extended, a supine posterior oblique scapular Y could also be used as a second option for a lateral shoulder position (see Chapter 19).

9. Inferosuperior axial projections—Lawrence or Westpoint method

10. Westpoint method or scapular Y position

11. B. Magnetic resonance imaging (MRI)

12. C. Ultrasound

Review Exercise D: Critique Radiographs of the Proximal Humerus and Shoulder Girdle

A. AP clavicle (Fig. C5-85)
   1. All of clavicle demonstrated

2. Rotation of body toward the right, superimposing sternal end over the spine and creating overall distortion of the clavicle and associated joints

3. Collimation much too loose and not evident at all; central ray centered too low (inferiorly), which also adds to distorted appearance of clavicle

4. Acceptable but slightly underexposed exposure factors

5. Missing (or not visible) anatomic marker

   Repeatable error(s): criteria 2 and 5

B. AP apical oblique axial shoulder (Fig. C5-86)
   1. All pertinent anatomic structures demonstrated but severely distorted
   2. Correct positioning of shoulder
   3. Evidence of acceptable side collimation (no evidence of top and bottom collimation). Excessive central ray angulation led to distortion of anatomic structures (see page 187 in text for correct appearance of this projection). Excessive object-image distance (OID) could also have added to this distortion.
   4. Acceptable but slightly underexposed exposure factors
   5. Missing (or not visible) anatomic marker

   Repeatable error(s): criteria 1, 3, and 5

C. AP scapula (Fig. C5-87)
   1. Lower margin of scapula cut off at bottom edge of radiograph
   2. Acceptable part positioning
   3. Collimation too loose or not evident; need to center central ray and cassette to include the entire scapula
   4. Underexposed scapula and blurring of ribs that is not evident from breathing technique
   5. Missing (or not visible) anatomic marker

   Repeatable error(s): criteria 1, 3, 4, and 5

D. AP shoulder and proximal humerus (Fig. C5-88)
   1. Majority of the shoulder girdle cut off and not demonstrated
   2. Correct part positioning for AP projection, but centering is off
   3. Evidence of collimation on one side only, indicating incorrect centering; central ray and film centering too lateral
   4. Acceptable but slightly underexposed exposure factors
   5. Acceptable; anatomic marker seen on radiograph

   Repeatable error(s): criteria 1 and 3
   Position: AP projection, external rotation

SELF-TEST

My Score = _____ %

This self-test should be taken only after completing all of the readings, review exercises, and laboratory activities for a particular section. The purpose of this test is not only to provide a good learning exercise but also to serve as a strong indicator of what your final unit evaluation grade will cover. It is strongly suggested that if you do not get at least a 90% to 95% grade on each self-test, you should review those areas in which you missed questions before going to your instructor for the final unit evaluation exam.

1. Select the term(s) that correctly describes the shoulder joint:

    A. Humeroscapular   C. Glenohumeral

    B. Scapulohumeral   D. B and C

2. Which specific joint is found on the lateral end of the clavicle?

    A. Scapulohumeral   C. Acromioclavicular

    B. Sternoclavicular   D. Glenohumeral

3. Which of the following is *not* an angle found on the scapula?

    A. Inferior angle   C. Lateral angle

    B. Medial angle   D. Superior angle

4. Which one of the following structures of the scapula extends most anteriorly?

    A. Glenoid cavity   C. Scapular spine

    B. Acromion   D. Coracoid process

5. True/False: The male clavicle is shorter and less curved than the female clavicle.

6. Which bony structure separates the supraspinous and infraspinous fossae?

    A. Scapular spine   C. Acromion

    B. Glenoid cavity   D. Superior border of scapula

7. Which one of the following structures is considered to be the most posterior?

    A. Scapular notch   C. Acromion

    B. Coracoid process   D. Glenoid process

8. What is the type of joint movement for the scapulohumeral joint?

    A. Plane   C. Ellipsoidal

    B. Spheroidal   D. Trochoidal

9. Identify the following structures labeled on Figs. 5-11 and 5-12.
   Answers may be used more than once:

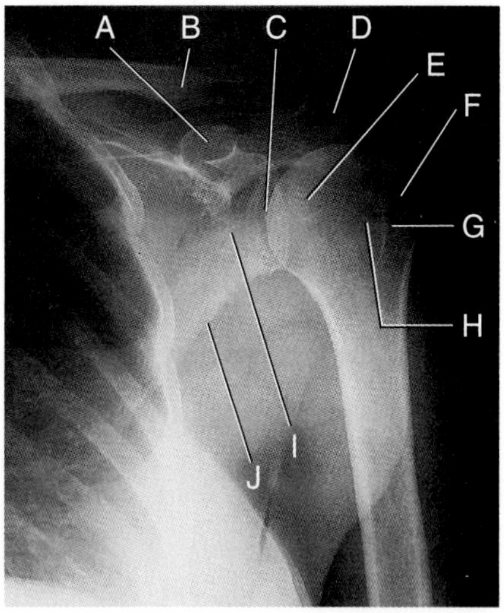

   _____ A.   1. Spine of scapula

   _____ B.   2. Lesser tubercle

   _____ C.   3. Coracoid process

   _____ D.   4. Lateral (axillary) border of scapula

   _____ E.   5. Scapulohumeral joint

   _____ F.   6. Clavicle

   _____ G.   7. Intertubercular groove

   _____ H.   8. Acromion of scapula

   _____ I.   9. Neck of scapula

   _____ J.   10. Greater tubercle

Fig. 5-11. Shoulder projection.

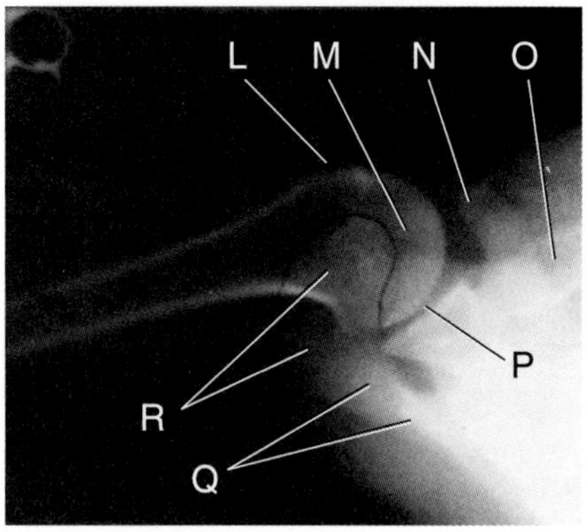

   K. Does Fig. 5-11 represent an (A) internal, (B) an external, or (C) a

       neutral rotation of the humerus? _____

   _____ L   11. Lateral extremity of clavicle

   _____ M.   12. Head of humerus

   _____ N   13. Glenoid cavity

   _____ O.

   _____ P.

   _____ Q.

   _____ R.

Fig. 5-12. Shoulder projection.

   S. What is the correct term and method for the projection seen on Fig. 5-12?

       A. Inferosuperior axial projection—Lawrence method

       B. Transthoracic lateral—Lawrence method

       C. Posterior oblique—Grashey method

10. Which one of the following technical considerations does not apply for adult shoulder radiography?

    A. Center and right automatic exposure control (AEC) chambers activated

    B. High-speed screen-film system

    C. 40 to 44 in (100 to 110 cm) SID

    D. 70 to 80 kVp (with grids)

11. True/False: Even though the amount of radiation exposure is minimal for most shoulder projections, gonadal
    shielding should be used for children and adults of child-bearing age.

12. True/False: The greatest technical concern during a pediatric shoulder study is voluntary motion.

13. Which one of the following imaging modalities/procedures best demonstrates osteomyelitis?

    A. Ultrasound

    B. Magnetic resonance imaging (MRI)

    C. Arthrography

    D. Nuclear medicine

14. Which one of the following imaging modalities/procedures provides a functional, or dynamic, study of the shoulder joint?

    A. Ultrasound

    B. Radiography

    C. Nuclear medicine

    D. MRI

15. Match the following pathologic indications or descriptions to the correct definition:

    _____ 1. Disability of the shoulder joint caused by chronic inflammation in and around the joint

    _____ 2. Lesion of the anteroinferior glenoid rim

    _____ 3. Chronic systemic disease with arthritic inflammatory changes throughout the body

    _____ 4. Superior displacement of distal clavicle

    _____ 5. Compression fracture of humeral head

    _____ 6. Traumatic injury to one more muscles of the shoulder joint

    _____ 7. Reduction in the quantity of bone

    A. Rotator cuff tear

    B. Osteoporosis

    C. Rheumatoid condition

    D. Idiopathic chronic adhesive capsulitis

    E. Bankart lesion

    F. Acromioclavicular joint or dislocation

    G. Hill-Sachs defect

16. Which one of the following projections/positions best demonstrates signs of impingement syndrome?

    A. AP and lateral shoulder

    B. Transaxillary

    B. Transaxillary with exaggerated, external rotation

    D. "Scapular Y," or Neer method

17. Which one of the following pathologic conditions produces narrowing of the joint space?

    A. Osteoarthritis

    B. Bursitis

    C. Osteoporosis

    D. Idiopathic chronic adhesive capsulitis

18. Which one of the following pathologic conditions may require a reduction in manual exposure factors?

    A. Bursitis

    B. Rheumatoid arthritis

    C. Rotator cuff tear

    D. Bankart lesion

19. Which basic projection of the shoulder requires that the humeral epicondyles be parallel to the cassette?

    A. External rotation

    B. Neutral rotation

    C. Internal rotation

    D. Grashey method

20. Where is the central ray centered for an AP projection of the shoulder?

    A. Acromion

    B. 1 inch (2.5 cm) superior to coracoid process

    C. 1 inch (2.5 cm) inferior to coracoid process

    D. 2 inches (5 cm) inferior to acromioclavicular joint

21. Which position of the shoulder and proximal humerus projects the lesser tubercle in profile medially?

    A. External rotation   C. Internal rotation

    B. Neutral rotation   D. Exaggerated rotation

22. What central ray angle should be used for the inferosuperior axiolateral (Lawrence) projection?

    A. 15° medially   C. 25° anteriorly and medially

    B. 25° medially   D. 35° to 45° medially

23. To best demonstrate the Hill-Sachs defect on the inferosuperior axiolateral projection, which additional positioning maneuver must be used?

    A. Angle central ray 35° medially   C. Use exaggerated internal rotation

    B. Use exaggerated external rotation   D. Abduct arm 120° rotation from midsagittal plane (MSP)

24. The inferosuperior axial projection (Westpoint method) requires a double central ray angulation of:

    A. 25° anterior and medial   C. 15° anterior and medial

    B. 5° medial and 15° anterior   D. 30° medial and 5° anterior

25. Which special projection of the shoulder places the glenoid cavity in profile for an "open" glenohumeral joint?

    A. Garth method   C. Fisk method

    B. Transthoracic lateral—Lawrence method   D. Grashey method

26. For the erect version of the tangential projection for the intertubercular groove, the patient leans forward

    _____ from vertical.

    A. 5° to 7°   C. 10° to 15°

    B. 20° to 25°   D. 35° to 45°

27. What is the major advantage of the supine, tangential version of the intertubercular groove projection over the erect version?

    A. Less radiation exposure   C. Less risk of motion

    B. Reduced object-image distance (OID)   D. Ability to use automatic exposure control (AEC)

28. Which one of the following projections best demonstrates the supraspinatus outlet region?

    A. Neer method   C. Inferosuperior axial—Lawrence method

    B. Fisk method   D. Inferosuperior axial—Westpoint method

29. With which one of the following projections is a breathing technique preferred?

    A. Grashey method   C. Scapular Y

    B. Transthoracic lateral   D. Garth method

30. How much caudad central ray angulation is required for the supraspinatus outlet tangential (Neer) projection?

    A. 10 to 15° caudad   C. 25° anteriorly and medially

    B. 45° caudad   D. None. Central ray is perpendicular

31. Which pathologic feature is best demonstrated with the Garth method?

   A. Bursitis   C. Scapulohumeral dislocations

   B. Rheumatoid arthritis   D. Signs of shoulder impingement

32. True/False: A posteroanterior (PA) axial projection of the clavicle requires a 15° to 20° caudal central ray angle.

33. True/False: A 72-inch (180-cm) source-image distance (SID) is recommended for acromioclavicular joint studies.

34. Match the correct patient dose ranges with the following types of projections (small- to average-size adult with accurate collimation):

   1. Thyroid dose for AP acromioclavicular joints   A. 1000 mrad or more

   2. Breast dose for AP shoulder   B. 40 to 100 mrad

   3. Thyroid dose for AP shoulder   C. 10 mrad or less

   4. Skin dose for AP shoulder

   5. Skin dose for transthoracic lateral

   6. Breast dose for AP acromioclavicular joints (two projections)

   7. Breast dose for scapular Y lateral

   8. Breast or thyroid dose for inferosuperior axiolateral shoulder

35. A radiograph of the Grashey method reveals that the anterior and posterior glenoid rims are not superimposed. The following positioning factors were used: erect position, body rotated 35° toward the affected side, central ray perpendicular to scapulohumeral joint space, and affected arm slightly abducted in neutral rotation. Which one of the following modifications will superimpose the glenoid rims during the repeat exposure?

   A. Angle central ray 10° to 15° caudad.   C. Place affected arm in external rotation position.

   B. Rotate body less toward affected side.   D. Rotate body more toward affected side.

36. **Situation:** A patient with a possible shoulder dislocation enters the emergency room. A neutral, AP projection of the shoulder has been taken, confirming a dislocation. Which additional projection should be taken?

   A. Grashey method   C. Garth method

   B. Inferosuperior axial projection—Lawrence method   D. AP, external rotation

37. A radiograph of an AP axial clavicle reveals that the clavicle is projected in the lung field below the top of the shoulder. The following positioning factors were used: erect position, central ray angled 15° cephalad, 40-inch (100-cm) SID, and respiration suspended at end of expiration. Which one of the following modifications should be made during the repeat exposure?

   A. Increase central ray angulation.   C. Reverse central ray angulation.

   B. Suspend respiration at end of inspiration.   D. Use 72-inch (180-cm) SID.

38. **Situation:** A patient with a possible acromioclavicular separation enters the emergency room. Which one of the following routines should be used?

   A. Acromioclavicular joint series: non–weight-bearing and weight-bearing projections

   B. AP neutral projection and Garth method

   C. AP neutral and transthoracic lateral projections

   D. AP internal and external projections

39. For the following critique questions, see Fig. C5-85, an AP clavicle radiograph, in your textbook.

A. Which positioning error(s) is/are visible on this AP left clavicle radiograph? More than one answer may be selected.

(a) All essential anatomic structures are not demonstrated.

(b) Central ray is centered incorrectly.

(c) Collimation is not evident.

(d) Exposure factors are incorrect.

(e) No anatomic marker is visible on the radiograph.

(f) Slight rotation toward the right is evident.

(g) Slight rotation toward the left is evident.

B. Which of the previous criteria are considered "repeatable errors?"_____

C. Which of the following modifications must be made during the repeat exposure? More than one answer may be selected.

(a) Increase collimation.

(b) Center central ray correctly.

(c) Decrease exposure factors.

(d) Increase exposure factors.

(e) Place anatomic marker on image receptor (IR) before exposure.

(f) Ensure that no rotation occurs to the right or left.

40. For the following critique questions, refer to the AP scapula radiograph, Fig. C5-87, in your textbook.

A. Which positioning error(s) is/are visible on this radiograph? More than one answer may be selected.

(a) All essential anatomic structures are not demonstrated.

(b) Central ray is centered incorrectly.

(c) Collimation is not evident.

(d) Exposure factors are incorrect.

(e) No anatomic marker is visible on radiograph.

(f) Excessive rotation toward the right is evident.

(g) Excessive rotation toward the left is evident.

B. Which of the previous criteria are considered "repeatable errors?"_____

C. Which of the following modifications must be made during the repeat exposure? More than one answer may be selected.

(a) Increase collimation.

(b) Center central ray more inferiorly.

(c) Decrease exposure factors.

(d) Increase exposure factors.

(e) Place anatomic marker on IR before exposure.

(f) Rotate body slightly toward the left.

(g) Rotate elbow slightly toward the right.

CHAPTER 6

Lower Limb

CHAPTER OBJECTIVES

After you have successfully completed **all** the activities in this chapter, you will be able to:

_____ 1. Identify the bones and specific features of the toes, foot, ankle, lower leg, knee, patella and distal femur.

_____ 2. On drawings and radiographs, identify specific anatomic features of the foot, ankle, leg, knee, patella, and distal femur.

_____ 3. Identify specific joints of the foot, ankle, leg, and knee according to the correct classification and movement type.

_____ 4. Match specific pathologic indications of the lower limb to the correct definition.

_____ 5. Match specific pathologic indications of the lower limb to the correct radiographic appearance.

_____ 6. Describe the basic and special projections of the toes, foot, ankle, calcaneus, knee, patella, intercondylar fossa, and femur, including central ray placement and angulation, correct film size and placement, part positioning, technical factors, and evaluation criteria.

_____ 7. List the various patient dose ranges for each projection of the lower limb.

_____ 8. Given various hypothetical situations, identify the correct modification of a position and/or exposure factors to improve the radiographic image.

_____ 9. Given various hypothetical situations, identify the correct position for a specific pathologic form or condition.

_____ 10. Given radiographs of specific lower limb projections, identify specific positioning and exposure factors errors.

POSITIONING AND FILM CRITIQUE

_____ 1. Using a peer, perform basic and special projections of the lower limb.

_____ 2. Using foot and knee phantoms, produce satisfactory radiographs of the lower limb (if equipment is available).

_____ 3. Critique and evaluate lower limb radiographs based on the four divisions of radiographic criteria: (1) structures shown, (2) position, (3) collimation and central ray, and (4) exposure criteria.

_____ 4. Distinguish between acceptable and unacceptable lower limb radiographs based on exposure factors, motion, collimation, positioning, or other errors.

Learning Exercises

Complete the following review exercises after reading the associated pages in the textbook as indicated by each exercise. Answers to each review exercise are given at the end of the review exercises.

PART I: Radiographic Anatomy

REVIEW EXERCISE A: Radiographic Anatomy of the Foot and Ankle (see textbook pp. 196-201)

1. Fill in the number of bones for the following:

    A. Phalanges _____   C. Tarsals _____

    B. Metatarsals _____   D. Total _____

2. What are two differences in the phalanges of the foot as compared with the phalanges of the hand?

    A. _____

    B. _____

3. Which tuberosity of the foot is palpable and a common site of foot trauma?

    _____

4. Where are the sesamoid bones of the foot most commonly located? _____

5. What is the largest and strongest tarsal bone? _____

6. What is the name of the joint found between the talus and calcaneus? _____

7. List the three specific articular facets found in the joint described in the previous question.

    A. _____   B. _____   C. _____

8. The small opening, or space, found between the talus and calcaneus is called the

    _____

9. Match the correct tarsal bone to the following characteristics. Answers may be used more than once:

    _____   1. Forms an aspect of the ankle joint   A. Calcaneus

    _____   2. The smallest of the cuneiforms   B. Talus

    _____   3. Found on the medial side of the foot between the talus   C. Cuboid
                and three cuneiforms

    _____   4. The largest of the cuneiforms   D. Navicular

    _____   5. Articulates with the second, third, and fourth metatarsal   E. Lateral cuneiform

    _____   6. The most superior tarsal bone   F. Intermediate cuneiform

    _____   7. Articulates with the first metatarsal   G. Medial cuneiform

    _____   8. Contains the sustentaculum tali

    _____   9. A tarsal found anterior to the calcaneus and lateral to the
                lateral cuneiform

    _____   10. Second largest tarsal bone

10. Identify the labeled structures found in Figs. 6-1 and 6-2:

A. _____

B. _____

C. _____

D. _____

E. _____

F. _____

G. _____

H. _____

I. _____

J. _____

K. _____

L. _____

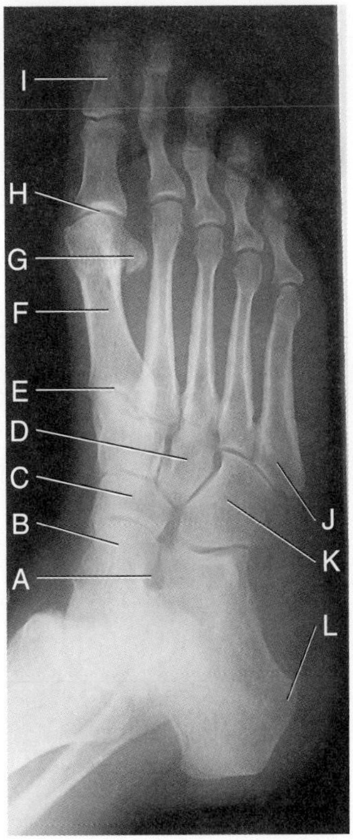

Fig. 6-1. Anatomy of the foot.

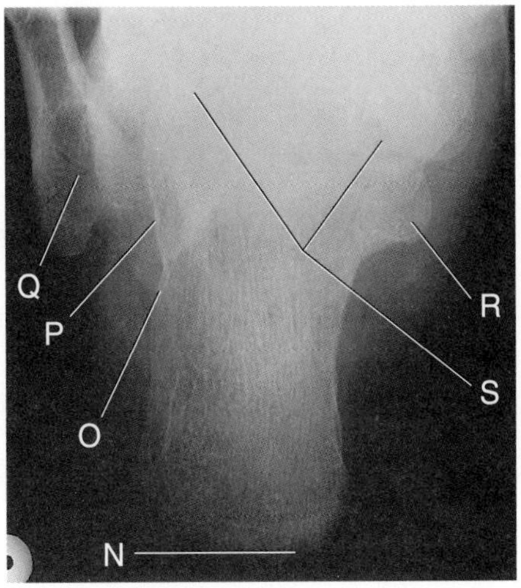

M. Fig. 6-1 represents a radiograph of which projection of

the foot?_____

N. _____

O. _____

P. _____

Q. _____

R. _____

S. _____

T. Fig. 6-2 represents a radiograph of which projection?

_____

Fig. 6-2. Anatomy of the foot.

11. True/False: The cuboid articulates with the four bones of the foot.

12. The calcaneus articulates with the talus and the:

    A. Navicular   C. Medial cuneiform

    B. Cuboid   D. Lateral cuneiform

13. List the two arches of the foot: (A) _____   (B) _____

14. Which three bones make up the ankle joint?

    A. _____   B. _____   C. _____

15. The three bones of the ankle form a deep socket into which the talus fits. This socket is called the _____

    _____

16. The distal, tibial joint surface forming the roof of the distal ankle joint is called the:

    A. Tibial plafond   C. Tibial plateau

    B. Articular facet   D. Ankle mortise

17. True/False: The medial malleolus is approximately 1/2 inch (1 cm) posterior to the lateral malleolus.

18. The ankle joint is classified as a synovial joint with _____ type movement.

19. Identify the structures labeled on Figs. 6-3 and 6-4:

    Fig. 6-3:

    A. _____

    B. _____

    C. _____

    D. _____

    E. _____

    Fig. 6-4:

    F. _____

    G. _____

    H. _____

    I. _____

    J. _____

    K. _____

    L. _____

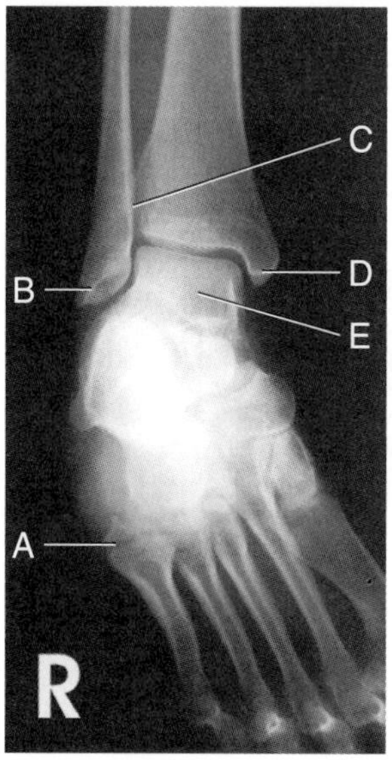

Fig. 6-3. Anatomy of the ankle. 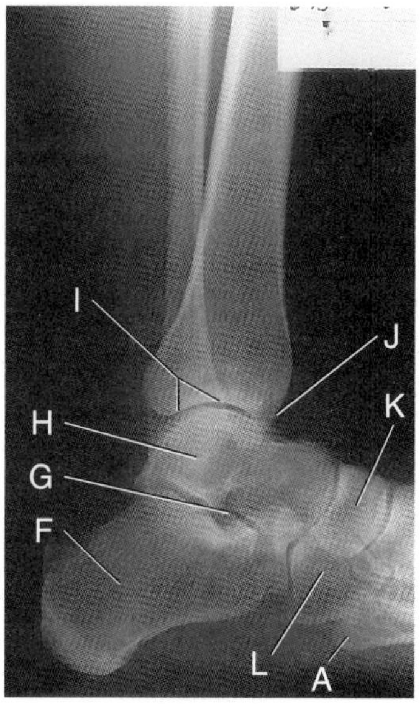   **Fig. 6-4.** Anatomy of the ankle.

    M. Fig. 6-3 represents a radiograph of which projection of the ankle? _____

REVIEW EXERCISE B: Radiographic Anatomy of the Lower Leg, Knee, and Distal Femur (see textbook pp. 202-208)

1. The _____ is the weight-bearing bone of the lower leg.

2. What is the name of the large prominence located on the midanterior surface of the proximal tibia that serves as a

    distal attachment for the patellar ligament? _____

3. What is the name of the small prominence located on the posterior border of the medial condyle of the femur that is

    an identifying mark to determine possible rotation of a lateral knee? _____

4. A small, triangular depression located on the tibia that helps form the distal tibiofibular joint is called the

    _____ .

5. The articular facets of the proximal tibia are also referred to as the _____ .

6. The articular facets slope _____ ° posteriorly.

    A. 25   C. 35

    B. 45   D. 10 to 15

7. The most proximal aspect of the fibula is the _____ .

8. The extreme, proximal end of the fibula is the _____ .

9. What is the name of the largest sesamoid bone in the body _____ ?

10. What are two other names for the patellar surface of the femur?

    A. _____   B. _____

11. What is the name of the depression located on the posterior aspect of the distal femur?

    _____

12. Why must the central ray be angled 5° to 7° cephalad for a lateral knee position?

    _____

13. The slightly raised area located on the lateroposterior aspect of the medial condyle is called the:

    A. Trochlear tubercle   C. Adductor tubercle

    B. Anterior crest   D. Tibial tuberosity

14. What are the two, palpable bony landmarks found on the distal femur?

    A. _____   B. _____

15. The general region of the posterior knee is called the _____ .

16. True/False: Flexion of 35° of the knee forces the patella firmly against the patellar surface of the femur.

17. True/False: The patella acts like a pivot to increase the leverage of a large muscle found in the anterior thigh.

18. True/False: The posterior surface of the patella is normally rough.

19. For which large muscle does the patella serve as a pivot to increase the leverage?

    _____

20. List the correct terms for the following joints:

    A. Between the patella and distal femur _____

    B. Between the two condyles of the femur and tibia _____

21. List the four major ligaments of the knee:

    A. _____   C. _____

    B. _____   D. _____

22. The crescent-shaped fibrocartilage disks that act as shock absorbers in the knee joint are called _____.

23. List the two bursae found in the knee joint.

    A. _____   B. _____

24. Match the correct bone to the following structures. Answers may be used more than once:

    _____ 1. Tibial plafond   A. Tibia

    _____ 2. Medial malleolus   B. Fibula

    _____ 3. Lateral epicondyle   C. Distal femur

    _____ 4. Patellar surface   D. Patella

    _____ 5. Articular facets

    _____ 6. Fibular notch

    _____ 7. Styloid process

    _____ 8. Base

    _____ 9. Intercondyloid eminence

    _____ 10. Neck

25. Match the correct joint classification or movement type with the following articulations:

    _____ 1. Ankle joint   A. Synarthrodial (gomphoses type)

    _____ 2. Patellofemoral   B. Ginglymus (hinge)

    _____ 3. Proximal tibiofibular   C. Sellar (saddle)

    _____ 4. Tarsometatarsal   D. Plane (gliding)

    _____ 5. Knee joint (femorotibial) E. Amphiarthrodial (syndesmosis type)

    _____ 6. Distal tibiofibular

26.   Identify the labeled structures on Figs. 6-5 through 6-7.

Fig. 6-5:

A. _____

B. _____

C. _____

D. _____

E. _____

F. _____

G. _____

H. _____

I. _____

Fig. 6-6:

J. _____

K. _____

L. _____

M. _____

N. _____

O. _____°

P. _____

Q. _____

R. _____

Fig. 6-7:

S. _____

T. _____

U. _____

V. _____

W. _____

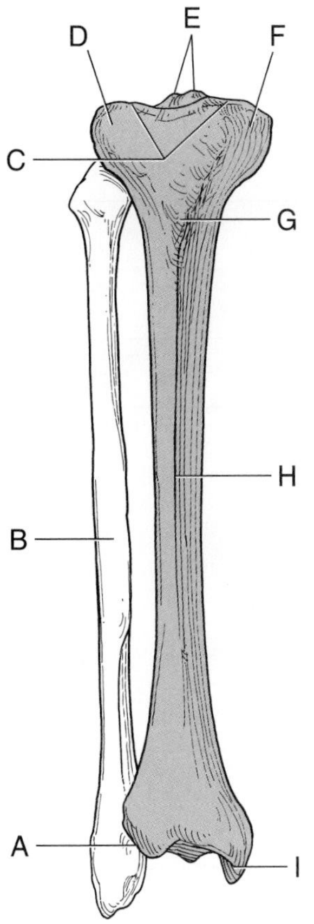

Fig. 6-5. Frontal view of tibia and fibula.

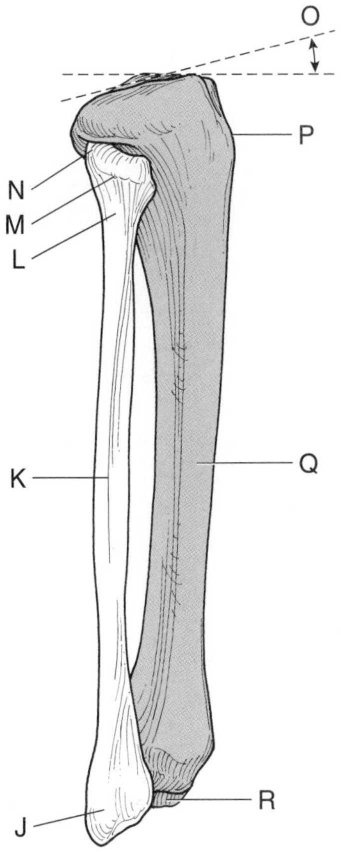

Fig. 6-6. Lateral view of tibia and fibula.

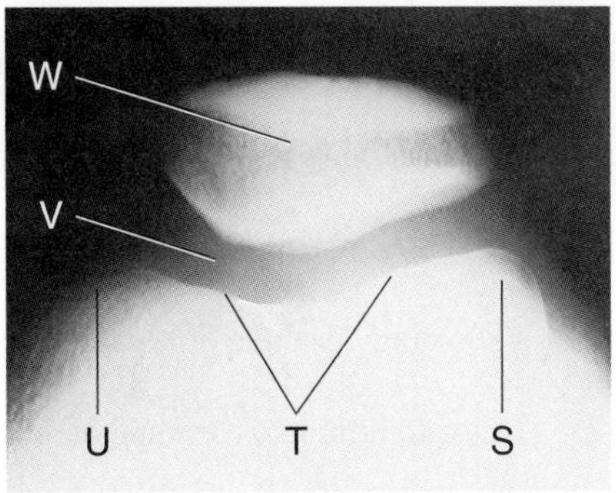

Fig. 6-7. Anatomy of the knee and patella.

X.   Which projection does the radiograph in Fig. 6-7 represent? _____

27. Identify the bony structures labeled on Figs. 6-8 and 6-9:

Fig. 6-8:

A. _____

B. _____

C. _____

D. _____

E. _____

F. _____

G. _____

H. _____

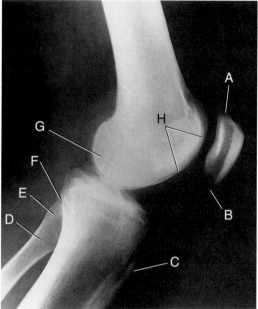

Fig. 6-8. True lateral radiograph of the knee.

Fig. 6-9

I. _____

J. _____

K. _____

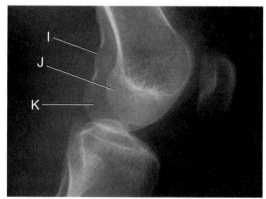

Fig. 6-9. Lateral radiograph of the knee.

28. Match the following foot and ankle movements to the correct definition:

_____ A. Inward turning or bending of ankle

_____ B. Decreasing the angle between the dorsum pedis and anterior lower leg

_____ C. Extending the ankle or pointing the foot and toe downward

_____ D. Outward turning or bending of ankle

1. Inversion (vargus)

2. Plantar flexion

3. Eversion (valgus)

4. Dorsiflexion

PART II: Radiographic Positioning

REVIEW EXERCISE C: Positioning of the Foot and Ankle (see textbook pp. 214-228)

1. True/False: The recommended source-to-image receptor distance (SID) for lower limb radiographs is 40 inches (100 cm).

2. True/False: To reduce scatter radiation during table top procedures, the Bucky tray should be positioned over the lower limb being radiographed.

3. True/False: With careful and close collimation, gonadal shielding does not have to be used during lower limb radiography.

4. True/False: When using digital radiography, lead masking should be placed on the regions of the imaging plate not within the collimation field.

5. True/False: A kilovoltage peak range between 50 and 70 should be used for lower limb radiography.

6. Match the following pathologic indications to the correct definition:

_____ A. An inflammatory condition involving the anterior, proximal tibia.   1.   Exostosis

_____ B. Also known as *osteitis deformans*   2.   Joint effusion

_____ C. Malignant tumor of the cartilage   3.   Bone cyst

_____ D. Inherited type of arthritis that commonly affects males   4.   Reiter's syndrome

_____ E. Benign, neoplastic bone lesion caused by overproduction of bone at a joint   5.   Osteoid osteoma

_____ F. Benign bone lesion usually developing in teens or young adults   6.   Ewing's sarcoma

_____ G. Most prevalent primary bone malignancy in pediatric patients   7.   Gout

_____ H. Benign, neoplastic bone lesion filled with clear fluid   8.   Paget's disease

_____ I. Accumulated fluid in the joint cavity   9.   Osgood-Schlatter disease

_____ J. Condition affecting the sacroiliac joints and lower limbs of young men, especially the posterosuperior margin of the calcaneus   10.   Chondrosarcoma

7. The formal name for "runner's knee" is _____

8. What is another term for *osteomalacia*? _____

9. Match the following radiographic appearances to the correct pathologic indication:

_____ A. Asymmetric erosion of joint spaces with calcaneal erosion   1.   Osteoid osteoma

_____ B. Uric acid deposits in joint spaces   2.   Ewing's sarcoma

_____ C. Well-circumscribed lucency   3.   Gout

_____ D. Small, round/oval density with lucent center   4.   Osgood-Schlatter disease

_____ E. Narrowed, irregular joint surfaces with sclerotic articular surfaces   5.   Osteoarthritis

_____ F. Fragmentation or detachment of the tibial tuberosity   6.   Osteomalacia

_____ G. Ill-defined area of bone destruction with surrounding "onion peel"   7.   Reiter's syndrome

_____ H. Decreased bone density and bowing deformities of weight-bearing limbs   8.   Bone cyst

10. Why is the central ray angled 10° to 15° toward the calcaneus for an anteroposterior (AP) projection of the toes?

_____

11. Where is the central ray centered for an AP oblique projection of the foot? _____

12. Which projection is best for demonstrating the sesamoid bones of the foot? _____

13. The foot should be dorsiflexed so that the plantar surface of the foot is _____° from vertical for the sesamoid projection.

14. Why should the central ray be angled 10° posterior for an AP projection of the foot?

    _____

15. If a foreign body is lodged in the plantar surface of the foot, which type of central ray angle should be used for the AP projection?

    A. 10° posterior   C. 10° anterior

    B. 15° posterior   D. None. Use a perpendicular central ray.

16. Rotation can be determined on a radiograph of an AP foot projection by the near-equal distance between the

    _____ metatarsals.

17. Which oblique projection of the foot best demonstrates the majority of the tarsal bones?

    _____

18. Which oblique projection of the foot best demonstrates the navicular and the first and second cuneiforms with

    minimal superimposition? _____

19. Which projection tends to place the foot into a truer lateral position—mediolateral or lateromedial?

    _____

20. Which type of study should be performed to best evaluate the condition of the longitudinal arches of the foot?

    _____

21. How much should the central ray be angled from the long axis of the foot for the plantodorsal projection of the

    calcaneus _____?

22. Which calcaneal structure should appear medially on a well-positioned plantodorsal

    projection? _____

23. Where is the central ray placed for a lateral projection of the calcaneus? _____

    _____

24. Which joint surface is *not* visualized with a correctly positioned AP projection of the ankle?

    A. Medial aspect of joint   C. Lateral aspect of joint

    B. Superior aspect of joint   D. All of the above aspects of the joint *are* visualized.

25. Why should AP, 45° oblique, and lateral ankle radiographs include the proximal metatarsals?

    _____

26. How much (if any) should the foot and ankle be rotated for a mortise projection of the ankle?

   _____

27. Which projection of the ankle best demonstrates a possible fracture of the lateral malleolus?

   _____

28. With a true lateral projection of the ankle, the lateral malleolus is:

   A. Projected over the anterior aspect of the distal tibia

   B. Projected over the posterior aspect of the distal tibia

   C. Directly superimposed over the distal tibia

   D. Directly superimposed over the medial malleolus

29. Which projections of the ankle require forced inversion and eversion movements?

   _____

REVIEW EXERCISE D: Positioning of the Tibia, Fibula, Knee, and Distal Femur (see textbook pp. 229-245)

1. What is the basic positioning routine for a study of the tibia and fibula? _____

2. Why is it important to include the knee joint for an initial study of tibia trauma, even if the patient's symptoms involve the middle and distal aspect?

   _____

3. To include both joints for a lateral projection of the tibia and fibula for an adult, the technologist may place the

   cassette _____ in relation to the part.

   A. Parallel   C. Diagonally

   B. Perpendicular   D. Transverse

4. What is the recommended central ray placement for an AP projection of the knee for a patient with thick thighs and buttocks (i.e., measuring greater than 24 cm)?

   A. 3° to 5° caudad   C. Central ray perpendicular to film

   B. 3° to 5° cephalad   D. Central ray perpendicular to patellar plane

5. Where is the central ray centered for an AP projection of the knee?

   A. ½ inch (1.25 cm) distal to apex of patella   C. Midpatella

   B. 1 inch (2½ cm) proximal to apex of patella   D. Level of tibial tuberosity

6. Which basic projection of a knee best demonstrates the proximal fibula free of superimposition?

   A. True AP   C. AP oblique, 45° medial rotation

   B. True lateral   D. AP oblique, 45° lateral rotation

7. Circle the correct choice. For the AP oblique projection of the knee, which rotation (medial [internal] or lateral [external]) best visualizes the lateral condyle of the tibia and the head and neck of the fibula?

8. What is the recommended central ray placement for a lateral knee position on a tall, slender male patient with a narrow pelvis?

    A. 3° to 5° caudad   C. Central ray perpendicular to IR

    B. 3° to 5° cephalad   D. Central ray perpendicular to patellar plane

9. How much flexion is recommended for a lateral projection of the knee?

    A. No flexion   B. 20° to 30°   C. 30° to 35°   D. 45°

10. Which positioning error is present if the distal borders of the femoral condyles are not superimposed on a

    radiograph of a lateral knee? _____

11. Which positioning error is present if the posterior portions of the femoral condyles are not superimposed on a

    lateral knee radiograph? _____

12. Which anatomic structure of the femur can be used to determine which rotation (overrotation or underrotation) is present on a slightly rotated lateral knee radiograph?

    _____

13. Which special projection of the knee best evaluates the knee joint for cartilage degeneration or deformities?

    _____

14. AP knee stress projections are performed to demonstrate:

    A. Patellar dislocation   C. Medial or collateral ligament damage

    B. Osgood-Schlatter disease   D. Osteoarthritis

15 Which one of the following special projections of the knee best demonstrates the intercondylar fossa?

    A. Holmblad   C. AP weight-bearing, bilateral projections

    B. Merchant   D. Settegast

16. How much flexion of the lower leg is required for the Camp-Coventry projection when the central ray is angled

    40° caudad? _____

17. Why is the posteroanterior (PA) axial projection for the intercondylar fossa recommended instead of an AP axial

    projection? _____

18. True/False: To place the interepicondylar line parallel to the image receptor for a PA projection of the patella, the lower limb must be rotated approximately 5° internally.

19. How much part flexion is recommended for a lateral projection of the patella?

    _____

20. The skin dose range for an AP knee projection is:

    A. 5 to 10 mrad   C. 50 to 60 mrad

    B. 20 to 30 mrad   D. More than 100 mrad

21. How much central ray angle from the long axis of the femora is required for a Merchant bilateral projection?

22. How much part flexion is required for the (A) Hughston method _____ and (B) Settegast

    method _____ ?

23. Which of these methods (Hughston or Settegast) is preferred and why?

    _____

24. Match the following characteristics, structures, and/or other names to the correct position for projections of the knee
    and/or patella. Use each answer only once:

    _____ 1. Patient on "all fours" on table

    _____ 2. Patient is prone, requires 90° knee flexion

    _____ 3. Patient is prone with 40° to 50° knee flexion and with equal 40°
                to 50° caudad CR angle

    _____ 4. Curved cassette preferred

    _____ 5. Patient is prone with 45° knee flexion and 10° to 20° cephalad
                CR angle from long axis of lower leg

    _____ 6. Patient is supine with cassette resting on midthighs of patient

    _____ 7. Patient is supine with 40° knee flexion and with with 30° caudad
                CR angle from horizontal

    A. Inferosuperior axial for
        patellofemoral joint

    B. Merchant method

    C. Hughston method

    D. Camp-Coventry method

    E. Settegast method

    F. Holmblad method

    G. Béclere method

25. To best utilize the anode-heel effect on a mediolateral hip projection, on which end (cathode or anode) should the

    hip be placed? _____

REVIEW EXERCISE E: Problem Solving for Technical and Positioning Errors

1. A radiograph of an AP foot reveals that the metatarsophalangeal joints are not open and the metatarsals are some-
    what foreshortened. What was the positioning error involved, and what modification should be made to improve this
    image on the repeat exposure?

    _____

2. A radiograph of a medial oblique foot reveals that the proximal first and second metatarsals are completely super-
    imposed. What type of positioning error led to this radiographic outcome?

    _____

3. A radiograph of a plantodorsal projection of the calcaneus reveals considerable foreshortening of the calcaneus.
    What type of positioning modification is needed on the repeat exposure?

    _____

4. A radiograph of an AP projection of the ankle reveals that the lateral surface of the ankle joint is totally open. (It
    should not be open on a true AP projection.) The technologist is positive that the ankle was in the correct, true AP
    position with the long axis of foot perpendicular to IR. What else could have led to this joint space being open?

    _____

5. A radiograph of an intended AP oblique-mortise projection reveals that the lateral malleolus is superimposed over the talus, and the distal tibiofibular joint is not well demonstrated. What is the most likely reason for this radiographic outcome?

_____

6. A radiograph of an AP knee demonstrates that the joint space is narrowed or not open at all. The patient is young and has no history of degenerative disease. What type of positioning modification may improve the outcome of this projection?

_____

7. A radiograph of an intended AP oblique with **medial** rotation of the knee to demonstrate the proximal fibula reveals that there is total superimposition of the proximal tibia and the fibula. What must be modified to correct this projection?

_____

8. A radiograph of a lateral recumbent knee reveals that the posterior border of the medial femoral condyle (identified by the adductor tubercle) is not superimposed but is slightly posterior to the lateral condyle. The fibular head is also completely superimposed by the tibia. What type of positioning error led to this radiographic outcome?

_____

9. **Situation:** A patient with trauma to the medial aspect of the foot comes to the emergency room. A heavy object was dropped on the foot near the base of the first metatarsal. Basic foot projections do not clearly demonstrate this region. What other projection of the foot could be used to better delineate this area?

_____

10. A radiograph of an AP and lateral tibia and fibula reveals that the ankle is not included on the AP projection, but both the knee and the ankle are included on the lateral projection. What should the technologist do in this situation?

_____

11. A radiograph obtained by using the Camp-Coventry method reveals that the distal femoral condyles and intercondylar fossa are asymmetric. Which specific positioning error is present?

_____

12. A radiograph of a lateral patella reveals that the patella is drawn tightly against the intercondylar sulcus. Which positioning modification should be performed to improve the quality of the image during the repeat exposure?

_____

13. **Situation:** A patient with a history of degenerative disease of the left knee joint comes to the radiology department. The orthopedic surgeon orders a radiographic study to determine the extent of damage to the joint space. Which projection(s) should be performed?

_____

14. **Situation:** A patient with a history of pain in the feet comes to the radiology department. The referring physician orders a study to examine the sesamoid bones. Which projection(s) would demonstrate these structures?

_____

15. **Situation:** A patient with a history of pain in the feet comes to the radiology department. The referring physician orders a study to evaluate the longitudinal arches of the feet. Which positioning routine should be used?

_____

REVIEW EXERCISE F: Critique Radiographs of the Lower Limbs (see textbook pp. 185-220)

The following questions relate to the radiographs found at the end of Chapter 6 of the textbook. Evaluate these radiographs for the radiographic criteria categories (*1* through *5*) that follow. Describe the corrections needed to improve the overall image. The major, or "repeatable," errors are specific errors that indicate the need for a repeat exposure, regardless of the nature of the other errors.

Comparing these radiographs with the correctly positioned and exposed radiographs in this chapter of the textbook will help you evaluate each of them for errors. Answers to each critique are given at the end of the laboratory activity.

NOTE: The critique exercises and detection of positioning errors is challenging, but studying the radiographs and answering the questions will help prepare you for your instructor's classroom and/or lab presentation, which will include slides of the same radiographs alongside the improved images. These learning experiences and the laboratory positioning exercises that follow also include critiques of additional radiographs provided by your instructor to prepare you for evaluating and critiquing the radiographs you take to help you avoid making mistakes as you begin your clinical work.

A. **Bilateral tangential patella (Fig. C6-146)**
   Description of possible error:

   1. Structures shown: _____

   2. Part positioning: _____

   3. Collimation and central ray: _____

   4. Exposure criteria: _____

   5. Markers: _____

   Repeatable error(s): _____

B. **AP foot (Fig. C6-147)**
   Description of possible error:

   1. Structures shown: _____

   2. Part positioning: _____

   3. Collimation and central ray: _____

   4. Exposure criteria: _____

   5. Markers: _____

   Repeatable error(s): _____

C. **Lateral ankle (Fig. C6-148)**
   Description of possible error:

   1. Structures shown: _____

   2. Part positioning: _____

   3. Collimation and central ray: _____

   4. Exposure criteria: _____

   5. Markers: _____

   Repeatable error(s): _____

D. **AP knee (Fig. C6-149)**
    Description of possible error:

    1. Structures shown: _____

    2. Part positioning: _____

    3. Collimation and central ray: _____

    4. Exposure criteria: _____

    5. Markers: _____

    Repeatable error(s): _____

E. **Lateral knee (Fig. C6-150)**
    Description of possible error:

    1. Structures shown: _____

    2. Part positioning: _____

    3. Collimation and central ray: _____

    4. Exposure criteria: _____

    5. Markers: _____

    Repeatable error(s): _____

F. **Lateral knee (Fig. C6-151)**
    Description of possible error:

    1. Structures shown: _____

    2. Part positioning: _____

    3. Collimation and central ray: _____

    4. Exposure criteria: _____

    5. Markers: _____

    Repeatable error(s): _____

PART III: Laboratory Activities (see textbook pp.189-220)

You must gain experience in positioning each part of the lower limb before performing the following exams on actual patients. You can get experience in positioning and radiographic evaluation of these projections by performing exercises using radiographic phantoms and practicing on other students (although you will not be taking actual exposures).

The following suggested activities assume that your teaching institution has an energized lab and radiographic phantoms. If not, perform Laboratory Exercises B and C, the radiographic evaluation and the physical positioning exercises. (Check off each step and projection as you complete it.)

LABORATORY EXERCISE A: Energized Laboratory

1. Using the foot/ankle radiographic phantom, produce radiographs of the basic routines for the following:

    _____   Foot

    _____   Ankle

    _____   Calcaneus

2. Using the knee radiographic phantom, produce radiographs of the following basic routines:

    _____   AP

    _____   AP oblique, medial rotation

    _____   Lateral (horizontal beam lateral if flexed knee is not available)

LABORATORY EXERCISE B: Radiographic Evaluation

1. Evaluate and critique the radiographs produced during the previous experiments, additional radiographs provided by your instructor, or both. Evaluate each radiograph for the following points. (Check off when completed.):

    _____   Evaluate the completeness of the study. (Are all of the pertinent anatomic structures included on the radiograph?)

    _____   Evaluate for positioning or centering errors (e.g., rotation, off centering).

    _____   Evaluate for correct exposure factors and possible motion. (Are the density and contrast of the images acceptable?)

    _____   Determine whether markers and an acceptable degree of collimation and/or area shielding are seen on the images.

LABORATORY EXERCISE C: Physical Positioning

1. On another person, simulate performing all basic and special projections of the lower limb as follows. (Check off each when completed satisfactorily.) Include the following six steps as described in the textbook.

   Step 1. Appropriate size and type of film holder with correct markers
   Step 2. Correct central ray placement and centering of part to central ray and/or film
   Step 3. Accurate collimation
   Step 4. Area shielding of patient where advisable
   Step 5. Use of proper immobilizing devices when needed
   Step 6. Approximate correct exposure factors, breathing instructions where applicable, and "making" exposure

Projections	Step 1	Step 2	Step 3	Step 4	Step 5	Step 6
• Positioning routine for a specific toe	——	——	——	——	——	——
• Basic foot routine	——	——	——	——	——	——
• Special projection for sesamoid bones	——	——	——	——	——	——
• Basic projections of the calcaneus	——	——	——	——	——	——
• Weight-bearing foot projections	——	——	——	——	——	——
• Basic ankle routine, including mortise and 45° oblique projections	——	——	——	——	——	——
• AP and lateral tibia and fibula	——	——	——	——	——	——
• Basic knee routine	——	——	——	——	——	——
• Special projections for intercondylar fossa	——	——	——	——	——	——
• Weight-bearing AP knee projections	——	——	——	——	——	——
• Special projections for patellofemoral joint space	——	——	——	——	——	——
• AP and lateral midfemur projections	——	——	——	——	——	——

ANSWERS TO REVIEW EXERCISES

Review Exercise A: Radiographic Anatomy of the Foot and Ankle

1. A. 14
   B. 5
   C. 7
   D. 26
2. A. Phalanges of the foot are smaller.
   B. The joint movements of the foot are more limited than those of the hand.
3. Tuberosity of base of the fifth metatarsal
4. The plantar surface of the foot near the first metatarsophalangeal joint
5. Calcaneus
6. Subtalar or talocalcaneal
7. A. Posterior facet
   B. Anterior facet
   C. Middle facet
8. Sinus tarsi or tarsal sinus
9. 1. B
   2. F
   3. D
   4. G
   5. E
   6. B
   7. G
   8. A
   9. C
   10. B
10. A. Sinus tarsi (tarsal sinus)
    B. Talus
    C. Navicular
    D. Lateral cuneiform
    E. Base of first metatarsal
    F. Body (shaft) of first metatarsal
    G. Sesamoid bone
    H. Metatarsophalangeal joint of first digit
    I. Distal phalanx of first digit
    J. Tuberosity at base of fifth metatarsal
    K. Cuboid
    L. Calcaneal tuberosity
    M. Anteroposterior (AP) 45° medial oblique
    N. Tuberosity of calcaneus
    O. Lateral process of calcaneus
    P. Peroneal trochlea (trohclear process)
    Q. Lateral malleolus of fibula
    R. Sustentaculum tali
    S. Talocalcaneal joint
    T. Plantodorsal (axial) projection of calcaneus
11. True
12. B. Cuboid
13. A. Longitudinal arch
    B. Transverse arch

14. A. Talus
    B. Tibia
    C. Fibula
15. Ankle mortise
16. A. Tibial plafond
17. False
18. Ginglymus or hinge
19. A. Tuberosity at base of fifth metatarsal (see fracture on radiograph in Fig. 6-3)
    B. Lateral malleolus of fibula
    C. Distal tibiofibular joint
    D. Medial malleolus
    E. Talus
    F. Calcaneus
    G. Sinus tarsi (tarsal sinus)
    H. Talus
    I. Tibial plafond
    J. Anterior tubercle
    K. Navicular
    L. Cuboid
    M. AP mortise, 15° to 20° medial rotation

Review Exercise B: Radiographic Anatomy of the Lower Leg, Knee, and Distal Femur

1. Tibia
2. Tibial tuberosity
3. Adductor tubercle
4. Fibular notch
5. Tibial plateau
6. D. 10 to 15
7. Apex or styloid process
8. Apex
9. Patella
10. A. Intercondylar sulcus
    B. Trochlear groove
11. Intercondylar fossa or notch
12. Because the medial condyle extends lower than the lateral condyle of the femur
13. C. Adductor tubercle
14. A. Medial epicondyle
    B. Lateral epicondyle
15. Popliteal region
16. False
17. True
18. False
19. Quadriceps femoris muscle
20. A. Patellofemoral
    B. Femorotibial
21. A. Fibular (lateral) collateral
    B. Tibial (medial) collateral
    C. Anterior cruciate
    D. Posterior cruciate
22. Medial and lateral menisci
23. A. Suprapatellar bursa
    B. Infrapatellar bursa

24. 1. A
    2. A
    3. C
    4. C
    5. A
    6. A
    7. B
    8. D
    9. A
    10. B
25. 1. B
    2. C
    3. D
    4. D
    5. B
    6. E
26. A. Fibular notch of tibia (also could be identified as distal tibiofibular joint)
    B. Body (shaft) of fibula
    C. Articular facets (or tibial plateau)
    D. Lateral condyle of tibia
    E. Intercondyloid eminence (tibial spine)
    F. Medial condyle of tibia
    G. Tibial tuberosity
    H. Anterior crest of body (shaft of tibia)
    I. Medial malleolus
    J. Lateral malleolus
    K. Body (shaft) of fibula
    L. Neck of fibula
    M. Head of fibula
    N. Apex or styloid process of fibula
    O. 10° to 20° angle
    P. Tibial tuberosity
    Q. Body (shaft) of tibia
    R. Medial malleolus
    S. Lateral condyle of femur
    T. Patellar surface of femur
    U. Medial condyle of femur
    V. Patellofemoral joint space
    W. Patella
    X. Tangential (patellofemoral joint)
27. A. Base of patella
    B. Apex of patella
    C. Tibial tuberosity
    D. Neck of fibula
    E. Head of fibula
    F. Apex or styloid process of fibula
    G. Superimposed medial and lateral condyles
    H. Patellar surface/intercondylar sulcus or trochlear groove
    I. Adductor tubercle
    J. Lateral femoral condyle
    K. Medial femoral condyle
28. A. 1
    B. 4
    C. 2
    D. 3

Review Exercise C: Positioning of the Foot and Ankle

1. True
2. False
3. False
4. True
5. True
6. A. 9
   B. 8
   C. 10
   D. 7
   E. 1
   F. 5
   G. 6
   H. 3
   I. 2
   J. 4
7. Chondromalacia patellae
8. Rickets
9. A. 7
   B. 3
   C. 8
   D. 1
   E. 5
   F. 4
   G. 2
   H. 6
10. Opens up the interphalangeal and metatarsophalangeal joints
11. Base of third metatarsal
12. Tangential projection
13. 15° to 20°
14. Opens up metatarsophalangeal and certain intertarsal joints
15. D. None. Use perpendicular central ray.
16. Second to fifth
17. AP oblique with medial rotation
18. AP oblique with lateral rotation
19. Lateromedial
20. AP and lateral weight-bearing projections
21. 40° cephalad
22. Sustentaculum tali
23. 1½ inches (4 cm) inferior to the medial malleolus
24. C. Lateral aspect of joint
25. To demonstrate a possible fracture of the fifth metatarsal tuberosity (a common fracture site)
26. 15° to 20° (medially)
27. 45° AP oblique with medial rotation
28. B. Projected over the posterior aspect of the distal tibia
29. AP stress projections

Review Exercise D: Positioning of the Tibia, Fibula, Knee, and Distal Femur

1. AP and lateral projections
2. A fracture may also be present at the proximal fibula in addition to the distal portion.

3. C. Diagonally
4. B. 3° to 5° cephalad
5. A. ½ inch (1.25 cm) distal to apex of patella
6. C. AP oblique, 45° medial rotation
7. Medial (internal)
8. B. 3° to 5° cephalad
9. B. 20° to 30°
10. Improper cephalad angle of the central ray
11. Overrotation or underrotation of the knee
12. Adductor tubercle on medial condyle
13. AP or PA weight-bearing knee
14. C Medial or collateral
15. A. Holmblad projections
16. 40° flexion
17. Distortion caused by central ray angle and increased OID for AP
18. True
19. 5° to 10°
20. B. 20 to 30 mrad
21. 30° from horizontal
22. A. 45° to 55°
    B. 90°
23. Hughston method. Acute knee flexion of 90° tends to draw the patella into the intercondylar sulcus, reducing the diagnostic value of this projection.
24. 1. F
    2. E
    3. D
    4. G
    5. C
    6. A
    7. B
25. Cathode end

Review Exercise E: Problem-Solving for Technical and Positioning Errors

1. Central ray is not angled correctly; adjust central ray angle to keep it perpendicular to metatarsals.
2. Overrotation of foot (toward the medial direction)
3. Increase cephalad angle of the central ray to correctly elongate the calcaneus.
4. Possibly a spread of the ankle mortise caused by ruptured ligaments
5. Underrotation of the ankle (toward the medial direction). The described appearance was that of a true AP ankle with little or no obliquity
6. Angling the central ray correctly to keep it parallel to the tibial plateau
7. The wrong oblique view of the knee was obtained. This description is that of a laterally or externally oblique view of the knee.

8. Underrotation of knee (excessive rotation of patella away from table top)
9. An AP lateral oblique projection with 30° of external rotation will separate the bases of the first and second metatarsal.
10. Repeat the AP projection to ensure the ankle joint is demonstrated.
11. Rotation of the affected limb
12. Decrease the amount of flexion of the knee to only 5° to 10°.
13. An AP or PA weight-bearing bilateral knee projection will best evaluate the joint spaces.
14. Tangential projection for the sesamoid bones
15. AP and lateral weight-bearing projections

Review Exercise F: Critique Radiographs of the Lower Limb

A. Bilateral tangential patella (Fig. C6-146)
   1. Portion of each patella superimposed over intercondylar sulcus of femur
   2. Excessive flexion of knee most likely cause of superimposition of patella over femur
   3. Evidence of collimation; correct central ray centering and IR placement; may be an error in central ray angle, which would have contributed to the superimposition
   4. Underexposed
   5. Anatomic side marker present
   Repeatable error(s): 1, 2, and 3 (possibly 4)
B. AP foot (Fig. C6-147)
   1. Proximal metatarsals and all tarsals totally obscured; metatarsophalangeal joints not open; fourth and fifth metatarsals partially superimposed (can compare with textbook Fig. 6-57, p. 218)
   2. Acceptable but superimposed part centering; obscured anatomic structures, indicating foot was not extended (plantar flexion) sufficiently and was rotated slightly externally
   3. Evidence of collimation; insufficient central ray angle, which could also have contributed to some of the distortion and closure of joint spaces and to obscuring of proximal metatarsals and tarsals
   4. Acceptable exposure factors, but lack of contrast
   5. Anatomic side marker only partially visible

Repeatable error(s): 1, 2, and possibly 3
C. Lateral ankle (Fig. C6-148)
   1. Joint space between tibia and talus not open; obscured anterior tubercle
   2. Excessive rotation of anterior foot toward cassette (overrotation)
   3. No evidence of collimation; correct central ray centering and film placement
   4. Acceptable exposure factors
   5. Anatomic side market present
   Repeatable error(s): 1 and 2
D. AP knee (Fig. C6-149)
   1. Joint space not totally open
   2. Leg rotated slightly medially (and note slight medial location of patella) (can compare with textbook Fig. 6-101, p. 231)
   3. No evidence of collimation; incorrect central ray angle, which led to

narrowing and closing of joint space; correct film placement
   4. Acceptable exposure factors
   5. Anatomic side marker not present; patient ID marker should be on top, away from fibular area.
   Repeatable error(s): 3 (not a repeatable error in most situations)
E. Lateral knee (Fig. C6-150)
   1. All pertinent anatomic structures included but patellofemoral joint not open* (presence of superimposition of patella over lateral condyle because of rotation)
   2. Rotation of anterior knee away from cassette (underrotation); almost total superimposition of proximal fibula; visibility of adductor tubercle identifies medial condyle as being posterior; overflexed knee (should be flexed only 15° to 20° rather than the almost 45° used in this radiograph)

   3. No evidence of collimation; correct central ray centering and film placement
   4. Acceptable exposure factors
   5. Anatomic side marker present
   Repeatable error(s): 1 and 2
F. Lateral knee (Fig. C6-151)
   1. Closure of patellofemoral joint space caused by positioning error
   2. Excessive rotation of anterior knee toward cassette (overrotation); separation of proximal fibula from tibia; outline of adductor tubercle on medial condyle also anterior to lateral condyle; knee slightly underflexed
   3. No evidence of collimation; correct central ray centering and film placement
   4. Acceptable exposure factors
   5. Anatomic side marker present
   Repeatable error(s): 1 and 2

SELF-TEST

This self-test should be taken only after completing all of the readings, review exercises, and laboratory activities for a particular section. The purpose of this test is not only to provide a good learning exercise but also to serve as a strong indicator of what your final evaluation grade will be. It is strongly suggested that if you do not get at least a 90% to 95% grade on this self-test, you should review those areas in which you missed questions before going to your instructor for the final evaluation exam for this chapter. There are 92 questions or blanks—each is worth 1.1 points.

1. Which of the following is not an aspect of the metatarsal?

    A. Head   C. Body

    B. Tail   D. Base

2. True/False: The distal portion of the fifth metatarsal is a common fracture site.

3. Where are the sesamoid bones of the foot most commonly located?

    A. Plantar surface near head of first metatarsal

    B. Plantar surface at first tarsometatarsal joint

    C. Dorsum aspect near base of first metatarsal

    D. Plantar surface near cuboid bone

4. What is the name of the tarsal bone found on the medial side of the foot between the talus and three cuneiforms?

    A. Calcaneus   C. Cuboid

    B. Lateral malleolus D. Navicular

5. Which tarsal bone is considered to be the smallest?

    A. Medial cuneiform   C. Intermediate cuneiform

    B. Navicular   D. Lateral cuneiform

6. What is another term for the talocalcaneal joint?

    A. Tarsometatarsal joint   C. Mortise joint

    B. Subtalar joint   D. Tibiocalcaneal joint

7. The distal tibial joint surface is called the:

    A. Medial malleolus   C. Lateral malleolus

    B. Tibial plafond   D. Anterior tubercle

8. True/False: The mortise of the ankle should be totally open and visible on a correctly positioned anteroposterior (AP) projection of the ankle.

9. Match the following structures or characteristics to the following bones of the foot and ankle (use each choice only once):

_____ 1. Trochlear process   A. Metatarsal

_____ 2. Lateral malleolus   B. Talus

_____ 3. The second largest tarsal bone   C. Tibia

_____ 4. Found between the navicular and base of first metatarsal   D. Calcaneus

_____ 5. Base   E. Sinus tarsi

_____ 6. Found between the calcaneus and talus   F. Medial cuneiform

_____ 7. Anterior tubercle   G. Fibula

10. Match the structures labeled on Fig. 6-10 (use each choice only once):

_____ A.   1. Talus

_____ B.   2. First metatarsal

_____ C.   3. Lateral malleolus

_____ D.   4. Distal tibiofibular joint

_____ E.   5. Medial malleolus

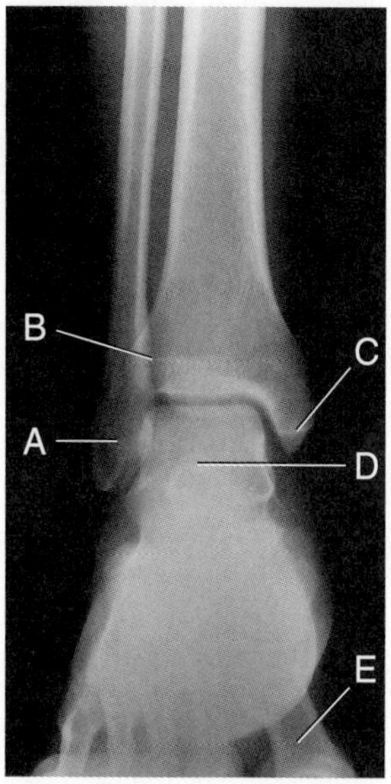

Fig. 6-10. Anatomy of the ankle.

F. What projection does this radiograph represent?

A. AP mortise ankle   C. AP ankle

B. AP stress ankle—inversion   D. AP stress ankle—eversion

11. Match the structures labeled on the radiographs in Figs. 6-11 through 6-13 (answers may be used more than once):

_____ A.   1. Distal phalanx, second digit

_____ B.   2. Proximal phalanx, first digit

_____ C.   3. Interphalangeal joint

_____ D.   4. First MP joint

_____ E.   5. Head of second metatarsal

_____ F.   6. Metatarsophalangeal joint, first digit

_____ G.   7. Base of first metatarsal

_____ H.   8. Proximal phalanx, second digit

_____ I.   9. Head of first metatarsal

_____ J.   10. Distal phalanx, first digit

_____ K.

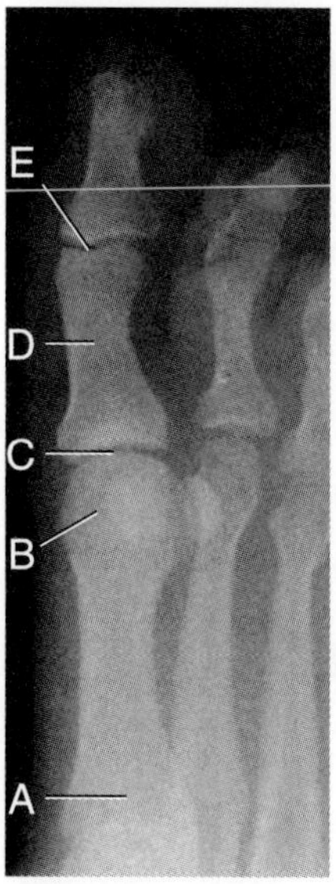

Fig. 6-11. Anatomy of the metatarsal bones and digits.

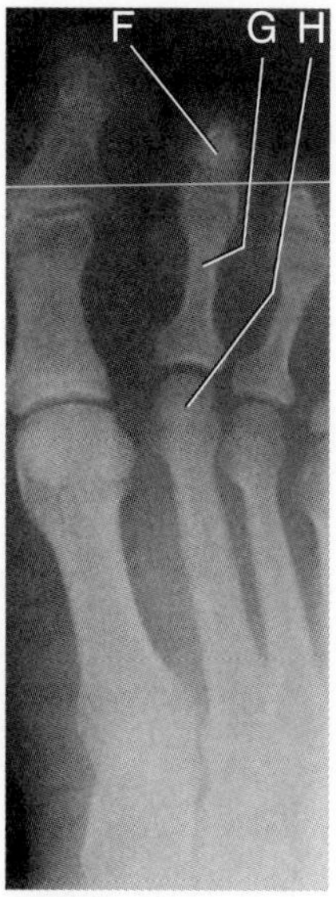

Fig. 6-12. Anatomy of the metatarsal bones and digits.

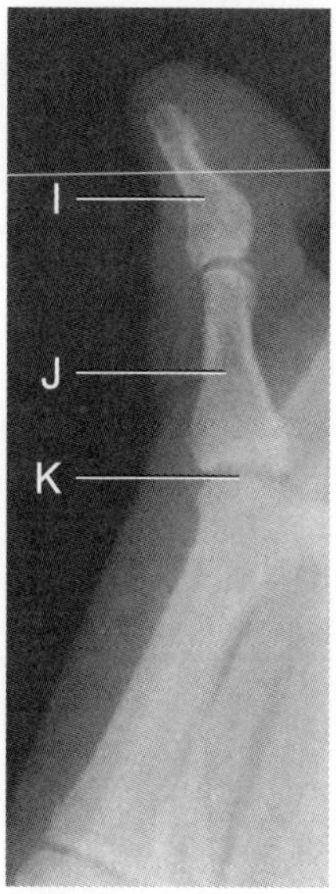

Fig. 6-13. Anatomy of the metatarsal bones and digits.

12. Which of the radiographs in the previous question represents an AP oblique projection of the toes?

    A. Fig. 6-11   C. Fig. 6-12

    B. Fig. 6-13   D. None of the above

13. What is the correct central ray centering placement for an AP projection of the toes?

    A. Affected MTP joint   C. Affected PIP joint

    B. Affected DIP joint   D. Head of affected metatarsal

14. Which type of central ray angle is required for an AP projection of the toes?

    A. None. Central ray is perpendicular.   C. 5° posterior

    B. 10° to 15° posterior   D. 20 to 25° posterior

15. Which of the following projections is used for the sesamoid bones of the foot?

    A. AP and lateral weight bearing   C. Tangential

    B. Camp-Coventry   D. AP mortise

16. How much foot rotation is required for the AP oblique, medial rotation projection of the foot?

    A. 3° to 5°   C. 15° to 20°

    B. 45°   D. 30° to 40°

17. What is another name for the AP projection of the foot?

    A. Mortise projection   C. Weight-bearing study

    B. Plantodorsal projection   D. Dorsoplantar projection

18. Which central ray angle and direction are generally required for the AP projection of the foot?

    A. 10° posterior   C. 15° posterior

    B. 10° anterior   D. None. Central ray is perpendicular.

19. Which projection of the foot best demonstrates the cuboid?

    A. AP   C. AP oblique—medial rotation

    B. AP oblique—lateral rotation   D. Lateromedial

20. What is another term for the intercondyloid eminence?

    A. Tibial plateaus   C. Tibial tuberosity

    B. Intercondylar fossa   D. Intercondylar tubercles

21. What is the name of the deep depression found on the posterior aspect of the distal femur?

    A. Intercondylar fossa   C. Patellar surface

    B. Intercondylar sulcus   D. Articular facets

22. A line drawn across the most distal aspect of the medial and lateral femoral condyles would be _____ from being at a right angle, or 90°, to the long axis of the femur.

    A. 5° to 7°   C. 0°

    B. 3° to 5°   D. 10° to 20°

23. True/False: The angle referred to in question 19 would be less on a tall, slender person.

24. The upper, or superior, portion of the patella is called the:

    A. Apex   C. Styloid process

    B. Base   D. Patellar head

25. Which two ligaments of the knee joint help stabilize the knee from the anterior and posterior perspective?

    A. Collaterals   C. Cruciate

    B. Patellar   D. Quadriceps femoris

26. Which structures serve as shock absorbers within the knee joint?

    A. Articular facets   C. Menisci

    B. Infrapatellar and suprapatellar bursae   D. Infrapatellar fat pads

27. Match the structures labeled on Figs 6-14 and 6-15 (use each choice only once):

    _____ A.   1. Medial condyle of tibia

    _____ B.   2. Neck of fibula

    _____ C.   3. Head of fibula

    _____ D.   4. Articular facets

    _____ E.   5. Patella

    _____ F.   6. Lateral condyle of femur

    _____ G.   7. Proximal tibiofibular joint

    _____ H.   8. Intercondyloid eminence

    _____ I.   9. Femorotibial joint space

    _____ J.   10. Lateral condyle of tibia

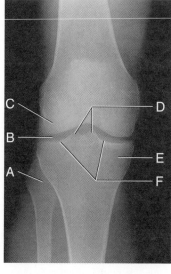
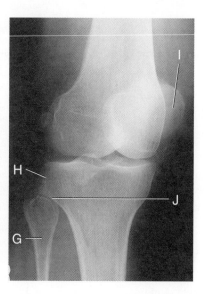

Fig. 6-14. AP radiograph of the knee   **Fig. 6-15.** Radiograph of the knee.

28. Which knee projection does Fig. 6-15 represent?

    A. AP

    B. AP oblique—medial rotation

    C. AP oblique—lateral rotation

    D. AP weight bearing

29. Match the parts labeled on Figs. 6-16 and 6-17. Answers may be used more than once:

    ____ A.   1. Adductor tubercle

    ____ B.   2. Head of fibula

    ____ C.   3. Medial femoral condyle

    ____ D.   4. Anterior aspect of medial condyle

    ____ E.   5. Lateral femoral condyle

    ____ F.   6. Anterior aspect of lateral condyle

    ____ G.   7. Tibial tuberosity

    ____ H.

    ____ I.

    ____ J

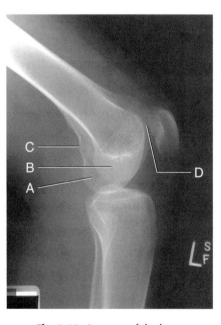

Fig. 6-16. Anatomy of the knee.

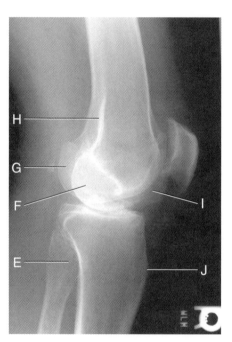

Fig. 6-17. Anatomy of the knee.

30. What is the *primary* positioning error present on Fig. 6-16?*

    A. Overangulation of central ray

    B. Underrotation toward image receptor

    C. Overrotation of knee toward image receptor

    D. Underangulation of central ray

31. True/False: The lateral knee position in Fig. 6-16 is excessively flexed.

32. What is the *primary* positioning error in Fig. 6-17?*

    A. Overangulation of central ray

    B. Underrotation toward image receptor

    C. Overrotation of knee toward image receptor

    D. Underangulation of central ray

*HINT: Two methods can be used to detect rotational errors on a lateral knee radiograph. Note the relative differences of the proximal fibula and superimposition by the tibia. In addition to identifying the medial or lateral femoral condyle by the structure C, the amount of superimposition of the fibular head also allows you to determine overrotation or underrotation of the knee if the radiograph is not a true lateral.

33. Which one of the following conditions may cause the tibial tuberosity to be pulled away from the tibial shaft?

    A. Gout

    B. Reiter's syndrome

    C. Osteomalacia

    D. Osgood-Schlatter disease

34. A condition that literally means "bone softening":

    A. Exostosis

    B. Paget's disease

    C. Osteoclastoma

    D. Osteomalacia

35. Which one of the following conditions may produce the radiographic appearance of a destructive lesion with irregular periosteal reaction?

    A. Osteogenic sarcoma

    B. Gout

    C. Bone cyst

    D. Osteoid osteoma

36. What is the common term for *chondromalacia patellae?*

    A. Brittle bone disease

    B. Runner's knee

    C. Degenerative joint disease

    D. Giant cell tumor

37. Where is the central ray placed for a plantodorsal projection of the calcaneus?

    A. Calcaneal tuberosity

    B. Sustentaculum tali

    C. Base of third metatarsal

    D. 1 inch (2½ cm) inferior to medial malleolus

38. Which ankle projection is best for demonstrating the mortise of the ankle?

    A. AP

    B. AP oblique (15° to 20° medial rotation)

    C. AP oblique (15° to 20° lateral rotation)

    D. Mediolateral

39. Which imaginary plane should be placed parallel to the IR for an AP projection of the knee?

    A. Intermalleolar

    B. Midcoronal

    C. Midsagittal

    D. Interepicondylar

40. Which joint space should be open or almost open for a well-positioned AP oblique knee projection with medial rotation?

    A. Both sides of knee joint

    B. Proximal tibiofibular

    C. Distal tibiofibular

    D. Patellofemoral

41. True/False: A 5° to 7° cephalad angle of the central ray for a lateral projection of the knee helps superimpose the distal borders of the medial and lateral condyles of the femur.

42. Why is a PA projection of the patella preferred to an AP projection?

    A. Less object-image distance (OID)

    B. Less distortion of patella

    C. Less magnification of patella

    D. All of the above

43. A projection is performed for the patellofemoral joint with the patient supine and the knee flexed 40°. The central ray is angled 30° caudad from horizontal. The cassette is resting on the lower legs supported by a special cassette-holding device. Which one of the following methods has been described?

    A. Camp-Coventry

    B. Settegast

    C. Hughston

    D. Merchant

44. What is the major disadvantage of the Settegast method?

    A. Requires use of specialized equipment   C. Requires overflexion of knee

    B. Requires AP positioning   D. Requires the use of a long OID

45. A radiograph of an AP knee reveals that the joint spaces are not equally open and the proximal fibula is superimposed over the tibia. Which specific positioning error lead to this radiographic outcome?

    A. Underangulation of central ray   C. Overangulation of central ray

    B. Lateral rotation of lower limb   D. Medial rotation of lower limb

46. A radiograph of the Camp-Coventry method was produced, but the intercondylar fossa is not open and is foreshortened. The following positioning factors were used: prone position, lower leg flexed 45°, and central ray angled 30° caudad and centered to the popliteal crease. Which of the following factors should be changed during the repeat exposure to produce a more diagnostic image?

    A. Decrease lower leg flexion to 30°   C. Increase CR angle to 45°

    B. Rotate lower limb 5° internally   D. Increase flexion of lower limb to 50° to 60°

47. A radiograph of a plantodorsal axial projection of the calcaneus reveals that the calcaneus is foreshortened. The following positioning factors were used: supine position, foot dorsiflexed perpendicular to image receptor, and central ray angled 30° cephalad and centered to base of third metatarsal. Which of the following factors should be changed during the repeat exposure to produce a more diagnostic image?

    A. Increase central ray angulation to 40°   C. Reduce dorsiflexion of foot

    B. Reverse direction of central ray angulation   D. Center central ray to sustentaculum tali

48. **Situation:** A patient with a possible fracture of the middle and distal femur enters the emergency room. The patient cannot be turned from the supine position. The physician orders a portable study because the patient is in a splint and in great pain. What specific positioning routine would be used with this patient?

    A. AP and lateral recumbent femur   C. AP projection only

    B. Lateral position only   D. AP and horizontal beam lateral position

49. For the following critique questions, refer to the bilateral patella radiograph in Fig. C6-146 in your textbook.

    A. Which positioning error(s) are visible on this radiograph? More than one answer may be selected.

       (a) All essential anatomic structures are not demonstrated.

       (b) Central ray is centered incorrectly.

       (c) Collimation is not evident.

       (d) Exposure factors are incorrect.

       (e) Central ray is angled incorrectly.

       (f) No anatomic marker is visible on the radiograph.

       (g) Excessive flexion of knees is evident.

       (h) Insufficient flexion of knees is evident.

    B. Which of the previous criteria are considered "repeatable errors?"* _____

C. Which of the following modifications must be made during the repeat exposure? More than one answer may be selected.

(a) Increase collimation.

(b) Center central ray correctly.

(c) Decrease exposure factors.

(d) Increase exposure factors.

(e) Alter central ray angulation.

(f) Place anatomic marker on image receptor before exposure.

(g) Decrease flexion of knees.

(h) Increase flexion of knees.

50. For the following critique questions, refer to the lateral ankle radiograph in Fig. C6-148 in your textbook.

A. Which positioning error(s) are visible on this radiograph? More than one answer may be selected.

(a) All essential anatomic structures are not demonstrated.

(b) Central ray is centered incorrectly.

(c) Collimation is not evident.

(d) Exposure factors are incorrect.

(e) No anatomic marker is visible on the radiograph.

(g) Excessive rotation of anterior foot toward cassette is evident.

(h) Excessive rotation of anterior foot away from cassette is evident.

B. Which of the previous criteria are considered "repeatable errors?" _____

C. Which of the following modifications must be made during the repeat exposure? More than one answer may be selected.

(a) Increase collimation.

(b) Center central ray correctly.

(c) Decrease exposure factors.

(d) Increase exposure factors.

(e) Place anatomic marker on image receptor before exposure.

(f) Rotate anterior foot away from image receptor.

(g) Rotate anterior foot toward image receptor

CHAPTER 7

Proximal Femur and Pelvis

CHAPTER OBJECTIVES

After you have successfully completed **all** the activities in this chapter, you will be able to:

_____ 1. Identify the bones and specific features of the proximal femur and pelvic girdle on drawings and radiographs.

_____ 2. Identify the location of the major landmarks of the pelvis and hip and describe two methods of locating the femoral head and neck on an anteroposterior (AP) hip and pelvis radiograph.

_____ 3. List the structural and functional differences of the greater and lesser pelvis and the structural difference between the male and female pelvis.

_____ 4. List the correct classification and movement type for the pelvic joints.

_____ 5. Identify the specific pediatric and geriatric applications for pelvis and hip radiographic examinations as described in the textbook.

_____ 6. Match specific pathologic indications of the pelvic girdle to the correct definition.

_____ 7. List specific pathologic indications of the shoulder girdle to the correct radiographic appearance.

_____ 8. Determine whether a pelvis or hip is in a true AP position based on the established radiographic criteria.

_____ 9. Identify and/or list the patient dose ranges for each projection of the hip and pelvis and know the approximate difference among patient doses when using a higher kilovoltage peak, lower milliamperage seconds technique.

_____ 10. List the basic projections, type and size of image receptor (IR), automatic exposure control (AEC) chamber selection, central ray location, and anatomic structures best demonstrated for radiographic examinations of the hips, pelvis, and sacroiliac (SI) joints.

_____ 11. Given various hypothetical clinical situations, identify the correct modification of a position and/or exposure factors to improve the radiographic image.

_____ 12. Given radiographs of specific shoulder girdle projections, identify positioning and exposure factors errors.

POSITIONING AND FILM CRITIQUE

_____ 1. Using a peer, position for the basic and special projections of the proximal femur and pelvic girdle.

_____ 2. Using a pelvic radiographic phantom, produce satisfactory radiographs of specific positions (if equipment is available).

_____ 3. Critique and evaluate pelvic girdle radiographs based on the four divisions of radiographic criteria: (1) structures shown, (2) position, (3) collimation and central ray, and (4) exposure criteria.

_____ 4. Distinguish between acceptable and unacceptable pelvic girdle radiographs based on exposure factors, motion, collimation, positioning, or other errors.

Learning Exercises

Complete the following review exercises after reading the associated pages in the textbook as indicated by each exercise. Answers to each review exercise are given at the end of the review exercises.

PART I: Radiographic Anatomy

REVIEW EXERCISE A: Radiographic Anatomy of the Hips and Pelvis (see textbook pp. 248-254)

1. The largest and strongest bone of the body is the _____ .

2. A small depression located in the center of the femoral head is the _____ .

3. The lesser trochanter is located on the _____ (medial or lateral) aspect of the proximal femur.

    It projects _____ (anteriorly or posteriorly) from the junction between the neck and shaft.

4. Because of the alignment between the femoral head and pelvis, the lower limb must be rotated _____° internally to place the femoral neck parallel to the plane of the film to achieve a true anteroposterior (AP) projection.

5. True/False: According to *Gray's Anatomy* reference textbook, the terms *pelvis* and *pelvic girdle* are **not** synonymous.

    A. List the **four** bones comprising the **pelvis:** _____

    B. List those **two** bones comprising the **pelvic girdle:** _____

    C. List two additional terms used for the bones in *B:*

        1. _____   2. _____

6. List the three divisions of the hip bone:

    A. _____   B. _____   C. _____

7. All three divisions of the hip bone eventually fuse at the _____ at the age of _____ .

8. What are the two important radiographic landmarks found on the ilium?

    A. _____   B. _____

9. Which bony landmark is found on the most **inferior** part of the posterior pelvis? _____

10. What is the name of the joint found between the superior rami of the pubic bones? _____

11. The _____ of the pelvis is the largest foramen in the skeletal system.

12. The upper margin of the greater trochanter is approximately (A) _____ above the level of the the superior border of the symphysis pubis, and the ischial tuberosity is about (B) _____ below.

13. An imaginary plane that divides the pelvic region into the greater and lesser pelvis is called the

    _____ .

14. List the alternate terms for the greater and lesser pelvis:

    A. Greater pelvis _____   B. Lesser pelvis _____

15. List the major function of the (A) the greater pelvis and (B) the lesser pelvis:

    A. Greater pelvis _____   B. Lesser pelvis _____

16. List the three aspects of the lesser pelvis, which also describe the birth route during the delivery process.

    A. _____   B. _____   C. _____

17. Match the following structures or characteristics to the correct hip bone:

    _____ 1. Possesses a large tuberosity found at the most inferior aspect of the pelvis   A. Ilium

    _____ 2. Lesser sciatic notch   B. Ischium

    _____ 3. Ala   C. Pubis

    _____ 4. Posterior superior iliac spine (PSIS)

    _____ 5. Possesses a slightly movable joint

    _____ 6. Anterior superior iliac spine (ASIS)

18. In the past, which radiographic examination was performed to measure the fetal head in comparison with the maternal pelvis to predict possible birthing problems?_____

19. Which other imaging modality has replaced the procedure listed in the previous question?

    _____

20. Indicate whether the following radiographic characteristics apply to a male or female in relation to an AP projection of the pelvis:

    _____ 1. Wide, more flared ilia   M. Male

    _____ 2. Pubic arch angle of 110°   F. Female

    _____ 3. A heart-shaped inlet

    _____ 4. Narrow ilia that are less flared

    _____ 5. Pubic arch angle of 75°

    _____ 6. A larger and more round-shaped inlet

21. List the joint classification, mobility type, and movement type for the joints of the pelvis. (Write *N/A* [not applicable] if the mobility or movement type does not apply.)

	CLASSIFICATION	MOBILITY TYPE	MOVEMENT
A. Hip	_____	_____	_____
B. Sacroiliac	_____	_____	_____
C. Symphysis pubis	_____	_____	_____
D. Acetabulum (union)	_____	_____	_____

22.   Identify the structures labeled on Figs. 7-1 and 7-2. Where indicated, use the following abbreviations to identify
with which bone of the pelvis each labeled part is associated: *IL*, ilium; *IS*, ischium; *P*, pubis.

	STRUCTURE	BONE
A.	_____	____
B.	_____	____
C.	_____	
D.	_____	____
E.	_____	____
F.	_____	
G.	_____	____
H.	_____	
I.	_____	
J.	_____	____
K.	_____	____
L.	_____	
M.	_____	
N.	_____	
O.	_____	____
P.	_____	____
Q.	_____	____
R.	_____	
S.	_____	
T.	_____	____
U.	_____	____
V.	_____	
W.	_____	____
X.	_____	____
Y.	_____	____
Z.	_____	____

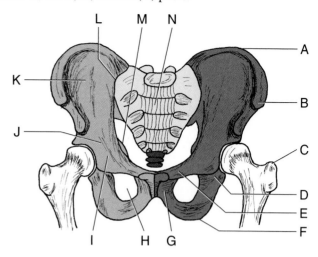

Fig. 7-1. Frontal view, pelvis.

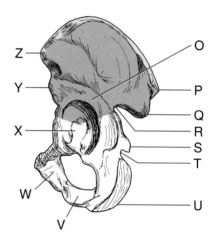

Fig. 7-2. Lateral view, pelvis.

PART II: Radiographic Positioning

REVIEW EXERCISE B: Positioning of the Hips, Pelvis, and Sacroiliac Joints (see textbook pp. 255-272)

1. Which two bony landmarks need to be palpated for hip localization?

   A. _____   B. _____

2. From the midpoint of the imaginary line created by the two landmarks identified in the previous question, where

   would the femoral neck be located? _____

3. A second method for locating the femoral head is to palpate the _____ and go _____

   inches/cm medial at the level of the _____ , which is _____
   inches/cm distal to the original palpation point.

4. To achieve a true AP position of the proximal femur, the lower limb must be rotated _____° internally.

5. Visualization of which structures on an AP pelvis or hip radiograph indicate whether the proximal head and neck
   are in position for a true AP projection?

   _____

6. Which physical sign may indicate that a patient has a hip fracture? _____

   _____

7. Which projection should be taken first and reviewed by a radiologist before attempting to rotate the hip into a lateral position (if trauma is suspected)?

   _____

8. Gonadal shielding should be used for all patients of reproductive age, unless _____

   _____

9. Should a gonadal shield be used for a hip study on a young female? _____ (yes or no). If *yes*, describe how it
   should be placed on the patient.

   _____

10. Should a gonadal shield be used for a hip study on a young male? _____ (yes or no). If *yes*, describe how it should
    be placed on the patient.

    _____

11. What is the advantage of using 90 kVp rather than 80 kVp range for hip and pelvis studies on younger patients?

    _____

12. What is the disadvantage of using 90 kVp for hip and pelvis studies, especially on older patients with some bone
    mass loss?

    _____

13. Which one of the following conditions is a common clinical indication for performing pelvic and hip examinations on a pediatric (newborn) patient?

   A. Osteoporosis C. Ankylosing spondylitis

   B. DDH D. Osteoarthritis

14. True/False: Geriatric patients are more prone to hip fractures because of their increased incidence of osteoporosis.

15. Which one of the following imaging modalities can be used on a newborn to assess hip joint stability during movement of the lower limbs?

   A. Sonography C. Magnetic resonance imaging

   B. Computed tomography D. Nuclear medicine

16. Which one of the following imaging modalities is most sensitive in diagnosing early signs of metastatic carcinoma of the pelvis?

   A. Sonography C. Magnetic resonance imaging

   B. Computed tomography D. Nuclear medicine

17. Match the following pathologic indications to the correct definition (use each choice only once):

   _____ A. A degenerative joint disease

   _____ B. Most common fracture in older patients because of high incidence of osteoporosis or avascular necrosis

   _____ C. A malignant tumor of the cartilage

   _____ D. A disease producing extensive calcification of the longitudinal ligament of the spinal column

   _____ E. A fracture resulting from a severe blow to one side of side of the pelvis

   _____ F. Malignancy spread to bone via the circulatory and lymphatic systems or direct invasion

   _____ G. Now referred to as *developmental dysplasia of the hip*

   1. Metastatic carcinoma

   2. Ankylosing spondylitis

   3. Congenital dislocation of hip

   4. Chondrosarcoma

   5. Proximal hip fracture

   6. Pelvic ring fracture

   7. Osteoarthritis

18. Where is the central ray placed for an AP pelvis projection? _____

19. Which ionization chambers should be activated when using automatic exposure control (AEC) for an AP pelvis projection?

   A. Center chamber only C. Center and upper left or right chambers

   B. Upper right and left chambers D. Upper left chamber only

20. Which specific positioning error is present when the left iliac wing is elongated on an AP pelvis radiograph?

   _____

21. Which specific positioning error is present when the left obturator foramen is more open than the right side?

   _____

22. Indicate whether the following projections are used for patients with traumatic injuries or nontraumatic injuries:

_____ A. Danelius-Miller projection   T.   Traumatic

_____ B. Unilateral frog-leg   NT.   Not traumatic

_____ C. Modified Cleaves (bilateral frog-leg)

_____ D. Clements-Nakayama

_____ E. Anterior pelvic bones

23. When gonadal shielding is *not* used, which gender (male or female) receives a greater gonadal dose with an AP

pelvis projection? _____

24. How many degrees are the femurs abducted (from the vertical plane) for the bilateral frog-leg projection?

_____

25. Where is the central ray placed for a unilateral frog-leg projection? _____

26. Which cassette size should be used for an adult bilateral frog-leg projection? _____

27. Where is the central ray placed for an AP bilateral frog-leg projection? _____

28. Which central ray angle is required for the "outlet" projection (Taylor method) for a female patient?

    A. 15° to 25° caudad   C. 20° to 35° cephalad

    B. 30° to 45° cephalad   D. None. Central ray is perpendicular.

29. Which type of pathologic feature is best demonstrated with the Judet method?

    A. Acetabular fractures   C. Proximal femur fractures

    B. Anterior pelvic bone fractures   D. Femoral neck fractures

30. How much obliquity of the body is required for the Judet method?

    A. None. Central ray is perpendicular   C. 30°

    B. 20°   D. 45°

31. True/False: Any orthopedic device or appliance of the hip should be seen in its entirety on an AP hip radiograph.

32. The axiolateral inferosuperior projection is designed for _____ (traumatic or nontraumatic) situations.

33. How is the unaffected leg positioned for the axiolateral hip projection? _____

_____

34. Which one of the following factors does **not** apply to an axiolateral projection of the hip?

    A. Cassette parallel to femoral neck   C. Use of gonadal shielding

    B. 80 to 90 kVp   D. Use of a stationary grid

35. True/False: An AP pelvis projection using 90 kVp and 8 mAs results in a patient dose of approximately 30% less than a projection using 80 kVp and 12 mAs (for both males and females).

36. True/False: During an axiolateral (inferosuperior) projection of the hip, a male patient receives more than 20 times the gonadal dose than a female.

37. The Clements-Nakayama method requires the CR to be angled _____° posteriorly from horizontal.

38. Which special projection of the hip demonstrates the **anterior** and posterior rims of the acetabulum and the ilioischial and iliopubic columns? (Include the proper name method.)

   A. _____

   B. Which central ray angle (if any) is used for this projection? _____

39. What is the name of a special AP axial projection of the pelvis used to assess trauma to pubic and ischial structures?

   (Include the proper name method.) _____.

40. Which SI joint is best demonstrated with the left posterior oblique (LPO) position (right or left)? _____

41. Does an anterior oblique projection demonstrate the downside or upside SI joint? _____

42. Which type of central ray angle is required for an AP projection of the SI joints? _____

43. Match the following projections with their corresponding proper name (use each choice only once):

   ____ 1. Axiolateral (inferosuperior)   A. Judet

   ____ 2. Modified axiolateral   B. Taylor

   ____ 3. Bilateral or unilateral frog-leg   C. Clements-Nakayama

   ____ 4. Modified frog-leg with affected side in contact with table top   D. Danelius-Miller

   ____ 5. AP axial for pelvic "outlet" bones   E. Modified Lauenstein and Hickey

   ____ 6. Posterior oblique for acetabulum   F. Modified Cleaves

44. True/False: The gonadal dose for female patients for posterior oblique projections of the SI joints is similar (±5 mrad) to the dose for anterior oblique projections of the SI joints.

REVIEW EXERCISE C: Problem Solving for Technical and Positioning Errors (see textbook pp. 261-271)

1. A radiograph of an AP pelvis projection reveals that the lesser trochanters are readily demonstrated on the medial side of the proximal femurs. The patient is ambulatory and has a history of general chronic pain in the hip regions. Which positioning modification needs to be made to prevent this positioning error?

   _____

   _____

2. A radiograph of an AP pelvis reveals that the right iliac wing is foreshortened as compared with the left side. Which specific positioning error has been made?

_____

3. A radiograph of a lateral frog-leg projection reveals that the greater trochanter is superimposed over the femoral neck. Based on the AP hip projection, the radiologist suspects a nondisplaced fracture of the femoral neck. What can the technologist do to better define this region?

_____

_____

4. A radiograph of an axiolateral (inferosuperior) projection reveals that the posterior aspect of the acetabulum and femoral head were cut off of the bottom of the image. The emergency room physician requests that the position be repeated. What can be done to avoid this problem on the repeat exposure?

_____

_____

5. A radiograph of an AP axial projection for anterior pelvic bones reveals that the pubic and ischial bones are not elongated sufficiently. The following factors were used for this study: 86 kVp, 7 mAs, Bucky, 20° to 30° central ray cephalad angle, and 40-inch (102-cm) source-image distance (SID). The female patient was placed in a supine position on the table. What must be changed to improve the quality of the image during the repeat exposure?

_____

_____

6. Bilateral oblique radiographs of the SI joints reveal that the right joint is open but the left one is not. The left iliac wing slightly overlaps the region of the left SI joint. The right posterior oblique (RPO) and LPO positions were performed. Which positioning error led to this radiographic outcome?

_____

_____

7. A radiograph of an AP pelvis reveals that overall the image is light and underexposed (underpenetrated). The following factors were used: 80 kVp, 40-inch (102-cm) SID, Bucky, and AEC with the center chamber activated. Which one of these factors should be changed to produce a darker and more diagnostic image?

_____

_____

8. A radiograph from a modified axiolateral projection reveals excessive grid lines on the image, which also appears underexposed. What can be done to avoid this problem during the repeat exposure?

_____

_____

9. **Situation:** A portable AP and lateral hip study is ordered for a patient who is in recovery after a hip replacement surgery. The radiograph of the AP hip reveals that the upper portion of the acetabular prosthesis is slightly cut off but is included on the lateral projection. Should the technologist repeat the AP projection? Why?

_____

_____

10. **Situation:** A patient with hip pain from a fall enters the emergency room. The physician orders a left hip study. When moved to the radiographic table, the patient complained loudly about the pain in the left hip. Which positioning routine should be used for this patient?

    _____

    _____

11. **Situation:** A patient has just been moved to his hospital room after a bilateral hip replacement surgery. The surgeon has ordered a postoperative hip routine for both hips. Which specific positioning routine should be used? (The patient can be brought to the radiology department.)

    _____

    _____

12. **Situation:** A patient with a possible pelvic ring fracture from a trauma enters the emergency room. The AP pelvis projection, which was taken to determine whether the right acetabulum is fractured, is inconclusive. Which other projection can be taken to better visualize the acetabulum?

    _____

    _____

REVIEW EXERCISE D: Critique Radiographs of the Proximal Femur and Pelvis (see textbook p. 272)

The following questions relate to the radiographs found at the end of Chapter 7 of the textbook. Evaluate these radiographs for positioning accuracy as well as exposure factors, collimation, and correct use of anatomical markers. Describe the corrections needed to improve the overall image. The major, or "repeatable," errors are specific errors that indicate the need for a repeat exposure, regardless of the nature of the other errors. Answers to each critique are given at the end of the laboratory activity.

A. **AP pelvis (83-year-old) (Fig. C7-76)**
    Description of possible error:

    1. Structures shown: _____

    2. Part positioning: _____

    3. Collimation and central ray: _____

    4. Exposure criteria: _____

    5. Markers: _____

    Repeatable error(s): _____

B. **Unilateral frog-leg (84-year-old) (Fig. C7-77)**
    Description of possible error:

    1. Structures shown: _____

    2. Part positioning: _____

    3. Collimation and central ray: _____

    4. Exposure criteria: _____

    5. Markers: _____

    Repeatable error(s): _____

C. **AP pelvis (57-year-old) (Fig. C7-78)**
   Description of possible error:

   1. Structures shown: _____

   2. Part positioning: _____

   3. Collimation and central ray: _____

   4. Exposure criteria: _____

   5. Markers: _____

   Repeatable error(s): _____

D. **Bilateral frog-leg (2-year-old) (Fig. C7-79)**
   Description of possible error:

   1. Structures shown: _____

   2. Part positioning: _____

   3. Collimation and central ray: _____

   4. Exposure criteria: _____

   5. Markers: _____

   Repeatable error(s): _____

PART III: Laboratory Exercises (see textbook pp. 261-271)

You must gain experience in positioning each part of the proximal femur and pelvis before performing the following exams on actual patients. You can get experience in positioning and radiographic evaluation of these projections by performing exercises using radiographic phantoms and practicing positioning on other students (although you will not be taking actual exposures).

The following suggested activities assume that your teaching institution has an energized lab and radiographic phantoms. If not, perform Laboratory Exercises B and C, the radiographic evaluation and the physical positioning exercises. (Check off each step and projection as you complete it.)

LABORATORY EXERCISE A: Energized Laboratory

1. Using the pelvic radiographic phantom, produce radiographs of the following basic routines:

   _____ AP pelvis

   _____ AP axial, SI joints

   _____ Posterior or anterior oblique for SI joints

   _____ Anterior oblique for acetabulum, Teufel method

   _____ AP axial, Taylor method

LABORATORY EXERCISE B: Radiographic Evaluation

1. Evaluate and critique the radiographs produced during the previous experiments, additional radiographs provided by your instructor, or both. Evaluate each radiograph for the following points. (Check off when completed.):

    _____ Evaluate the completeness of the study. (Are all of the pertinent anatomic structures included on the radiograph?)

    _____ Evaluate for positioning or centering errors (e.g., rotation, off centering).

    _____ Evaluate for correct exposure factors and possible motion. (Are the density and contrast of the images acceptable?)

    _____ Determine whether markers and an acceptable degree of collimation and/or area shielding are visible on the images.

LABORATORY EXERCISE C: Physical Positioning

On another person, simulate performing all basic and special projections of the proximal femur and pelvic girdle as follows. (Check off each when completed satisfactorily.) Include the following six steps as described in the textbook.

Step 1. Appropriate size and type of film holder with correct markers
Step 2. Correct central ray placement and centering of part to central ray and/or film
Step 3. Accurate collimation
Step 4. Area shielding of patient where advisable
Step 5. Use of proper immobilizing devices when needed
Step 6. Approximate correct exposure factors, breathing instructions when applicable, and "making" exposure

Projections	Step 1	Step 2	Step 3	Step 4	Step 5	Step 6
• AP pelvis	_____	_____	_____	_____	_____	_____
• AP hip, unilateral	_____	_____	_____	_____	_____	_____
• Unilateral frog-leg	_____	_____	_____	_____	_____	_____
• Bilateral frog-leg	_____	_____	_____	_____	_____	_____
• Axiolateral (inferosuperior)	_____	_____	_____	_____	_____	_____
• Modified axiolateral	_____	_____	_____	_____	_____	_____
• Anterior oblique for acetabulum	_____	_____	_____	_____	_____	_____
• AP axial for anterior pelvic bones	_____	_____	_____	_____	_____	_____
• AP axial for SI joints	_____	_____	_____	_____	_____	_____
• Posterior obliques, SI joints	_____	_____	_____	_____	_____	_____
• Anterior obliques, SI joints	_____	_____	_____	_____	_____	_____

ANSWERS TO REVIEW QUESTIONS

Review Exercise A: Anatomy of Hips and Pelvis

1. Femur
2. Fovea capitis
3. Medial, posteriorly
4. 15 to 20
5. True
   A. Right and left hip bones, sacrum and coccyx
   B. Right and left hip bones
   C. Ossa coxae and/or innominate bones
6. A. Ilium
   B. Ischium
   C. Pubis
7. Acetabulum, mid teens
8. A. Crest of ilium (iliac crest)
   B. Anterior superior iliac spine (ASIS)
9. Ischial tuberosity
10. Symphysis pubis
11. Obturator foramen
12. A. 1 inch (2½ cm)
    B. 1½ to 2 inches (4 to 5 cm)
13. Brim
14. A. False pelvis
    B. True pelvis
15. A. Supports the lower abdominal organs and fetus
    B. Forms the actual birth canal
16. A. Inlet
    B. Cavity
    C. Outlet
17. 1. B
    2. B
    3. A
    4. A
    5. C
    6. A
18. Cephalopelvimetry
19. Sonography (ultrasound)
20. 1. F
    2. F
    3. M
    4. M
    5. M
    6. F
21. A. Synovial, diarthrodial, spheroidal
    B. Synovial, amphiarthrodial, N/A
    C. Cartilaginous, amphiarthrodial, N/A
    D. Cartilaginous, amphiarthrodial, N/A
22. A. Crest, IL
    B. ASIS, IL
    C. Greater trochanter
    D. Body, IS
    E. Superior ramus, P
    F. Ischial tuberosity, IS
    G. Inferior ramus, P

H. Obturator foramen
I. Body, P
J. Body, IL
K. Wing (ala), IL
L. Right sacroiliac (SI) joint
M. Ischial spine, IS
N. Sacrum
O. Body, IL
P. Posterior superior iliac spine (PSIS), IL
Q. Posterior inferior iliac spine, IL
R. Greater sciatic notch, IL
S. Ischial spine, IS
T. Lesser sciatic notch, IS
U. Ischial tuberosity, IS
V. Ramus, IS
W. Inferior ramus, P
X. Acetabulum, IS, IL, P
Y. Anterior inferior iliac spine, IL
Z. ASIS, IL

Review Exercise B: Positioning of Hips, Pelvis, and Sacroiliac Joints

1. A. ASIS
   B. Symphysis pubis
2. Approximately 2½ inches (6 to 7 cm) below the midpoint of the line
3. ASIS, 1 to 2 inches (3 to 5 cm), symphysis pubis and greater trochanter, 3 to 4 inches (8 to 10 cm)
4. 15 to 20
5. Lesser trochanter should not be visible, or should only be slightly visible, on the radiograph.
6. The patient's foot is rotated externally.
7. AP pelvis
8. It covers anatomic structures of primary interest.
9. Yes. Use a shaped ovarian shield with top of shield at level of ASIS and bottom at symphysis pubis.
10. Yes. The top of the shield should be placed at the inferior margin of the symphysis pubis.
11. It reduces patient dose by about 30%.
12. It reduces radiographic contrast.
13. B. DDH (Development dysphasia of hip)
14. True
15. A. Sonography
16. D. Nuclear medicine
17. A. 7
    B. 5
    C. 4
    D. 2
    E. 6
    F. 1

G. 3
18. Midway between ASIS and symphysis pubis
19. B (upper right and left chambers)
20. Rotation toward left side
21. Right rotation
22. A. T
    B. NT
    C. NT
    D. T
    E. T
23. Female (nearly 3 times more)
24. 40° to 45°
25. Midfemoral neck
26. 35 × 43 cm (14 × 17 inches) crosswise
27. 1 inches (2½ cm) superior to the symphysis pubis
28. B. 30° to 45° cephalad
29. A. Acetabular fractures
30. D. 45°
31. True
32. Traumatic
33. It is flexed and elevated to prevent it from being superimposed over the affected hip.
34. C (use of gonadal shielding)
35. True
36. True
37. 15 to 20
38. A. Posterior oblique projection of acetabulum (Judet method)
    B. 0°(perpendicular)
39. AP axial outlet projection (Taylor method)
40. Right
41. Downside
42. 30° to 35° cephalad
43. 1. D
    2. C
    3. F
    4. E
    5. B
    6. A
44. True

Review Exercise C: Problem-Solving for Technical and Positioning Errors

1. Rotate the lower limbs 15° to 20° internally to place the proximal femurs into a true AP position. (With general chronic pain, the lower limbs can usually be rotated safely.)
2. The patient is rotated toward the left—left posterior oblique (LPO).
3. Repeat the exposure using a 20° to 25° cephalad central ray angle. (It will separate the greater trochanter from the femoral neck.)

4. If possible, elevate the patient at least 2 inches or 5 cm by placing sheets or blankets beneath the pelvis.

5. A larger central ray angle is required. Female patients require a central ray angle of 30° to 45°.

6. The right posterior oblique (RPO) position was performed with too much obliquity. The obliques must be no more than 30° of rotation.

7. When using automatic exposure control (AEC) for an AP pelvis projection, both the center and left or right ionization chambers must be activated. The center chamber is over the less dense pelvic cavity, which may lead to an underexposed image.

8. Ensure that the central ray is centered to near the midline of the grid cassette and the face of the cassette is perpendicular to the central ray.

9. Yes. Any orthopedic appliance or prosthesis must be seen in its entirety in both projections.

10. AP pelvis and axiolateral left hip. The AP pelvis radiograph should be taken initially without leg rotation; the radiograph must be reviewed by the physician and checked for fractures or dislocations before attempting an internal rotation of the left leg for the axiolateral (inferosuperior) projection.

11. AP pelvis and modified axiolateral—Clements-Nakayama method

12. Posterior oblique—Judet method

Review Exercise D: Critique Radiographs of the Proximal Femur and Pelvis

A. AP pelvis (83-year-old) (Fig. C7-76)
   1. Both hands of patient superimposed over hips obscuring hip detail; watch on left wrist
   2. Slight rotation **toward the right** with left side of pelvis elevated; no internal rotation of legs (which is acceptable in this case because of evidence of right hip fracture)
   3. No evidence of collimation (but only slight collimation should be visible for this projection); pelvis slightly off center to the left and centered a little high
   4. Acceptable exposure factors
   5. Anatomic side marker present (but a better placement would be to the mid lateral margin away from the hip region)
      Repeatable error(s): criteria 1

B. Unilateral frog-leg (84-year-old) (Fig. C7-77)
   1. Distal part of orthopedic prosthesis cut off—needs to be seen in its entirety
   2. Correct part positioning
   3. Excellent collimation; correct centering but a larger cassette is required
   4. Acceptable exposure factors
   5. Anatomic side marker cut off
      Repeatable error(s): criteria 1

C. AP pelvis (57-year-old) (Fig. C7-78)
   1. Superior iliac wings cut off (but this may be acceptable if patient history indicates hip region is area of interest)
   2. Rotation of pelvis toward the right (and note the elongation of the right ilium); to viewer's right, film

incorrectly placed for viewing; lesser trochanters visible and femoral necks severely foreshortened, indicating the legs were not rotated internally for a true AP projection
   3. Acceptable collimation; central ray centering/film placement too high (which cut off upper iliac wings)
   4. Acceptable exposure factors
   5. Anatomic side marker present (but better placement would have been higher up under patient ID blocker, away from hip region)
      NOTE: Radiograph is incorrectly placed for viewing and should be flipped right to left.
      Repeatable error(s): criteria 1 and 2

D. Bilateral frog-leg (2-year-old) (Fig. C7-79)
   1. Left hip (assuming that this is the left side because the side marker is not visible) obscured by artifact (superimposition of patient's hand)
   2. Tilted pelvis (and note that the gonadal shield placement is useless for either males *or* females—a serious error for a small child)
   3. No visible collimation, which should be visible for this pediatric patient; central ray centering/film placement too high for pelvis centering but acceptable for bilateral hip projection
   4. Very low contrast (may have been caused by not using a grid)
   5. No visible anatomic side marker
      Repeatable error(s): criteria 1

SELF-TEST

My Score = _____%

This self-test should be taken only after completing all of the readings, review exercises, and laboratory activities for a particular section. The purpose of this test is not only to provide a good learning exercise but also to serve as a strong indicator of what your final evaluation grade for this chapter will cover. It is strongly suggested that if you do not get at least a 90% to 95% grade on each self-test, you should review those areas in which you missed questions before going to your instructor for the final evaluation exam. There are 85 questions or blanks—each is worth 1.2 points.)

1. List the four bones of the pelvis:

   A. _____   C. _____

   B. _____   D. _____

2. List the three divisions of the hip bone:

   A. _____   B. _____   C. _____

3. *Innominate bone* is another name for:

   A. One half of pelvic girdle   C. Ossa coxae

   B. Hip bone   D. All of the above

4. What is the largest foramen in the body? _____

5. Which one of the following landmarks is **not** a palpable bony landmark?

   A. Greater trochanter   C. Ischial tuberosity

   B. Lesser trochanter   D. Anterior superior iliac spine (ASIS)

6. What are the two aspects of the ischium?

   A. _____   B. _____

7. What is the name of the imaginary plane that separates the greater from the lesser pelvis?

   _____

8. Match the following structures or characteristics to the correct division of the pelvis:

   _____ 1. True pelvis   A. Greater pelvis

   _____ 2. Supports the lower abdominal organs B. Lesser pelvis

   _____ 3. Formed primarily by the ala of the ilium

   _____ 4. Cavity

   _____ 5. False pelvis

   _____ 6. Forms the actual birth canal

   _____ 7. Found below the pelvic brim

9. What is the name of the outdated radiographic procedure that measures the fetal head and dimensions of the maternal pelvis? _____

10. Identify the labeled structures found on the following radiographs.

Fig. 7-3:

A. _____

B. _____

C. _____

D. _____

E. _____

F. _____

G. _____

H. _____

I. _____

J. Is this a male or female pelvis? _____

Fig. 7-4:

K. _____

L. _____

M. _____

N. _____

O. Which projection of the hip is represented on

   this radiograph? _____

Fig. 7-5

P. _____

Q. _____

R. _____

S. _____

T. _____

U. _____

V. _____

W. Which projection of the hips is represented

   on this radiograph? _____

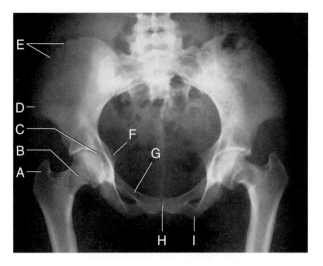

Fig. 7-3. AP pelvis radiograph.

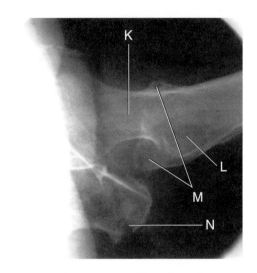

Fig. 7-4. Lateral hip radiograph.

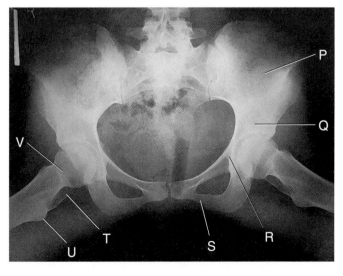

Fig. 7-5. Bilateral hip radiograph.

11.   Indicate whether the following characteristics are those of a male or female pelvis:

_____   1.   Heart-shaped inlet   F.   Female

_____   2.   Acute pubic arch (less than 90°)   M.   Male

_____   3.   More flared iliac wings

_____   4.   Obtuse pubic arch (greater than 90°)

_____   5.   Larger and more rounded inlet

_____   6.   Less flared iliac wings

12.   Which one of the following structures is considered to be the most posterior?

A.   Ischial spines   C.   Symphysis pubis

B.   ASIS   D.   Acetabulum

13.   The small depression near the center of the femoral head where a ligament is attached is called the

_____ .

14.   A geriatric patient with an externally rotated lower limb may have:

A.   A normal hip joint   C.   Fractured proximal femur

B.   Osteoarthritis   D.   Slipped capital femoral epiphyses (SCFE)

15.   Which one of the following pathologic indications may result in the early fusion of the sacroiliac (SI) joints?

A.   Chondrosarcoma   C.   Developmental dysplasia of the hip

B.   Metastatic carcinoma   D.   Ankylosing spondylitis

16.   Match the following radiographic appearances with the following pathologic indications (use each choice only once):

_____   1.   Usually, consists of numerous, small lytic lesions   A.   Pelvic ring fracture

_____   2.   Increased hip joint space and misalignment   B.   DDH

_____   3.   Bilateral radiolucent lines across bones and   C.   Osteoarthritis
                misalignment of SI joints

_____   4.   Early fusion of SI joints and "bamboo spine"   D.   SCFE

_____   5.   Epiphyses appears shorter and epiphyseal plate wider   E.   Ankylosing spondylitis

_____   6.   Hallmark sign of spurring and narrowing of joint space   F.   Metastatic carcinoma

17.   Which one of the following radiographic signs indicates whether the proximal femurs are in position for a true AP projection?

A.   Appearance of the greater trochanter in profile

B.   Limited view of fovea capitis

C.   Limited view of the lesser trochanter in profile

D.   Symmetric appearance of iliac wings

18. The gonadal dose for an average-size male with a routine axiolateral (inferosuperior) lateral trauma hip projection

    is in the _____ mrad range.

    A. 50 to 100   C. 10 to 50

    B. 200 to 500   D. 600 to 800

19. True/False: The female gonadal dose for an AP pelvis is in the 50 to 100 mrad range, which is about 3 times greater than the dose for a male when no gonadal shields are used.

20. Which one of the following projections/methods is often used to evaluate a pediatric patient for congenital hip dislocation?

    A. Bilateral frog-leg   C. Taylor method

    B. Clements-Nakayama   D. Judet

21. What type of central ray angle is required when using the Taylor method for a female patient?

    A. None. Central ray is perpendicular.   C. 20° to 25° cephalad

    B. 10° to 15° caudad   D. 30° to 45° cephalad

22. True/False: The modified Cleaves method is designed for nontraumatic hip projections.

23. True/False: Centering for the AP pelvis projection is 1 inch, or 21/2 cm, superior to the symphysis pubis.

24. True/False: The Clements-Nakayama method is considered a nontraumatic lateral hip projection.

25. Which position of the pelvic girdle is designed to demonstrate the acetabulum? _____

26. Which one of the following projections/methods is used to evaluate the pelvic inlet for possible fracture?

    A. Danelius-Miller   C. Taylor method

    B. AP axial projection   D. Clements-Nakayama

27. Where is the central ray centered for posterior oblique projections of the SI joints?

    _____

28. Does the AP axial projection for SI joints of a male generally require more or less central ray angle than the same

    projection for a female? _____

29. Does a right anterior oblique (RAO) position for SI joints demonstrate the right or left SI joints?

    _____

30. **Situation:** An initial AP pelvis radiograph reveals possible fractures involving the lower pelvis. The emergency room physician asks for another projection to better demonstrate this area of the pelvis. The patient is traumatized and must remain in a supine position. Which projection should be taken?

    _____

31.   A radiograph of an axiolateral (inferosuperior) projection of a hip demonstrates a soft tissue density that is visible across the affected hip and acetabulum. This artifact is obscuring the image of the proximal femur. What is the most likely cause of the artifact, and how can it be prevented from showing up on the repeat exposure?

_____

_____

32.   **Situation:** An SI study is ordered for a patient with severe pelvic pain. Because the table is so hard and the patient has lower pelvic discomfort, the patient refuses to lie on the back. Which positioning routine should the technologist use? (Include central ray angle and direction if applicable.)

_____

33.   A radiograph of an AP hip reveals that the lesser trochanter is not visible. Should the technologist repeat the projection? (yes or no). If _yes,_ what should be modified to improve the image during the repeat exposure?

_____

_____

34.   **Situation:** A young patient with a clinical history of SCFE comes to the radiology department. Which projection(s) are most often taken for this condition?

_____

_____

35.   A radiograph produced using the Taylor method demonstrates that the anterior pelvic bones of a female patient are foreshortened. The following positioning factors were used: supine position, 40-inch (100-cm) source-image distance (SID), and central ray angled 30° caudad and centered 1 to 2 inches (3 to 5 cm) distal to symphysis pubis. Which one of the following modifications should be made during the repeat exposure?

   A.   Increase central ray angle.   C.   Center central ray at level of ASIS.

   B.   Reverse central ray angle.   D.   Place patient prone on table.

36.   For the following critique questions, refer to the unilateral frog-leg radiograph in Fig. C7-77 on p. 272 in the textbook:

   A.   Which positioning error(s) are visible on this radiograph? More than one answer may be selected.

      (a) All essential anatomic structures are not demonstrated.

      (b) Central ray is centered incorrectly.

      (c) Collimation is not evident.

      (d) Exposure factors are incorrect.

      (e) No anatomic marker is visible on the radiograph.

   B.   Which of the above criteria are considered "repeatable errors?" _____

   C.   Which of the following modifications must be made during the repeat exposure? More than one answer may be selected.

      (a) Increase collimation.

      (b) Center central ray to femoral neck.

      (c) Decrease exposure factors.

      (d) Increase exposure factors.

      (e) Reposition anatomic marker on image receptor (IR) before exposure.

      (f) Use larger IR.

37. For the following critique questions, refer to the AP pelvis radiograph in Fig. C7-78 on p. 272 in the textbook.

    A. Which positioning error(s) are visible on this radiograph? More than one answer may be selected.

        (a) All essential anatomic structures are not demonstrated.

        (b) Central ray is centered incorrectly.

        (c) Collimation is not evident.

        (d) Exposure factors are incorrect.

        (e) No anatomic marker is visible on the radiograph.

        (f) Slight rotation toward the right is evident.

        (g) Slight rotation is evident.

        (h) Proximal femurs are not placed in a true AP position.

    B. Which of the previous criteria are considered "repeatable errors?"_____

    C. Which of the following modifications must be made during the repeat exposure? More than one answer may be selected.

        (a) Increase collimation.

        (b) Center central ray correctly.

        (c) Decrease exposure factors.

        (d) Increase exposure factors.

        (e) Place anatomic marker on IR before exposure.

        (f) Rotate body slightly toward the left.

        (g) Rotate body slightly toward the right.

        (h) Rotate proximal femurs 15° to 20° internally.

CHAPTER 8

Cervical and Thoracic Spine

After you have completed **all** the activities of this chapter, you will be able to:

_____ 1. Identify specific anatomic structures of the cervical and thoracic spine using drawings and radiographs.

_____ 2. Identify specific features of the cervical and thoracic vertebrae that distinguish them from other aspects of the vertebral column.

_____ 3. Identify the location, angulation, classification, and type of movement for specific joints of the cervical and thoracic spine.

_____ 4. List additional terms for the first, second, and seventh cervical vertebrae.

_____ 5. Identify topographic landmarks that can be palpated to locate specific thoracic and cervical vertebrae.

_____ 6. Match specific pathologic indications of the cervical and thoracic spine to the correct definition.

_____ 7. Identify which radiographic projection and/or procedure best demonstrates specific pathologic indications.

_____ 8. Identify structures that are best demonstrated with each position of the cervical and thoracic spine.

_____ 9. List the patient dose ranges, including thyroid and female breast doses, for specific projections of the cervical and thoracic spine.

_____ 10. Identify basic and special projections of the cervical and thoracic spine and list the correct size and type of image receptor (IR) and the central ray location, direction, and angulation for each position.

_____ 11. Given various hypothetical situations, identify the correct modification of a position and/or exposure factors to improve the radiographic image.

_____ 12. Given radiographs of specific cervical and thoracic spine projections, identify positioning and exposure factors errors.

POSITIONING AND FILM CRITIQUE

_____ 1. Using a peer, position for basic and special projections of the cervical and thoracic spine.

_____ 2. Using appropriate radiographic phantoms, produce satisfactory radiographs of specific positions (if equipment is available).

_____ 3. Critique and evaluate cervical and thoracic spine radiographs based on the four divisions of radiographic criteria: (1) structures shown, (2) position, (3) collimation and central ray, and (4) exposure criteria.

_____ 4. Distinguish between acceptable and unacceptable spine radiographs based on exposure factors, motion, collimation, positioning, or other errors

Learning Exercises

Complete the following review exercises after reading the associated pages in the textbook as indicated by each exercise. Answers to each review exercise are given at the end of the exercises.

PART I: Radiographic Anatomy

REVIEW EXERCISE A: Radiographic Anatomy of the Cervical and Thoracic Spine (see textbook pp. 274-284)

1. List the number of bones found in each division in the **adult** vertebral column:

   A. Cervical _____   D. Sacrum _____

   B. Thoracic _____   E. Coccyx _____

   C. Lumbar _____   F. Total _____

   Refer to Fig. 8-1 to answer questions 2 through 4.

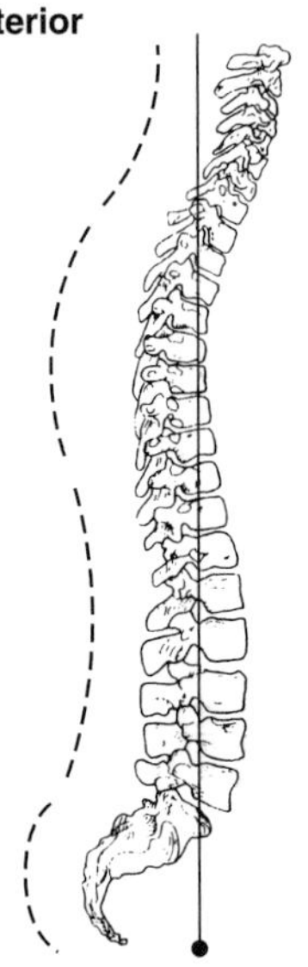

2. List the two **primary** or **posterior convex** curves seen in the vertebral column:

   A. _____

   B. _____

3. Indicate which two portions of the vertebral column are classified as **secondary** or **compensatory** curves:

   A. _____

   B. _____

4. Match the correct aspect(s) of the vertebral column with the following characteristics (may be more than one answer):

   _____ 1. Convex curve (with respect to posterior)   A. Cervical spine

   _____ 2. Concave curve (with respect to posterior)   B. Thoracic spine

   _____ 3. Secondary curve   C. Lumbar spine

   _____ 4. Primary curve   D. Sacrum

   _____ 5. Develops as child learns to hold head erect

5. An abnormal, or exaggerated, "sway back" lumbar curvature is called _____.

6. An abnormal lateral curvature seen in the thoracolumbar spine is called _____.

7. The two main parts of a typical vertebra are the _____ and the _____.

8. The _____ are two bony aspects of the vertebral arch that extend posteriorly from each pedicle to join at the midline.

9. The _____ foramina are created by two small notches on the superior and inferior aspects of the pedicles.

Posterior   **Anterior**

Centerline of gravity

Fig. 8-1. Lateral view, spinal column.

10. The opening, or passageway, for the spinal cord is the _____.

11. The spinal cord begins with the (A) _____ of the brain and extends down to the

    (B) _____ vertebra, where it tapers and ends. This tapered ending is called the

    (C) _____ .

12. Which structures pass through the intervertebral foramina? _____

13. Identify the following structures labeled on these drawings of typical thoracic vertebrae (Fig. 8-2):

Superior view

A. _____

B. _____

C. _____

D. _____

E. _____

F. _____

Lateral view

G. _____

H. _____

I. _____

J. _____

K. _____

Lateral oblique view

L. _____

M. _____

N. _____

O. _____

P. _____

Q. The joints between the ribs and vertebrae at *N* are called:

   _____

R. The joints between the ribs and vertebrae at *P* are called:

   _____

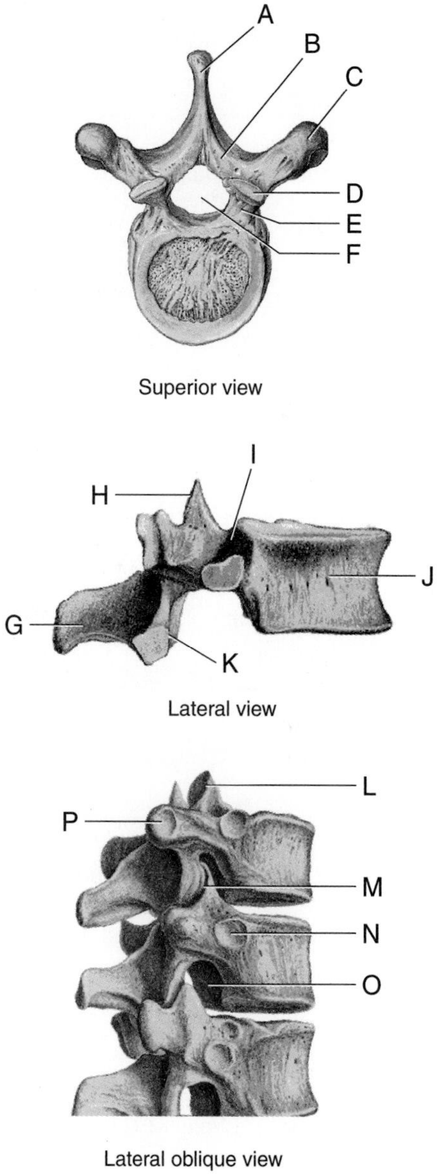

Superior view

Lateral view

Lateral oblique view

Fig. 8-2. Typical thoracic vertebra.

14. Which one of the following joints is found between the superior and inferior articular processes?

    A. Intervertebral joints   C. Zygapophyseal joints

    B. Articular joints   D. Intervertebral facets

15. True/False: Only T1, T11, and T12 have **full** facets for articulation with ribs.

16. True/False: The zygapophyseal joints of **all** cervical vertebrae are visualized only in a true lateral position.

17. List the outer and inner aspects of the intervertebral disk:

    A. Outer aspect _____   B. Inner aspect _____

18. The condition involving a "slipped disk" is correctly referred to as _____

    _____ .

19. List the additional names for the following cervical vertebrae:

    A. C1 _____

    B. C2 _____

    C. C7 _____

20. List three features that make the cervical vertebrae unique:

    A. _____   B. _____

    C. _____

21. A short column of bone found between the superior and articular processes in a typical cervical vertebra is called

    _____ .

22. What is the term for the same structure, identified in the previous question, for the C1 vertebra?

    _____

23. The zygapophyseal joints for the second through seventh cervical vertebrae are at a (A) _____° angle to the mid-

    sagittal plane; the thoracic vertebrae are at a (B) _____° angle to the midsagittal plane.

24. What is the name of the joint found between the superior articular processes of C1 and the occipital condyles of the

    skull? _____

25. The modified body of C2 is called the _____ or _____ .

26. A lack of symmetry of the zygapophyseal joints between C1 and C2 may be caused by injury or may be associated

    with _____ .

27. List the unique feature of all thoracic vertebrae that distinguishes them from other vertebrae:

    _____ .

28. Which specific thoracic vertebrae are classified as typical thoracic vertebrae (i.e., they least resemble cervical or

    lumbar vertebrae)? _____ .

29. Identify the labeled structures on the radiographs of the cervical spine in Figs. 8-3 and 8-4. (Indicate the specific structure and the vertebra of which it is a part.)

STRUCTURE   VERTEBRA

A. _____   _____

B. _____   _____

C. _____   _____

D. _____   _____

E. _____   _____

F. _____   _____

G. _____   _____

H. _____   _____

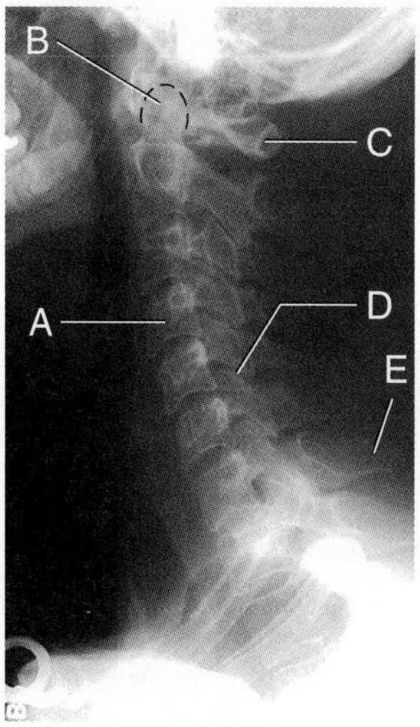

Fig. 8-3. Lateral view, cervical spine.

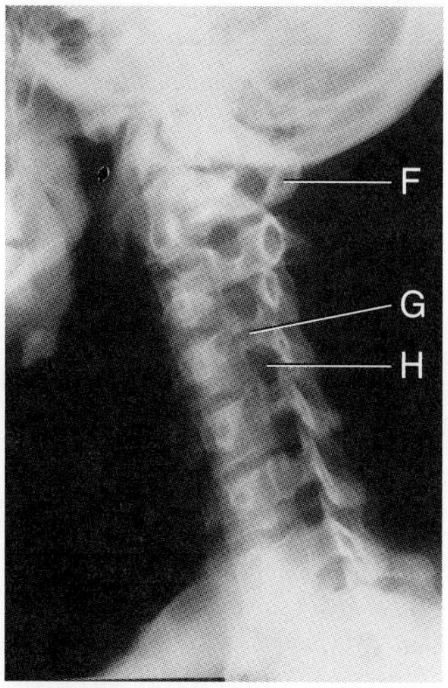

Fig. 8-4. 45-degree oblique view, cervical spine.

30. For the central ray to pass through and "open" the intervertebral spaces on a 45° posterior oblique projection of the

cervical vertebrae, which central ray angle (if any) would be required? _____

PART II: Radiographic Positioning

REVIEW EXERCISE B: Positioning of the Cervical and Thoracic Spine (see textbook pp. 286-304)

1. Name the following parts of the sternum and the associated topographic landmarks where indicated:

    A. Upper portion of sternum: _____

    B. Superior margin of this upper section (landmark): _____

    C. Main center portion of sternum: _____

    D. Joint between top and center portions (landmark): _____

    E. Most inferior aspect of sternum (landmark): _____

2. Match the following topographic landmarks to the correct vertebral level (use each choice only once):

    _____ 1. Gonion   A. T1

    _____ 2. Xiphoid process (tip)   B. T2-3

    _____ 3. Thyroid cartilage   C. C1

    _____ 4. Jugular notch   D. T4-5

    _____ 5. Sternal angle   E. T10

    _____ 6. Mastoid tip   F. C4-6

    _____ 7. Vertebra prominens   G. T7

    _____ 8. 3 to 4 inches (8 to 10 cm) below jugular notch H. C3

3. In addition to the gonads, which other radiosensitive organs are of greatest concern during cervical and thoracic spine radiography?

_____

4. List the two advantages of using higher kilovoltage peak exposure factors for spine radiography, especially on an anteroposterior (AP) thoracic spine radiograph:

   A. _____   B. _____

5. True/False: When using digital imaging for spine radiography, it is important to use close collimation, grids, and lead masking.

6. True/False: If close collimation is used during conventional radiography of the spine, the use of lead masking is generally not required.

7. True/False: To a certain degree, magnetic resonance imaging (MRI) and computed tomography (CT) are replacing myelography as the imaging modalities of choice for the diagnosis of a ruptured intervertebral disk.

8. True/False: Nuclear medicine is often performed to diagnose bone tumors of the spine.

9. To ensure that the intervertebral joint spaces are open for lateral thoracic spine projections, it is important to:

   A. Keep the vertebral column parallel to the image receptor (IR)
   B. Use a small focal spot
   C. Use a breathing technique
   D. Angle the central ray cephalad

10. For lateral and oblique projections of the cervical spine, it is important to minimize magnification and maximize detail by doing what? (More than one answer may be used):

   A. Keeping vertebral column parallel to film holder
   B. Using a small focal spot
   C. Increasing source-image receptor distance (SID)
   D. Using a breathing technique

11. Match the following pathologic indication of the spine to the correct definition (use each choice only once):

   ____ A. Fracture through the pedicles and anterior arch of C2
   ____ B. Inflammation of the vertebrae
   ____ C. Abnormal or exaggerated convex curvature of the thoracic spine
   ____ D. Comminuted fracture of the vertebral body with posterior fragments displaced into the spinal canal
   ____ E. Avulsion fracture of the spinous process of C7
   ____ F. Abnormal lateral curvature of the spine
   ____ G. A form of rheumatoid arthritis
   ____ H. Impact fracture from axial loading of the anterior and posterior arch of C1
   ____ I. Mild form of scoliosis and kyphosis developing during adolescence
   ____ J. Produces the "bow tie" sign

   1. Ankylosing spondylitis
   2. Clay shoveler's fracture
   3. Unilateral subluxation
   4. Kyphosis
   5. Scheuermann's disease
   6. Scoliosis
   7. Jefferson fracture
   8. Teardrop burst fracture
   9. Hangman's fracture
   10. Spondylitis

12. List the conventional radiographic examination/projections performed for the following pathologic indications:

    A. Scoliosis: _____

    B. Teardrop burst fracture: _____

    C. Jefferson fracture: _____

    D. Scheuermann's disease: _____

    E. Unilateral subluxation of cervical spine: _____

    F. HNP: _____

13. Which two landmarks must be aligned for an AP "open mouth" projection? _____

14. What is the purpose of the 15° to 20° angle for the AP axial projection of the cervical spine?

    _____

15. For an AP axial of the C spine, a plane through the tip of the mandible and _____ should be parallel to the angled central ray.

    A. Mastoid process   C. Base of skull

    B. Gonion   D. External auditory meatus (EAM)

16. What are two important benefits of a SID longer than 40 to 44 inches (100 to 112 cm) for the lateral cervical spine projection?

    A. _____   B. _____

17. What central ray angulation must be used with a posterior oblique projection of the cervical spine?

    _____

18. Which foramina are demonstrated with a left posterior oblique (LPO) position of the cervical spine?

    _____

19. Which foramina are demonstrated with a left anterior oblique (LAO) position of the cervical spine?

    _____

20. In addition to extending the chin, which additional positioning technique can be performed to ensure that the mandible is not superimposed over the upper cervical vertebrae for the oblique projections?

    _____

21. What is the recommended SID for a lateral projection of the cervical spine?

    _____

22. The lateral projection of the cervical spine should be taken during _____ (inspiration, expiration, or suspended respiration). Why?

    _____

23. Which specific projection must be taken first if trauma to the cervical spine is suspected and the patient is in a

    supine position on a backboard?_____

24. The proper name of the method for performing the cervicothoracic (swimmer's lateral) projection is the

_____ .

25. Where should the central ray be placed for a cervicothoracic (swimmer's lateral) projection?

_____

26. Which region of the spine must be demonstrated with a cervicothoracic (swimmer's lateral) projection?

_____

27. Which one of the following projections is considered a "functional study" of the cervical spine?

   A. AP "wagging jaw" projection   C. Fuchs or Judd method

   B. AP "open mouth" position   D. Hyperextension and flexion lateral positions

28. When should the Judd or Fuchs method be performed?

_____

29. Which AP projection of the cervical spine demonstrates the entire **upper** cervical spine with one single projection?

_____

30. Which two things can be done to produce equal density along the entire thoracic spine for the AP projection (especially for a patient with a thick chest)?_____

_____

31. What is the purpose of using a breathing technique for a lateral projection of the thoracic spine?

_____

32. Which zygapophyseal joints are demonstrated in a right anterior oblique (RAO) projection of the thoracic spine?

_____

33. Which one of the following projections provides the greatest skin dose for the patient?

   A. AP thoracic spine projection   C. Swimmer's lateral projection

   B. Lateral cervical spine projection   D. Fuchs or Judd method

34. Which of the following results in the lowest midline and skin doses for the patient? (Note dose relationship to milliamperage seconds.)

   A. AP thoracic spine at 90 kVp, 7 mAs   C. Lateral thoracic spine at 80 kVp, 50 mAs

   B. AP thoracic spine at 80 kVp, 12 mAs   D. Oblique thoracic spine at 80 kVp, 20 mAs

35. True/False: The thyroid dose used during a posterior oblique cervical spine projection is more than 10 times greater than the dose used for an anterior oblique projection of the cervical spine.

36. Which one of the following structures is best demonstrated with an AP axial vertebral arch projection?

   A. Spinous processes of lumbar spine   C. Zygapophyseal joints of thoracic spine

   B. Articular pillar (lateral masses) of cervical spine   D. Cervicothoracic spine region

37. What central ray angle must be used with the AP axial—vertebral arch projection?

    A. 15° to 20° cephalad   C. 20° to 30° caudad

    B. 5° to 10° cephalad   D. None. Central ray is perpendicular to IR.

REVIEW EXERCISE C: Problem Solving for Technical and Positioning Errors (see textbook pp. 286-304)

1. A radiograph of an AP "open mouth" projection of the cervical spine reveals that the base of the skull is superimposed over the upper dens. Which **specific** positioning error is present on this radiograph?

    _____

2. A radiograph of an AP axial projection of the cervical spine reveals that the intervertebral disk spaces are not open. The following positioning factors were used: extension of the skull, central ray angled 10° cephalad, central ray centered to the thyroid cartilage, and no rotation or tilt of the spine. Which of these factors need to be modified to produce a more diagnostic image?

    _____

3. A radiograph of an right posterior oblique (RPO) cervical spine projection reveals that the lower intervertebral foramina are *not* open. The upper intervertebral foramina are well visualized. What positioning error most likely led to this radiographic outcome?

    _____

4. A radiograph on a lateral projection of the cervical spine reveals that C7 is not clearly visible. The following factors were used: erect position, 44-inch (112-cm) SID, arms down by the patient's side, and exposure made during inspiration. Which two of these factors should be changed to produce a more diagnostic image during the repeat exposure?

    _____

5. A radiograph of an AP "chewing" or "wagging jaw" projection taken at 75 kVp, 20 mAs, and 1/2 second demonstrates that part of the image of the mandible is still visible and obscuring the upper cervical spine. Which modification needs to be made to produce a more diagnostic image during the repeat exposure?

    _____

6. A radiograph of a lateral thoracic spine reveals that lung markings and ribs make it difficult to visualize the vertebral bodies. The following factors were used: recumbent position, 40-inch (102-cm) SID, short exposure time, and exposure made during full expiration. Which one of these factors need to be modified to produce a more diagnostic image during the repeat exposure?

    _____

7. A radiograph of an AP projection of the thoracic spine reveals that the upper thoracic spine is greatly overexposed but the lower vertebrae are well visualized. The head of the patient was placed at the anode end of the table. What can be modified during the repeat exposure to produce a more diagnostic image?

    _____

8. **Situation:** A patient with a possible cervical spine injury enters the emergency room. The patient is on a backboard. Which projection of the cervical spine should be taken first?

    _____

    _____

9. **Situation:** A patient who has been in a motor vehicle accident enters the emergency room. The basic projections of the cervical spine reveal no subluxation (partial dislocation) or fracture. The physician wants the spine evaluated for whiplash injury. Which additional projections would best demonstrate this type of injury?

_____

10. **Situation:** A patient comes to the radiology department for a cervical spine series. An AP "open mouth" radiograph indicates that the base of the skull and lower edge of the front incisors are superimposed, but the top of the dens is not clearly demonstrated. What should the technologist do to demonstrate the upper portion of the dens? (A horizontal beam lateral has ruled out a C-spine fracture or subluxation.)

_____

REVIEW EXERCISE D: Critique Radiographs of the Cervical and Thoracic Spine (see textbook p. 306)

The following questions relate to the radiographs found at the end of Chapter 8 of the textbook. Evaluate these radiographs for the radiographic criteria categories (1 through 5) that follow. Describe the corrections needed to improve the overall image. The major, or "repeatable," errors are specific errors that indicate the need for a repeat exposure, regardless of the nature of the other errors.

A. **AP open mouth (Fig. C8-91)**
    Description of possible error:

1. Structures shown: _____

2. Part positioning: _____

3. Collimation and central ray: _____

4. Exposure criteria: _____

5. Markers: _____

Repeatable error(s): _____

B. **AP open mouth (Fig. C8-92)**
    Description of possible error:

1. Structures shown: _____

2. Part positioning: _____

3. Collimation and central ray: _____

4. Exposure criteria: _____

5. Markers: _____

Repeatable error(s): _____

C. **AP axial projection (Fig. C8-93)**
    Description of possible error:

1. Structures shown: _____

2. Part positioning: _____

3. Collimation and central ray: _____

    4.   Exposure criteria: _____

    5.   Markers: _____

    Repeatable error(s): _____

D.   **Oblique (RPO) (Fig. C8-94)**
     Description of possible error:

    1.   Structures shown: _____

    2.   Part positioning: _____

    3.   Collimation and central ray: _____

    4.   Exposure criteria: _____

    5.   Markers: _____

    Repeatable error(s): _____

E.   **Lateral (trauma) (Fig. C8-95)**
     Description of possible error:

    1.   Structures shown: _____

    2.   Part positioning: _____

    3.   Collimation and central ray: _____

    4.   Exposure criteria: _____

    5.   Markers: _____

    Repeatable error(s): _____

F.   **Lateral (nontrauma) (Fig. C8-96)**
     Description of possible error:

    1.   Structures shown: _____

    2.   Part positioning: _____

    3.   Collimation and central ray: _____

    4.   Exposure criteria: _____

    5.   Markers: _____

    Repeatable error(s): _____

PART III: Laboratory Exercises (see textbook pp. 292-304)

You must gain experience in positioning each part of the cervical and thoracic spine before performing the following exams on actual patients. You can get experience in positioning and radiographic evaluation of these projections by performing exercises using radiographic phantoms and practicing positioning critique on other students (although you will not be taking actual exposures).

The following suggested activities assume that your teaching institution has an energized lab and radiographic phantoms. If not, perform Laboratory Exercises B and C, the radiographic evaluation and the physical positioning exercises. (Check off each step and projection as you complete it.)

LABORATORY EXERCISE A: Energized Laboratory

1. Using the radiographic phantom, produce radiographs of the following basic routines:

    A. AP, lateral, and oblique cervical spine

    B. AP, lateral, and oblique thoracic spine

LABORATORY EXERCISE B: Radiographic Evaluation

1. Evaluate and critique the radiographs produced during the previous experiments, additional radiographs provided by your instructor, or both. Evaluate each radiograph for the following points. (Check off when completed.):

    _____ Evaluate the completeness of the study. (Are all of the pertinent anatomic structures included on the radiograph?)

    _____ Evaluate for positioning or centering errors (e.g., rotation, off centering).

    _____ Evaluate for correct exposure factors and possible motion. (Are the density and contrast of the images acceptable?)

    _____ Determine whether markers and an acceptable degree of collimation and/or area shielding are visible on the images.

LABORATORY EXERCISE C: Physical Positioning

On another person, simulate performing all basic and special projections of the cervical and thoracic spine as follows. (Check off each when completed satisfactorily.) Include the following six steps as described in the textbook.

Step 1. Appropriate size and type of film holder with correct markers
Step 2. Correct central ray placement and centering of part to central ray and/or film
Step 3. Accurate collimation
Step 4. Area shielding of patient where advisable
Step 5. Use of proper immobilizing devices when needed
Step 6. Approximate correct exposure factors, breathing instructions where applicable, and "making" exposure

PROJECTIONS	STEP 1	STEP 2	STEP 3	STEP 4	STEP 5	STEP 6
• Cervical spine series (AP axial, AP C1-2, obliques, lateral)	____	____	____	____	____	____
• Thoracic spine series (AP and lateral)	____	____	____	____	____	____
• Swimmer's lateral	____	____	____	____	____	____
• Hyperextension and flexion laterals	____	____	____	____	____	____
• AP "chewing" or "wagging jaw"	____	____	____	____	____	____
• AP (Fuchs) for dens	____	____	____	____	____	____
• PA (Judd) for dens	____	____	____	____	____	____
• Thoracic spine obliques	____	____	____	____	____	____

ANSWERS TO REVIEW EXERCISES

Review Exercise A: Radiographic Anatomy of the Cervical and Thoracic Spine

1. A. 7
   B. 12
   C. 5
   D. 1
   E. 1
   F. 26
2. A. Thoracic
   B. Sacral
3. A. Cervical
   B. Lumbar
4. 1. B and D
   2. A and C
   3. A and C
   4. B and D
   5. A
5. Lordosis
6. Scoliosis
7. Body, vertebral arch
8. Lamina
9. Intervertebral
10. Vertebral (spinal) canal
11. A. Medulla oblongata
    B. Lower border of L1
    C. Conus medullaris
12. Spinal nerves and blood vessels
13. A. Spinous process
    B. Lamina
    C. Transverse process
    D. Facet of superior articular process
    E. Pedicle
    F. Vertebral foramen
    G. Spinous process
    H. Facet of superior articular process
    I. Pedicle
    J. Body
    K. Inferior articular process
    L. Superior articular process
    M. Zygapophyseal joint
    N. Facet for head of rib articulation
    O. Intervertebral foramen
    P. Facet for rib articulation
    Q. Costovertebral joints
    R. Costotransverse joints
14. C. Zygapophyseal joints
15. True
16. False (between C1 and C2 visualized on a frontal or AP projection)
17. A. Annulus fibrosus
    B. Nucleus pulposus
18. Herniated nucleus pulposus (HNP)
19. A. C1: Atlas
    B. C2: Axis
    C. C7: Vertebra prominens

20. A. Transverse foramina
    B. Bifid spinous process
    C. Overlapping vertebral bodies
21. Articular pillar
22. Lateral mass
23. A. 90
    B. 70 to 75
24. Atlanto-occipital articulation
25. Dens or odontoid process
26. Rotation of the skull
27. Presence of facets for articulation with ribs
28. T5 to T8
29. A. Body, C4
    B. Dens (odontoid), C2
    C. Posterior arch and tubercle, C1
    D. Zygapophyseal joint, C5-6
    E. Spinous process (vertebra prominens), C7
    F. Posterior arch and tubercle, C1
    G. Pedicle, C4
    H. Intervertebral foramen, C4-5
30. 15° to 20° cephalad

Review Exercise B: Positioning of the Cervical and Thoracic Spine

1. A. Manubrium
   B. Jugular (suprasternal) notch
   C. Body
   D. Sternal angle
   E. Xiphoid process
2. 1. H
   2. E
   3. F
   4. B
   5. D
   6. C
   7. A
   8. G
3. Thyroid gland, parathyroid glands, and female breasts
4. A. Increase in exposure latitude
   B. Decrease in patient dose
5. True
6. False (Lead masking should be used even if close collimation is used.)
7. True
8. True
9. A. Keep vertebral column parallel to image receptor (IR)
10. B. Using a small focal spot
    C. Increasing SID
11. A. 9
    B. 10
    C. 4
    D. 8
    E. 2
    F. 6

G. 1
H. 7
I. 5
J. 3
12. A. Erect (AP/PA) and lateral spine including bending laterals
    B. Lateral cervical
    C. AP open mouth C1-2, tomography—following lateral projection
    D. Scoliosis series
    E. Lateral cervical spine
    F. Lateral of affected spine
13. Lower margin of upper incisors and base of skull
14. To open up the intervertebral disk spaces
15. C. Base of skull
16. A. Compensates for increased object-image distance (OID), reduces magnification
    B. Less divergence of x-ray beam to reduce shoulder superimposition of C7
17. 15° to 20° cephalad
18. Right intervertebral foramina (upside)
19. Left intervertebral foramina (downside)
20. Rotate the skull into a near lateral position
21. 60 to 72 inches (150 to 180 cm)
22. Expiration, for maximum shoulder depression
23. Lateral, horizontal beam projection
24. Twining method
25. To T1; 1 inch (2.5 cm) above the jugular notch, or at vertebra prominens
26. C4 to T3
27. D. Hyperextension and flexion lateral positions
28. If unable to demonstrate the upper portion of the dens with the AP "open mouth" projection
29. AP "wagging jaw" projection (Ottonello method)
30. Correct use of anode-heel effect; use of wedge filter
31. To blur out rib and lung markings that obscure detail of thoracic vertebrae
32. Right (downside)
33. C. Swimmer's lateral projection
34. A. At 90 kVp, 7mAs
35. True; anterior oblique ≈5 mrad Posterior oblique ≈69 mrad
36. B. Articular pillar (lateral masses)
37. C. 20° to 30° caudad

Review Exercise C: Problem-Solving for Technical and Positioning Errors

1. Excessive extension of the skull
2. Increase central ray angulation to 15° to 20°.
3. The shoulders are incorrectly rotated. They need to be rotated 45°.
4. Initiate exposure during suspended expiration and increase SID to 72 inches (183 cm).
5. Reduce milliamperage and increase exposure time to produce more blurring of the mandible
6. Use of a breathing technique to blur lung markings and ribs more effectively
7. Utilize a wedge filter with thicker part of filter placed over the upper thoracic spine to equalize the density along the thoracic spine
8. Lateral, horizontal beam lateral
9. Hyperextension and flexion lateral positions
10. Perform either the Fuchs or Judd method.

Review Exercise D: Critique Radiographs of the Cervical and Thoracic Spine

A. AP open mouth (Fig. C8-91)
   1. Upper aspect of dens obscured by base of skull
   2. Overextension of skull causing superimposition of base of skull over dens
   3. Collimation too loose, resulting in excessive exposure to face, eyes and neck region; correct central ray and IR placement
   4. Acceptable exposure factors
   5. No evidence of anatomic side marker
      Repeatable error(s): criteria 1 and 2
B. AP open mouth (Fig. C8-92)
   1. Upper aspect of dens and joint space obscured by front incisors
   2. Overflexion of skull causing superimposition of front incisors over top of dens
   3. Collimation too loose, resulting in excessive exposure to face, eyes, and neck region; slightly low central ray and IR
   4. Acceptable exposure factors
   5. No evidence of anatomic side marker
      Repeatable error(s): criteria 1 and 2
C. AP axial projection (Fig. C8-93)
   1. Distorted vertebral bodies and intervertebral joint spaces; base of skull superimposed over upper cervical spine
   2. Overextension of skull and/or excessive central ray cephalic angle, which probably led to poor definition of vertebral bodies and joint spaces
   3. Evidence of collimation; slightly low central ray centering but correct IR placement
   4. Acceptable exposure factors
   5. Evidence of anatomic side marker
      Repeatable error(s): criteria 1 and 2
      NOTE: Unsure of the origin of the artifact seen on lower, left cervical spine region
D. Oblique (RPO) (Fig. C8-94)
   1. Intervertebral joint spaces and foramina not clearly demonstrated; superimposition of mandible over upper cervical spine
   2. Appears that body is underrotated from AP position (with appearance of upper rib cage suggesting underrotation rather than overrotation), an error that led to narrowing and obscuring of the intervertebral foramina; can place the skull into lateral position to remove mandible from the upper C-spine (department option)
   3. No evidence of collimation; insufficient or incorrect central ray angulation (and foreshortened cervical spine)—may have led to closure of disk spaces
   4. Acceptable exposure factors
   5. No evidence of anatomic side marker
      Repeatable error(s): criteria 1, 2, and 3
E. Lateral (trauma) (Fig. C8-95)
   1. Aspect of C1 and dens cut off; C7-T1 not demonstrated
   2. Need to depress shoulders (because chin cannot be adjusted as a result of the trauma)
   3. No evidence of collimation except along anterior, upper margin; central ray centered too posteriorly, causing upper cervical spine to be cut off; IR placement centered too low
   4. Acceptable exposure factors (poor contrast resulting from using a nongrid technique)
   5. No evidence of anatomic side marker
      Repeatable error(s): criteria 1, 2, and 3
F. Lateral (nontrauma) (Fig. C8-96)
   1. Only six cervical demonstrated vertebrae; slight superimposition of posterior aspect of mandible over anterior arch of C1
   2. Need to depress shoulders more to demonstrate C7-T1; need to extend chin further
   3. Evidence of collimation (but it could be tighter); correct central ray centering and IR placement
   4. Radiography slightly underexposed (difficult to evaluate in this printed version).
   5. No evidence of anatomic side marker
      Repeatable errors: criteria 1 and 2

SELF-TEST

My Score = _____%

This self-test should be taken only after completing all of the readings, review exercises, and laboratory activities for a particular section. The purpose of this test is not only to provide a good learning exercise but also to serve as a strong indicator of what your final evaluation grade will cover. It is strongly suggested that if you do not get at least a 90% to 95% grade on each self-test, you should review those areas in which you missed questions before going to your instructor for the final evaluation exam for this chapter. (There are 110 questions or blanks—each is worth 0.9 points.)

1. At which vertebral level does the solid spinal cord terminate? _____

2. How many segments make up the sacrum in the neonate? _____

3. Which of the following divisions of the spine is described as possessing a primary curve? (There may be more than one correct answer.)

    A. Thoracic   B. Lumbar   C. Cervical   D. Sacral

4. True/False: The lumbar possesses a concave posterior spinal curvature.

5. An abnormal or exaggerated thoracic curvature with increased convexity is called _____.

6. An abnormal or exaggerated lateral curvature is called _____.

7. What is the correct term for the condition involving a "slipped disk?" _____

8. Which foramina are created by the superior and inferior vertebral notches? _____

9. Which joints are found between the superior and inferior articular processes? _____

10. Which one of the following structures makes up the inner aspect of the intervertebral disk?

    A. Annulus fibrosus   B. Annulus pulposus   C. Nucleus pulposus   D. Nucleus fibrosus

11. True/False: The carotid artery and certain nerves pass through the cervical transverse foramina.

12. True/False: The thoracic spine possesses facets for rib articulations and bifid spinous processes.

13. The intervertebral foramina for the cervical spine lie at a _____ ° angle to the midsagittal plane.

14. Which ligament holds the dens against the anterior arch of C1? _____

15. The large joint space between C1 and C2 is the called the _____.

16. Two partial facets found on the thoracic vertebrae are called _____.

17. Which of the following thoracic vertebrae do **not** possess a facet for the costotransverse joint? (There may be more than one correct answer.)

    A. T1   B. T7   C. T11   D. T12

18. What are two distinctive features of all cervical vertebrae that make them different from any other vertebrae?

    A. _____   B. _____

19. What is the one feature of all thoracic vertebrae that makes them different from all other vertebrae?

    _____

20. Which position of the thoracic spine best demonstrates the intervertebral foramina?

_____

21. Identify the following structures labeled on Figs. 8-5, 8-6, and 8-7.
    Include the specific vertebra of which it is a part where indicated:

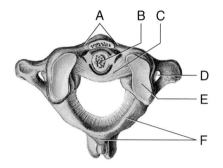

Fig. 8-5. Superior view.

	STRUCTURE	*VERTEBRA*

Fig. 8-5

A. _____   _____

B. _____   _____

C. _____   _____

D. _____   _____

E. _____   _____

F. _____   _____

Fig. 8-6

G. _____   _____

H. _____   _____

I. _____   _____

J. _____   _____

K. _____   _____

L. _____   _____

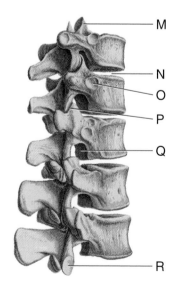

Fig. 8-6. Posterolateral view, cervical spine.

Fig. 8-7

M. _____   _____

N. _____   _____

O. _____   _____

P. _____   _____

Q. _____   _____

R. _____   _____

S. Which vertebrae are represented by this drawing?

_____

T. How can these specific vertebrae be identified?

_____

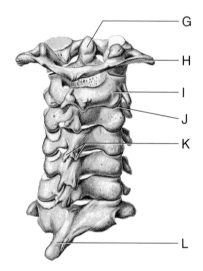

Fig. 8-7. Lateral view.

22. Identify the following structures and vertebrae labeled on this AP "open mouth" cervical spine radiograph (Fig. 8-8):

	STRUCTURE	VERTEBRA
A.	_____	_____
B.	_____	_____
C.	_____	_____
D.	_____	_____
E.	_____	_____
F.	_____	_____
G.	_____	_____

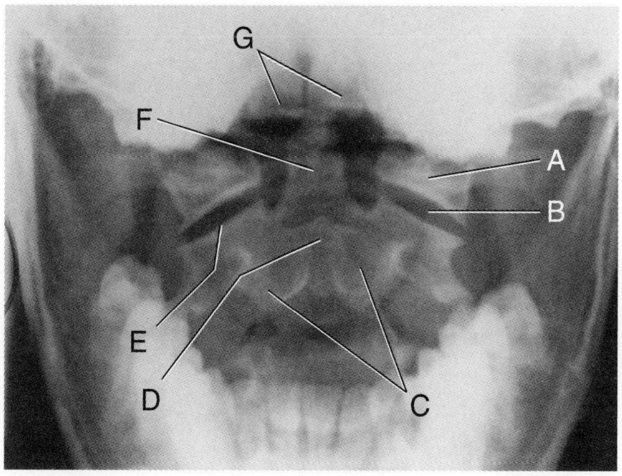

Fig. 8-8. AP "open mouth" cervical spine radiograph.

23. Which position or projection of the cervical spine best demonstrates the zygapophyseal joints?

_____

24. Which specific joint spaces are visualized with a left anterior oblique (LAO) projection of the thoracic spine?

_____

25. Match the following topographic landmarks to the correct vertebral level (use each choice only once):

_____ 1. Vertebra prominens	A. T2-3
_____ 2. Jugular notch	B. T1
_____ 3. 3 to 4 inches (8 to 10 cm) below jugular notch	C. T7
_____ 4. Gonion	D. C3
_____ 5. Sternal angle	E. C4-5
_____ 6. Thyroid cartilage	F. T4-5

26. Which of the following imaging modalities is not normally performed to rule out a herniated nucleus pulposus (HNP)?

A. Computed tomography (CT)   C. Magnetic resonance imaging (MRI)

B. Myelography   D. Nuclear medicine

27. An avulsion fracture of the spinous processes of C6 is called a:

A. Hangman's fracture   C. Jefferson fracture

B. Clay shoveler's fracture   D. Teardrop burst fracture

28. Scheuermann's disease is a form of:

A. Scoliosis and/or kyphosis   C. Arthritis

B. Subluxation   D. Fracture

29. True/False: HNP most frequently develops at the L2-3 vertebral level.

30. Which two things can be done to minimize the effects of scatter radiation on lateral projections of the thoracic and lumbar spine?

    A. _____   B. _____

31. Which position or projection best demonstrates the zygapophyseal joints between C1 and C2? _____

32. How much and in which direction (caudad or cephalad) should the central ray be angled for:

    A. An AP axial projection of the cervical spine? _____

    B. An anterior oblique projection of the cervical spine? _____

    C. A posterior oblique projection of the cervical spine? _____

33. Which one of the following projections of the cervical spine demonstrates the left intervertebral foramen?

    A. Left posterior oblique (LPO)   C. Lateral projection

    B. LAO   D. Right anterior oblique (RAO)

34. In addition to using a long source-image distance (SID), list the two positioning maneuvers you can use to lower the shoulders enough to visualize the C7 for a lateral projection of the cervical spine.

    A. _____   B. _____

35. Which position or projection demonstrates the lower cervical and upper thoracic spine (C4 to T3) in a lateral perspective?

    _____

36. List the two positions or projections that will project the dens in the center of the foramen magnum.

    A. _____   B. _____

37. A lateral cervical spine radiograph demonstrates that the zygapophyseal joint spaces are not superimposed. Which type of positioning error(s) may lead to this radiographic outcome?

    _____

38. A radiograph of a lateral thoracic spine projection reveals that the intervertebral foramina and intervertebral joint spaces are not clearly demonstrated. Which type of problems can lead to this radiographic outcome?

    _____

39. **Situation:** A patient who was involved in a motor vehicle accident 3 days ago is experiencing severe neck pain and comes to the radiology department for a cervical spine series. The patient is not wearing a cervical collar. Should the technologist take a horizontal beam lateral radiograph and have it cleared before proceeding with the study?

    _____

40. **Situation:** A patient with a possible Jefferson fracture enters the emergency room. Which specific radiographic position best demonstrates this type of fracture?

_____

41. What dose range would be received by the breasts of a slightly larger-than-average female during a lateral thoracic spine projection taken at 80 kVp and 50 mAs with proper collimation?

   A. 300 to 500 mrad   C. 100 to 200 mrad

   B. 1 to 50 mrad   D. No detectable contribution (NDC)

42. The breast dose used for a posterior oblique thoracic spine projection is approximately _____ that used for an anterior oblique projection.

   A. The same as   C. 2 times greater than

   B. One half   D. 4 times greater than

43. What skin dose range would be received by an average-size male patient during a lateral thoracic spine projection?

   A. 300 to 400 mrad   C. 1 to 2 rad

   B. 10 to 50 mrad   D. 900 to 1000 mrad

44. Compare the thyroid dose used during a posterior oblique cervical spine projection with that used during an anterior oblique projection.

   A. No significant difference   C. 10 to 15 times greater

   B. 4 times greater   D. About one quarter the amount

45. For the following critique questions, refer to the AP open mouth radiograph in Fig. C8-91 on p. 306 in the textbook.

   A. Which positioning error(s) are visible on this radiograph? More than one answer may be selected.

      (a) All essential anatomic structures are not demonstrated.

      (b) Central ray is centered incorrectly.

      (c) Collimation is not evident.

      (d) Exposure factors are incorrect.

      (e) No anatomic marker is visible on the radiograph.

      (f) Excessive extension of the skull is evident.

      (g) Excessive flexion of the skull is evident.

   B. Which of the previous criteria are considered "repeatable errors?" _____

   C. Which of the following modifications must be made during the repeat exposure? More than one answer may be selected.

      (a) Increase collimation.

      (b) Center central ray to femoral neck.

      (c) Decrease exposure factors.

      (d) Increase exposure factors.

      (e) Reposition anatomic marker on IR before exposure.

      (f) Increase skull flexion.

      (g) Increase skull extension.

46. For the following critique questions, refer to the AP axial cervical spine radiograph in Fig. C8-93 in the textbook.

   A. Which positioning error(s) are visible on this radiograph? More than one answer may be selected.

      (a) All essential anatomic structures are not demonstrated.

      (b) Central ray is centered incorrectly.

      (c) Central ray is angled incorrectly.

      (d) Collimation is not evident.

      (e) Exposure factors are incorrect.

      (f) No anatomic marker is visible on the radiograph.

      (g) Excessive extension of skull is evident.

      (h) Excessive flexion of skull is evident.

   B. Which of the above criteria are considered as "repeatable errors?" _____

   C. Which of the following modifications must be made during the repeat exposure? (more than one answer may be selected)

      (a) Increase collimation.

      (b) Increase central ray cephalic angulation.

      (c) Decrease central ray cephalic angulation.

      (d) Increase skull flexion.

      (e) Increase skull extension.

      (f) Place anatomic marker on IR before exposure.

CHAPTER 9

Lumbar Spine, Sacrum, and Coccyx

CHAPTER OBJECTIVES

After you have completed **all** the activities in this chapter, you will be able to:

_____ 1. Identify specific anatomic structures of the lumbar spine, sacrum, and coccyx on drawings and radiographs.

_____ 2. Identify the anatomic structures that make up the "Scotty dog" sign.

_____ 3. Identify the classification and type of movement of the joints found in the lumbar spine.

_____ 4. List topographic landmarks that can be palpated to locate specific aspects of the lumbar spine, sacrum, and coccyx.

_____ 5. Define specific types of pathologic features of the spine as described in the textbook.

_____ 6. Identify radiographic appearances related to these specific types of pathologic spine features.

_____ 7. Identify basic and special projections of the lumbar spine, sacrum, and coccyx, including the correct size and type of image receptor (IR), central ray location, direction, and angulation of the central ray for each projection.

_____ 8. Identify which structures are best seen with specific projections of the lumbar spine.

_____ 9. List the patient dose ranges for skin, midline, and gonadal doses for specific spine projections.

_____ 10. Identify the approximate difference in patient doses between anteroposterior (AP) compared with posteroanterior (PA) projections and anterior compared with posterior oblique positions of the lumbar spine.

_____ 11. Given various hypothetical situations, identify the correct modification of a position and/or exposure factors to improve the radiographic image.

_____ 12. Given radiographs of specific lumbosacral spine projections or positions, identify positioning and exposure factors errors.

POSITIONING AND FILM CRITIQUE

_____ 1. Using a peer, position for basic and special projections of the lumbosacral spine.

_____ 2. Using a lumbar spine radiographic phantom, produce satisfactory radiographs of specific positions (if equipment is available).

_____ 3. Critique and evaluate lumbar spine radiographs based on the four divisions of radiographic criteria: (1) structures shown, (2) position, (3) collimation and central ray, and (4) exposure criteria.

_____ 4. Distinguish between acceptable and unacceptable lumbosacral spine radiographs based on exposure factors, motion, collimation, positioning, or other errors.

Learning Exercises

Complete the following review exercises after careful study of the associated pages in the textbook as indicated by each exercise.

After completing each of these individual exercises, check your answers with the answer sheets that follow before continuing to the next exercise.

PART I: Radiographic Anatomy

REVIEW EXERCISE A: Anatomy of the Lumbar Spine, Sacrum, and Coccyx (see textbook pp. 308-313)

1. A portion of the lamina located between the **superior and inferior** articular processes is called the

    _____ .

2. The superior and inferior vertebral notches join together to form the:

    A. Vertebral foramen   C. Pedicle

    B. Intervertebral foramina   D. Lamina

3. Which radiographic position best demonstrates the structure identified in the previous question?

    _____ .

4. Identify the parts of a typical lumbar vertebra as labeled on Fig. 9-1:

    A. _____

    B. _____

    C. _____

    D. _____

    E. _____

    F. The central ray projection labeled *F* in this drawing would demonstrate the

       _____

       _____

    G. The central ray projection labeled *G* would demonstrate the

       _____

       _____

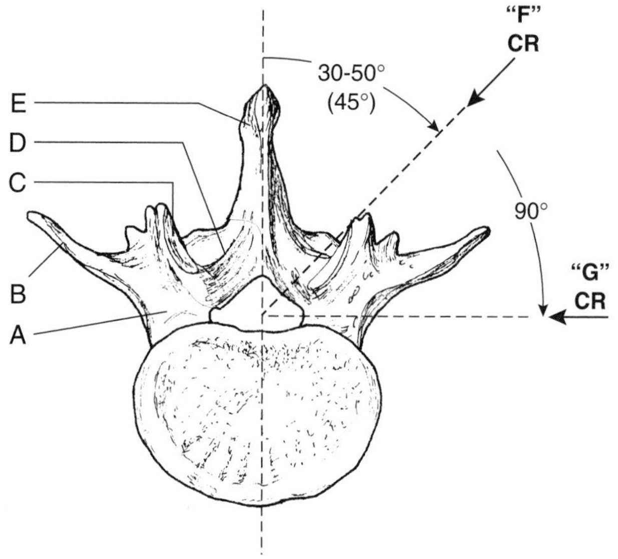

Fig. 9-1. Typical L3 vertebra.

5. Would the degree of angle to demonstrate the structures identified in *F* in the previous question be greater or lesser

    for the lower lumbar vertebrae as compared with the upper? _____ .

6. The small foramina found in the sacrum are called _____ .

7. The anterior and superior aspect of the sacrum that forms the posterior wall of the pelvic inlet is called the

    _____ .

8. What is another term for the sacral horns? _____ .

9. The sacroiliac joints lie at an oblique angle of _____° to the coronal plane.

10. What is the formal term for the "tail bone?" _____.

11. What is the name for the upper broad aspect of the coccyx? _____.

12. List the structure classification and movement classification and type for the following joints of the vertebrae:

	CLASSIFICATION	*MOBILITY TYPE*	*MOVEMENT*
A. Zygapophyseal	_____	_____	_____
B. Intervertebral	_____	_____	_____

13. Identify the following structures labeled on the radiographs of the lumbar spine (Figs. 9-2 through 9-4):

A. _____

B. _____

C. _____

D. _____

E. _____

F. _____

G. _____

H. _____

I. _____

J. _____

K. _____

Fig. 9-2. Anteroposterior.   **Fig. 9-3.** Lateral.

Parts of "Scotty dog" image, which should be visible on an oblique lumbar spine (Figs. 9-4 and 9-5):

L. _____

M. _____

N. _____

O. _____

P. _____

Q. _____

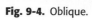

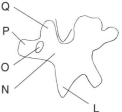

Fig. 9-4. Oblique.   **Fig. 9-5.** "Scotty dog."

14. List which specific zygapophyseal joint or intervertebral foramen is demonstrated with the following lumbar spine positions:

    A. Left posterior oblique (LPO): _____.

    B. Right anterior oblique (RAO): _____.

    C. Lateral: _____.

    D. Right posterior oblique (RPO): _____.

    E. Left anterior oblique (LAO): _____.

15. The degree of obliquity required for an oblique projection at the T12/L1 level is approximately

    _____, whereas the L5/S1 level spine requires a _____ oblique.

    Therefore, a _____ oblique is performed for the general lumbar spine.

PART II: Radiographic Positioning

REVIEW EXERCISE B: Topographic Landmarks and Positioning of Lumbar Spine, Sacrum, and Coccyx (see textbook pp. 314-332)

1. Match the following topographical landmarks to the correct vertebral level (use each choice only once):

    _____ 1. ASIS   A. L2-3

    _____ 2. Xiphoid process   B. L4-5

    _____ 3. Lower costal margin   C. S1-2

    _____ 4. Iliac crest   D. Tip of coccyx

    _____ 5. Symphysis pubis   E. T9-10

2. True/False: The use of higher kilovoltage peak (kVp) and lower milliamperage seconds (mAs) for lumbar spine radiography improves radiographic contrast but increases patient dose.

3. True/False: Placing a lead blocker mat behind the patient for lateral lumbar spine positions improves image quality.

4. True/False: Gonadal shielding should always be used for male and female patients for studies of the lumbar spine, sacrum, and coccyx.

5. True/False: The anteroposterior (AP) projection of the lumbar spine opens the intervertebral joint spaces better than the posteroanterior (PA) projection.

6. True/False: The knees and hips should be extended for an AP projection of the lumbar spine.

7. True/False: An increased source-image distance (SID) of 44 or 46 inches (112 to 117 cm) is advantageous for AP and lateral projections of the lumbar spine.

8. True/False: The use of lead blocker mat and close collimation must not be used when performing digital imaging of the lumbar spine.

9. Select the imaging modality that best demonstrates the following pathologic feature or condition (answers may be used more than once):

   _____ A.   Osteoporosis   1.   Magnetic resonance imaging (MRI)

   _____ B.   Soft tissues of lumbar spine   2.   Computed tomography (CT)

   _____ C.   Structures within subarachnoid space   3.   Myelography

   _____ D.   Inflammatory conditions such as Paget's disease 4.   Bone densitometry

   _____ E.   Compression fractures of the lumbar spine   5.   Nuclear medicine

10. Match the following pathologic indications to the correct definition or statement (use each choice only once):

    _____ A.   Lateral curvature of the vertebral column   1.   Spina bifida

    _____ B.   Fracture of the vertebral body caused by   2.   Herniated nucleus
               hyperflexion force   pulposus (HNP)

    _____ C.   Congenital defect in which the posterior   3.   Chance fracture
               elements of the vertebrae fail to unite

    _____ D.   Most common at the L4-5 level and   4.   Spondylolisthesis
               may result in sciatica

    _____ E.   Forward displacement of one vertebra   5.   Compression fracture
               onto another vertebra

    _____ F.   Inflammatory condition that is most   6.   Spondylolysis
               common in males in their 30s

    _____ G.   Dissolution and separation of the pars interarticularis   7.   Ankylosing spondylitis

    _____ H.   A type of fracture that rarely causes neurologic deficits   8.   Scoliosis

11. With a 35 × 43 cm (14 × 17 inches) image receptor (IR), the central ray is centered at the level of the

    _____ for AP and lateral lumbar spine projections.

12. Which two structures can be evaluated to determine whether rotation is present on a radiograph of an AP projection of the lumbar spine?

    A. _____   B. _____

13. How much obliquity is required to properly visualize the zygapophyseal joints at the L5-S1 level?

    _____.

14. Which specific set of zygapophyseal joints are demonstrated with an LAO position?

    _____.

15. The _____, which is the eye of the "Scotty dog," should be near the center of the vertebral body on a correctly obliqued lumbar spine.

16. Which positioning error has been committed if the structures in the previous question are projected too far posterior with a 45° oblique position of the lumbar spine? _____.

17. Which position or projection of the lumbar spine series best demonstrates a possible compression fracture?

    _____.

18. A patient with a wide pelvis and narrow thorax may require a central ray angle of _____°

    _____ (caudad or cephalad) for a lateral position of the lumbar spine.

19. How should the spine of a patient with scoliosis be positioned for a lateral position of the lumbar spine?

    _____.

20. Why should the knees and hips be flexed for an AP lumbar spine projection?

    _____.

21. True/False: The female ovarian dose used for a PA lumbar spine projection is approximately 30% less than the dose used for an AP projection.

22. Where is the central ray centered for a lateral L5-S1 projection of the lumbar spine? _____

    _____.

23. What type of central ray angulation is required for an AP axial L5-S1 projection on a male patient?

    _____.

24. True/False: A PA or AP projection for a scoliosis series frequently includes one erect and one recumbent position for comparison.

25. True/False: The lower margin of the cassette must include the symphysis pubis for a scoliosis series.

26. True/False: A PA projection for a scoliosis series requires only about one tenth the dose to the breasts as the AP projection, even if good collimation is used.

27. The typical skin dose range of the lateral projection of a scoliosis series on a small to average female is:

    A.   1000 to 1200 mrad   C.   200 to 400 mrad

    B.   500 to 700 mrad   D.   Less than 100 mrad

28. Which side of the patient should be elevated for the second exposure for the Ferguson scoliosis series (by having

    patient stand on a block with one foot)? _____.

29. During the AP (PA) right and left bending projections of the lumbar spine, the _____ must remain stationary during positioning.

30. Which projections should be taken to evaluate flexibility following spinal fusion surgery?

    _____.

31. How much central ray angulation is required for an AP projection of the sacrum for a typical male patient?

_____.

32. If a patient cannot lie on the back for the AP sacrum because it is too painful, what alternate projection can be taken

to achieve a similar view of the sacrum? _____

_____.

33. Where is the central ray centered for an AP projection of the coccyx? _____.

34. True/False: The AP projections of the sacrum and coccyx can be taken as one single projection to decrease gonadal
dose.

35. Patients should be asked to empty their urinary bladders before performing which projection(s) of the vertebral column?

_____.

36. In addition to good collimation, what should be done to minimize overall "fogging" on a lateral lumbar spine or lat-

eral sacrum and coccyx radiograph? _____.

REVIEW EXERCISE C: Problem Solving for Technical and Positioning Errors (see textbook pp. 314-332)

1. A radiograph of an AP projection of the lumbar spine reveals that the spinous processes are not midline to the

vertebral column. Which specific positioning error is present on this radiograph? _____

_____.

2. A radiograph of an LPO projection of the lumbar spine reveals that the downside pedicles are projected over the anterior portion of the vertebral bodies. Which specific positioning error is present on this radiograph?

_____

_____.

3. A radiograph of a lateral projection of a female lumbar spine reveals that the mid-to-lower intervertebral joint
spaces are not open. The technologist supported the midsection of the spine with sponges to straighten the spine.
What can be done to improve this image during the repeat exposure?

_____

_____.

4. A radiograph of a lateral L5-S1 projection reveals that the joint space is *not* open. The technologist did support the
middle aspect of the spine with a sponge. What else can the technologist do to open up the joint space during the repeat exposure?

_____

_____.

5. A radiograph of an AP axial projection of the coccyx reveals that the distal tip is superimposed over the symphysis pubis. What must the technologist do to eliminate this problem during the repeat exposure?

_____

6. A radiograph of an oblique position of the lumbar spine reveals that the downside pedicle and zygapophyseal joint are posterior in relation to the vertebral body. What modification of the position must be made during the repeat exposure to produce a more diagnostic image?

_____

7. **Situation:** A patient comes to the radiology department for a follow-up study for a compression fracture of L3. The radiologist requests that collimated projections be taken of L3. Which projections and what centering would provide a quality study of L3 and the intervertebral joint spaces?

_____

_____.

8. **Situation:** A young female patient comes to the radiology department for a scoliosis series. She has had repeated radiation exposure over a period of time and is rightfully concerned about the radiation. What three things can the technologist do to minimize the dose received by the patient's breasts?

   A. _____

   B. _____

   C. _____

9. **Situation:** A patient with an injury to the coccyx enters the emergency room. When attempting the AP projection, the patient complains that it is too uncomfortable to lie on his back, and he is unable to stand. What other options are available to complete the study?

_____

10. **Situation:** A patient with a clinical history of spondylolisthesis at the L5-S1 level comes to the radiology department. Which specific lumbar spine position would be most diagnostic in demonstrating the extent of this condition?

_____

REVIEW EXERCISE D: Critique Radiographs of the Lumbar Spine, Sacrum, and Coccyx (see textbook p. 333)

The following questions relate to the radiographs found at the end of Chapter 9 of the textbook. Evaluate these radiographs for the radiographic criteria categories *(1* through *5)* that follow. Describe the corrections needed to improve the overall image. The major, or "repeatable," errors are specific errors that indicate the need for a repeat exposure, regardless of the nature of the other errors.

A.   Lateral lumbar spine (Fig. C9-80)

    1.   Structures shown: _____

    2.   Part positioning: _____

    3.   Collimation and central ray: _____

    4.   Exposure criteria: _____

    5.   Markers: _____

    Repeatable error(s): _____

B.   AP lumbar spine (Fig. C9-81)

    1.   Structures shown: _____

    2.   Part positioning: _____

    3.   Collimation and central ray: _____

    4.   Exposure criteria: _____

    5.   Markers: _____

    Repeatable error(s): _____

C.   Lateral L5-S1 (Fig. C9-82)

    1.   Structures shown: _____

    2.   Part positioning: _____

    3.   Collimation and central ray: _____

    4.   Exposure criteria: _____

    5.   Markers: _____

    Repeatable error(s): _____

D. Oblique lumbar spine (Fig. C9-83)

1. Structures shown: _____

2. Part positioning: _____

3. Collimation and central ray: _____

4. Exposure criteria: _____

5. Markers: _____

Repeatable error(s): _____

E. Oblique lumbar spine (Fig. C9-84)

1. Structures shown: _____

2. Part positioning: _____

3. Collimation and central ray: _____

4. Exposure criteria: _____

5. Markers: _____

Repeatable error(s): _____

PART III: Laboratory Exercises (see textbook pp. 319-332)

You must gain experience in positioning each part of the lumbar spine, sacrum, and coccyx before performing the following exams on actual patients. You can get experience in positioning and radiographic evaluation of these projections by performing exercises using radiographic phantoms and practicing on other students (although you will not be taking actual exposures).

The following suggested activities assume that your teaching institution has an energized lab and radiographic phantoms. If not, perform Laboratory Exercises B and C, the radiographic evaluation and the physical positioning exercises. (Check off each step and projection as you complete it.)

LABORATORY EXERCISE A: Energized Laboratory

1. Using the abdomen/lumbosacral radiographic phantom, produce radiographs of the following basic routines:

_____ AP lumbar spine   _____ AP sacrum   _____ Posterior oblique lumbar spine

_____ Lateral lumbar spine   _____ AP coccyx   _____ Anterior oblique lumbar spine

_____ Lateral L5-S1   _____ Lateral sacrum and coccyx   _____ AP axial L5-S1

LABORATORY EXERCISE B: Radiographic Evaluation

1. Evaluate and critique the radiographs produced during the previous experiments, additional radiographs provided by your instructor, or both. Evaluate each radiograph for the following points. (Check off when completed.):

    _____   Evaluate the completeness of the study. (Are all of the pertinent anatomic structures included on the radiograph?)

    _____   Evaluate for positioning or centering errors (e.g., rotation, off centering).

    _____   Evaluate for correct exposure factors and possible motion. (Are the density and contrast of the images acceptable?)

    _____   Determine whether markers and an acceptable degree of collimation and/or area shielding are visible on the images.

LABORATORY EXERCISE C: Physical Positioning

On another person, simulate performing all basic and special projections of the lumbar spine, sacrum, and coccyx as follows. (Check off each when completed satisfactorily.) Include the following six steps as described in the textbook.

Step 1. Appropriate size and type of film holder with correct markers
Step 2. Correct central ray placement and centering of part to central ray and/or film
Step 3. Accurate collimation
Step 4. Area shielding of patient where advisable
Step 5. Use of proper immobilizing devices when needed
Step 6. Approximate correct exposure factors, breathing instructions where applicable, and "making" exposure

Projections	Step 1	Step 2	Step 3	Step 4	Step 5	Step 6
• AP lumbar spine	____	____	____	____	____	____
• Lateral lumbar spine	____	____	____	____	____	____
• Lateral L5-S1	____	____	____	____	____	____
• AP sacrum	____	____	____	____	____	____
• AP coccyx	____	____	____	____	____	____
• Lateral sacrum and coccyx	____	____	____	____	____	____
• Posterior oblique lumbar spine	____	____	____	____	____	____
• Anterior oblique lumbar spine	____	____	____	____	____	____
• AP axial L5-S1	____	____	____	____	____	____

Spinal fusion series:

	Step 1	Step 2	Step 3	Step 4	Step 5	Step 6
• AP (PA) R and L bending	____	____	____	____	____	____
• Lateral hyperextension and hyperflexion	____	____	____	____	____	____

Scoliosis series:

	Step 1	Step 2	Step 3	Step 4	Step 5	Step 6
• PA (AP) and lateral erect	____	____	____	____	____	____
• AP (Ferguson method)	____	____	____	____	____	____

ANSWERS TO REVIEW EXERCISES

Review Exercise A: Anatomy of the Lumbar Spine, Sacrum, and Coccyx

1. Pars interarticularis
2. B. Intervertebral foramina
3. Lateral position
4. A. Pedicle
   B. Transverse process
   C. Superior articular process and facet
   D. Lamina
   E. Spinous process
   F. Zygapophyseal joints
   G. Intervertebral foramina
5. Greater (50° for lower and 30° for upper)
6. Pelvic sacral foramina
7. Promontory
8. Cornu
9. 30°
10. Coccyx
11. Base
12. A. Synovial, diarthrodial, plane, or gliding
    B. Cartilaginous, amphiarthrodial (slightly moveable), none
13. A. Intervertebral disk space, L1-2
    B. Spinous process, L2
    C. Transverse process, L3
    D. Region of lamina (body), L4
    E. Left ala of sacrum
    F. Left sacroiliac joint
    G. Body of L1
    H. Pedicles of L2
    I. Intervertebral foramina, L3-4
    J. Intervertebral disk space, L5-S1
    K. Sacrum
    L. Inferior articular process, L3 (leg)
    M. Zygapophyseal joint, L4-5
    N. Pars interarticularis, L3 (neck)
    O. Pedicle, L3 (eye)
    P. Transverse process, L3 (nose)
    Q. Superior articular process, L3 (ear)
14. A. Left zygapophyseal joints
    B. Left zygapophyseal joints
    C. Intervertebral foramina
    D. Right zygapophyseal joints
    E. Right zygapophyseal joints
15. 50°, 30°, 45°

Review Exercise B: Topographic Landmarks and Positioning of the Lumbar Spine, Sacrum, and Coccyx

1. 1. C
   2. E
   3. A
   4. B
   5. D
2. False
3. True
4. False (not female when shield obscures essential anatomy)
5. False (Posteroanterior [PA] would open spaces better.)
6. False (should be flexed)
7. True
8. False
9. A. 4
   B. 1
   C. 1
   D. 5
   E. 2
10. A. 8
    B. 3
    C. 1
    D. 2
    E. 4
    F. 7
    G. 6
    H. 5
11. Iliac crest
12. A. Sacroiliac (SI) joints are equidistant from the spine.
    B. Spinous process should be midline to the vertebral column.
13. 30°
14. Right (upside)
15. Pedicle
16. Excessive obliquity
17. Lateral
18. 5 to 10, caudad
19. With the sag or convexity of the spine closest to the image receptor (IR)
20. Reduces lumbar curvature which opens the intervertebral disk space
21. True
22. 1¹⁄₅ inches (4 cm) inferior to iliac crest and 2 inches (5 cm) posterior to ASIS.
23. 30° cephalad
24. True
25. False (lower margin 1 to 2 inches [3 to 5 cm] below iliac crest)
26. True
27. A 1000 to 1200 mrad
28. The convex side of the spine
29. Pelvis
30. Hyperextension and hyperflexion projections
31. 15° cephalad
32. A PA (prone) with 15° caudad central ray angle
33. 2 inches (5 cm) superior to the symphysis pubis
34. False (need different central ray angles for anteroposterior [AP] projections; can combine lateral but not AP projections)
35. AP of sacrum and coccyx
36. Place lead blocker on table top behind patient.

Review Exercise C: Problem-Solving for Technical and Positioning Errors

1. Rotation of the spine
2. Insufficient rotation or obliquity of the spine (should be to midvertebral bodies).
3. If the patient has a wide pelvis, the central ray can be angled 5° to 10° caudad.
4. Place additional support beneath the spine, or use a 5° to 10° caudad angle.
5. An increase in central ray angle is required to separate the coccyx from the symphysis pubis.
6. Decrease obliquity of the body and spine.
7. AP or PA and collimated lateral projections would provide the best view of the L3 region. The central ray should be about 2 inches (5 cm) above the iliac crest.
8. A. Use high kilovoltage peak technique
   B. Perform a PA rather than an AP projection
   C. Use breast shields
9. Perform a PA rather than an AP projection and reverse the direction of the central ray from caudad to cephalad.
10. A lateral L5-S1 position would demonstrate the degree of forward displacement of L5 onto S1.

Review Exercise D: Critique Radiographs of the Lumbar Spine, Sacrum, and Coccyx

A. Lateral lumbar spine (Fig. C9-80)
   1. Posterior elements of upper lumbar spine cut off
   2. Patient too far posterior
   3. Evident and acceptable collimation (could be collimated a little more tightly if centering were correct); central ray centering too anterior, causing posterior elements to become cut off
   4. Acceptable but slightly underexposed exposure factors

5. Anatomic side marker cut off
Repeatable errors: criteria 1, 2, and 3
B. AP lumbar spine (Fig. C9-81)
1. Metallic artifacts obscuring aspects of lumbar spine
2. Part positioning acceptable but centered slightly to left
3. Acceptable collimation; acceptable central ray centering and IR placement
4. Overexposed exposure factors
5. No evidence of anatomic side marker
Repeatable errors: criteria 1 and 4
C. Lateral L5-S1 (Fig. C9-82)
1. All pertinent anatomic structures included
2. Excellent part and central ray centering

3. Additional collimation needed; S1 joint space not open; may need waist support or central ray caudal angle
4. Underexposed L5-S1 joint space region
5. Evidence of anatomic side marker (Better placement would have been up and posterior to spine.)
Repeatable errors: criteria 3 and 4
D. Oblique lumbar spine (Fig. C9-83)
1. Posterior elements of upper lumbar spine cut off
2. Overobliqued upper aspect of lumbar spine (eye of "Scotty dog"—pedicles posterior and not centered to body)
3. Evidence of collimation; central ray centered too anterior, posterior elements of lumbar spine to become cut off

4. Acceptable exposure factors
5. Evidence of anatomic side marker
Repeatable errors: criteria 1, 2, and 3
E. Oblique lumbar spine (Fig. C9-84)
1. Entire lumbar spine demonstrated
2. Underobliqued lumbar spine (pedicles or eyes of "Scotty dogs" too anterior)
3. Collimation too loose and not evident (should be visible on sides); central ray centering and IR placement correct
4. Acceptable but slightly overexposed exposure factors
5. No evidence of anatomic side marker
Repeatable error: criteria 2

SELF-TEST

This self-test should be taken only after completing all of the readings, review exercises, and laboratory activities for a particular section. The purpose of this test is not only to provide a good learning exercise but also to serve as a strong indicator of what your final evaluation grade will cover. It is strongly suggested that if you do not get at least a 90% to 95% grade on each self-test, you should review those areas in which you missed questions before going to your instructor for the final evaluation exam for this chapter (There are 70 questions or blanks in this chapter—each is worth 1.4 points.)

1. Compared with the spinous processes of the cervical and thoracic spine, the lumbar spinous processes are:

    A.   Smaller   C.   Larger and more blunt

    B.   Pointed downward more   D.   Absent

2. The anterior ridge of the upper sacrum is called the:

    A.   Median sacral crest   C.   Promontory

    B.   Cornua   D.   Sacral horns

3. Each sacroiliac joint is obliqued posteriorly _____°.

    A.   20   C.   45

    B.   30   D.   50

4. The angle of the midlumbar spine zygapophyseal joints in relation to the midsagittal plane is _____°.

5. Where is the pars interarticularis found?

    A.   Superior and inferior aspect of the pedicle   C.   Between the superior and inferior articular processes

    B.   Between the intervertebral disk and vertebral   D.   Between the lamina and body spinous processes

6. Identify the labeled parts of the sacrum and coccyx on the following drawings (Figs. 9-6 through 9-7):

    A. _____

    B. _____

    C. _____

    D. _____

    E. _____

    F. _____

    G. _____

    H. _____

    I. _____

    J. _____

    K. _____

    L. _____

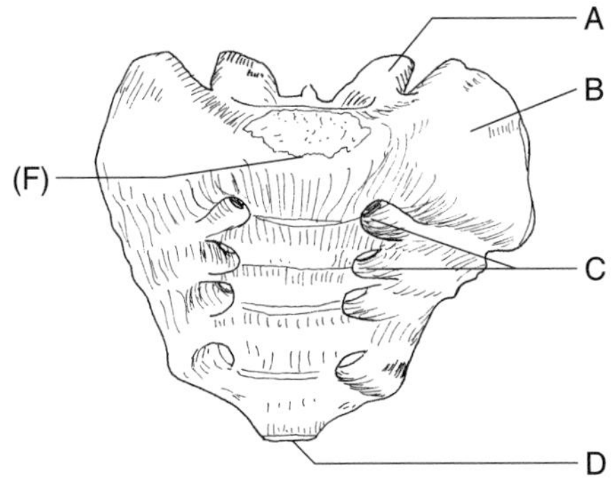

Fig. 9-6. Sacrum.

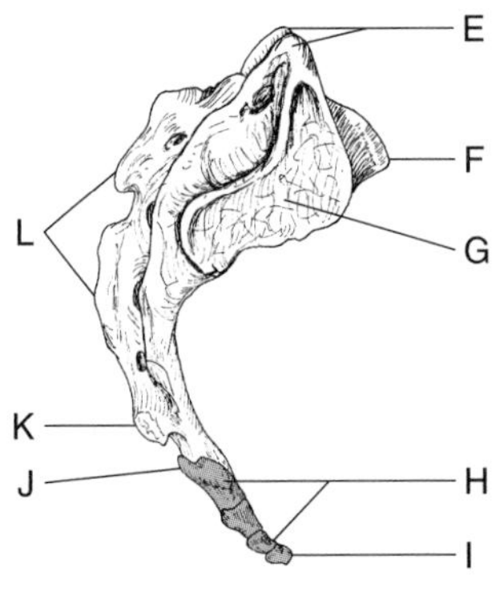

Fig. 9-7. Sacrum and coccyx.

7. Identify the labeled parts on these radiographs
    of individual vertebrae (see Figs. 9-8 and 9-9).

    A. _____

    B. _____

    C. _____

    D. _____

    E. _____

    F. _____

    G. _____

    H. _____

    I. _____

    J. _____

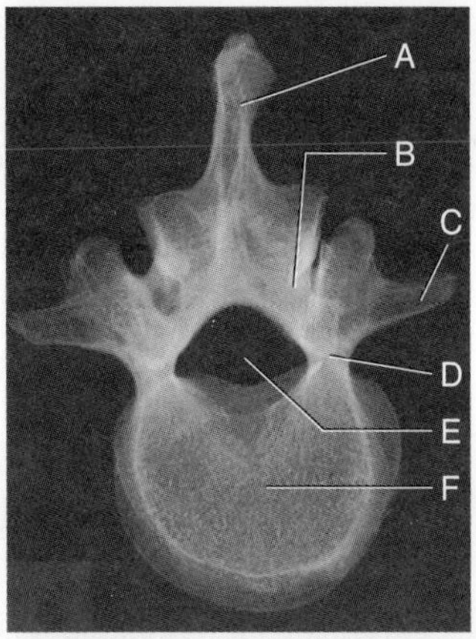

Fig. 9-8. Individual vertebrae
(A through F).

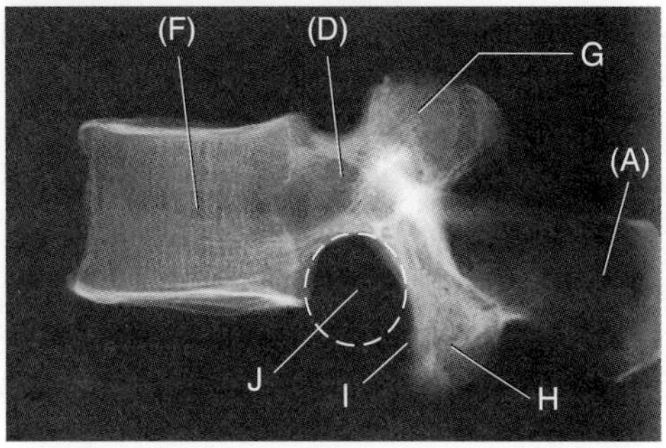

Fig. 9-9. Individual vertebrae (G through K).

8. What are the characteristics of the vertebra in Fig. 9-9 that identify it as a lumbar vertebra rather than a thoracic?

    _____.

9. The zygapophyseal joints of the lumbar spine are classified as _____ type joints with

    _____ type joint movement.

10. List the correct terms of the lumbar vertebra that correspond to the
    following parts of the "Scotty dog" as seen on an oblique radiograph
    of the lumbar spine (Fig. 9-10).

    A. _____

    B. _____

    C. _____

    D. _____

    E. _____

    F. _____

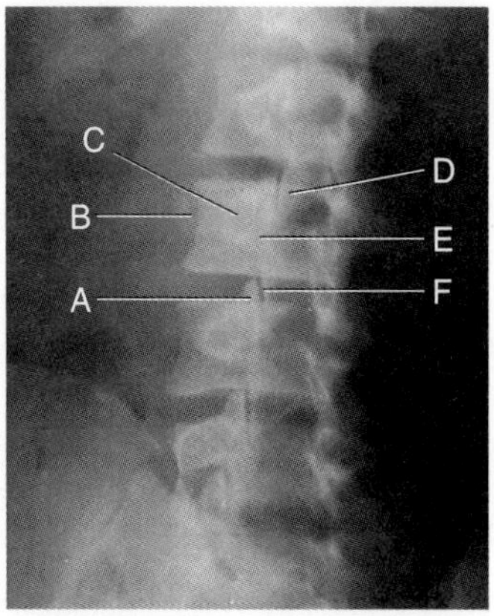

Fig. 9-10. Oblique lumbar spine.

11. The ear and front leg make up the _____ joint best seen in the oblique position.

12. Which one of the following topographic landmarks corresponds to the L2-3 level?

    A. Xiphoid process   B. Lower costal margin   C. Iliac crest   D. ASIS

13. True/False: It is possible to shield females for an anteroposterior (AP) projection of the sacrum or coccyx if the gonadal shields are correctly placed.

14. True/False: The female gonadal dose is approximately that of the midline dose and is almost the same for either AP or posteroanterior (PA) projections of the lumbar spine.

15. Why should the knees and hips be flexed for an AP projection of the lumbar spine? _____

_____.

16. True/False: The use of a lead blocker mat for lateral positions of the lumbar spine should not be used with digital imaging.

17. True/False: The efficiency of computed tomography (CT) and magnetic resonance imaging (MRI) of the spine is reducing the number of myelograms being performed.

18. Anterior wedging and loss of vertebral body height is characteristic of:

    A. Chance fracture   C. Compression fracture

    B. Spina bifida   D. Spondylolysis

19. Which one of the following conditions is often diagnosed with prenatal ultrasound?

    A. Scoliosis   C. Spondylolisthesis

    B. Spina bifida   D. Ankylosing spondylitis

20. Which one of the following conditions usually requires an increase in manual exposure factors?

    A. Ankylosing spondylitis   C. Spina bifida

    B. Spondylolysis   D. Spondylolisthesis

21. Where is the central ray centered for an AP projection of the lumbar spine with an 30 × 35 cm (11 × 14 inches)

    image receptor (IR)? _____.

22. Which set of zygapophyseal joints of the lumbar spine are best demonstrated with a left anterior oblique (LAO)

    position? _____.

23. How much obliquity is required to demonstrate the zygapophyseal joint space between L1-2?

_____.

24. Describe the body build that may require central ray angulation to open the intervertebral joint spaces with a lateral projection of the lumbar spine, even if the patient has some support under the waist?

_____.

25. What type of central ray angulation should be utilized for the lateral L5-S1 projection if the waist is not supported?

    A. Central ray perpendicular to film   C. 10° to 15° cephalad

    B. 5° to 10° caudad   D. 3° to 5° cephalad

26. What type of central ray angulation should be utilized for an AP axial projection for L5-S1 on a female patient?

    A. 35° cephalad   C. 5° to 8° caudad

    B. 30° cephalad   D. Central ray perpendicular to film

27. Where is the central ray centered for an AP axial projection for L5-S1? _____.

28. True/False: The center ionization chamber should be utilized when using automatic exposure control (AEC) for either a lateral lumbar spine or a lateral L5-S1 projection

29. Which projection or method is designed to demonstrate the degree of scoliosis deformity between the primary and

    compensatory curves as part of a scoliosis study? _____

    _____.

30. Which projections are designed to measure anteroposterior movement at the site of a spinal fusion?

    _____.

31. Where is the central ray centered for an AP projection of the sacrum? _____

    _____.

32. What two things can be done to reduce the high amounts of scatter reaching the IR during a lateral projection of the sacrum and coccyx?

    A.   _____   B.   _____

33. Why should a single, lateral projection of the sacrum and coccyx be performed rather than separate laterals of the

    sacrum and coccyx? _____.

34. The skin dose on a lateral sacrum and/or coccyx projection on an average-size patient is in the _____ range.

    A.   200 to 500 mrad   C.   1000 to 1500 mrad
    B.   500 to 700 mrad   D.   1500 to 2000 mrad

35. A radiograph of an AP projection of the lumbar spine reveals that the sacroiliac (SI) joints are *not* equidistant from the spine. The right ala of the sacrum appears larger, and the left SI joint is more open than the left. Which specific

    positioning error is evident on this radiograph? _____

    _____.

36. A radiograph of an LPO projection of the lumbar spine reveals that the downside pedicles are projected toward the posterior aspect of the vertebral bodies. What must be done to correct this error during the repeat exposure?

    _____.

37. An AP projection of the sacrum reveals that the sacrum is foreshortened and the foramina are not open. What posi-

    tioning error led to this radiographic outcome? _____

    _____.

38. **Situation:** A patient with a possible compression fracture of L3 enters the emergency room. Which projection(s) of

    the lumbar spine best demonstrates the extent of this injury? _____

    _____.

39. **Situation:** A patient with a clinical history of spondylolisthesis of L5-S1 region comes to the radiology department. What basic (i.e., routine) and special (i.e., optional) projections should be included in this study? (HINT: If

    the obliques are included, what angle of obliquity should be used?) _____

    _____.

40. For the following critique questions, refer to the oblique lumbar spine radiograph (Fig. C9-83) in your textbook:

    A. Which positioning error(s) are visible on this radiograph? More than one answer may be selected.

        (a) All essential anatomic structures are not demonstrated.

        (b) Central ray is centered incorrectly.

        (c) Collimation is not evident.

        (d) Exposure factors are incorrect.

        (e) No anatomic marker is visible on the radiograph.

        (f) Excessive obliquity of the spine is evident.

        (g) Insufficient obliquity of the spine is evident.

    B. Which of the previous criteria are considered "repeatable errors?" _____

    C. Which of the following modifications must be made during the repeat exposure? More than one answer may be selected.

        (a) Center central ray to long aspect of spine.

        (b) Use closer collimation.

        (c) Decrease exposure factors.

        (d) Increase exposure factors.

        (e) Place anatomic side marker on IR before exposure.

        (f) Decrease obliquity of lumbar spine.

        (g) Increase obliquity of lumbar spine.

CHAPTER 10

Bony Thorax—Sternum and Ribs

CHAPTER OBJECTIVES

After you have completed **all** the activities in this chapter, you will be able to:

_____ 1. Identify specific anatomic structures of the sternum and ribs using drawings and radiographs.

_____ 2. Classify ribs as either true, false, or floating ribs.

_____ 3. Classify specific joints in the bony thorax according to their structural classification, mobility classification, and movement type.

_____ 4. Define specific types of pathologic features of the bony thorax as described in the textbook.

_____ 5. Identify basic and special projections of the ribs and sternum, including the correct size and type of image receptor (IR) and the location, direction, and angulation of the central ray for each position.

_____ 6. Identify which structures are best seen with specific projections of the ribs and sternum.

_____ 7. Identify the technical considerations important in radiography of the ribs and sternum, including breathing instructions, general body position, kilovoltage peak range, and other imaging options.

_____ 8. Identify patient dose ranges for skin, midline, thyroid, and breast for specific projection of the ribs and sternum.

_____ 9. Given various hypothetical situations, identify the correct modification of a position and/or exposure factors to improve the radiographic image.

_____ 10. Given radiographs of specific bony thorax projections or positions, identify specific positioning and exposure factors errors.

POSITIONING AND FILM CRITIQUE

_____ 1. Using a peer, position for basic and special projections of the bony thorax.

_____ 2. Using a chest radiographic phantom, produce satisfactory radiographs of specific positions (if equipment is available).

_____ 3. Critique and evaluate cranial radiographs based on the four divisions of radiographic criteria: (1) structures shown, (2) position, (3) collimation and central ray, and (4) exposure criteria.

_____ 4. Distinguish between acceptable and unacceptable bony thorax radiographs based on exposure factors, motion, collimation, positioning, or other errors.

Learning Exercises

The following review exercises should be completed only after careful study of the associated pages in the textbook as indicated by each exercise.

After completing each of these individual exercises, check your answers with the answer sheets that follow before continuing to the next exercise.

PART I: Radiographic Anatomy

REVIEW EXERCISE A: Anatomy of Bony Thorax, Sternum, and Ribs (see textbook pp. 336-338)

1. List the three structures that make up the bony thorax:

    A. _____   B. _____   C. _____

2. Identify the parts of the sternum and ribs labeled in Fig. 10-1.

    A. _____

    B. _____

    C. _____

    D. _____

    E. _____

    F. _____

    G. _____

    H. _____

    I. _____

    J. _____

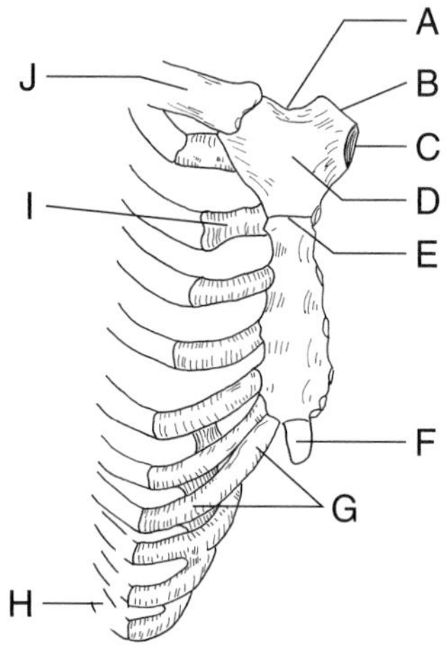

    Fig. 10-1. Sternum and ribs.

3. List the two secondary names for the long, middle aspect of the sternum:

    A. _____   B. _____

4. The most distal aspect of the sternum does not ossify until a person reaches the approximate age of _____.

5. The total sternum length on an average adult is about _____ inches (_____ cm).

6. A. The xiphoid end of the sternum is at the approximate level of the _____ vertebra.

    B. The sternal angle is at the level of _____ .

7. What is the name of the joint that connects the upper limb to the bony thorax (the only **bony** connection between

    the bony thorax and upper limbs)? _____.

8. What is the name of the section of cartilage that connects the anterior end of the rib to the sternum?

    _____.

9.   What distinguishes a true rib from a false rib? _____

_____.

10.   True/False: The eleventh and twelfth ribs are classified as false *and* floating ribs.

11.   True/False: The anterior end of the ribs is called the vertebral end.

12.   Which aspect of the ribs articulates with the transverse process of the thoracic vertebrae?

  A.   Head   C.   Neck

  B.   Costal angle   D.   Tubercle

13.   List the three structures found within the costal groove of each rib:

  A.   _____   B.   _____   C.   _____

14.   Answer the following questions as you study this chest
    radiograph (Fig. 10-2).

  A.   Which end of the ribs are most superior—the posterior
       vertebral ends or the anterior sternal ends?

       _____

  B.   Approximately how much difference in height is there
       between these two ends of the ribs?

       _____

  C.   Which ribs articulate with the upper lateral aspect of the
       manubrium of the sternum?

       _____

  D.   The bony thorax is widest at the lateral margins

       of which ribs? _____

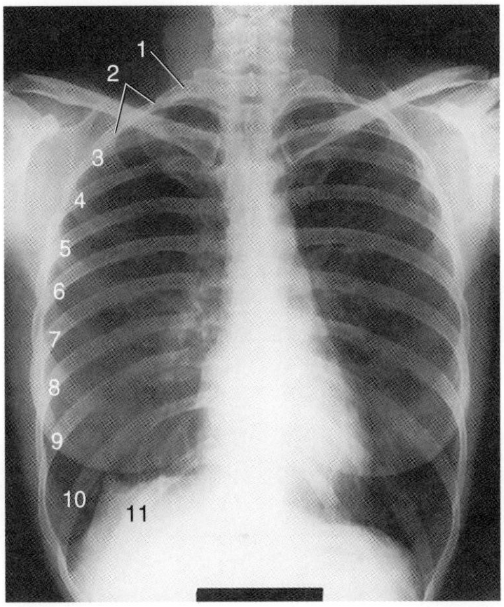

Fig. 10-2. Chest radiograph.

  E.   How many posterior ribs are shown above the diaphragm? _____.
       (Recall from Chapter 2 that a **minimum** of 10 posterior ribs must be seen on an average inspiration
       posteroanterior [PA] chest projection.)

15.   Match the following joints with the correct movement type:

  A.   Movable—diarthrodial (plane or gliding)   B.   Immovable—synarthrodial

  _____   1.   First sternocostal

  _____   2.   First through twelfth costovertebral joints

  _____   3.   First through tenth costochondral unions (between costocartilage and ribs)

  _____   4.   First through tenth costotransverse joints (between ribs and transverse processes of T vertebrae)

  _____   5.   Second through seventh sternocostal joints (between second through seventh ribs and sternum)

  _____   6.   Sixth through tenth interchondral joints (between anterior sixth through tenth costal cartilage)

16. The joints from the previous question that have diarthrodial movement are classified as _____.

17. Classify the following group of ribs labeled as *A, B,* and *C,* and identify the number of the ribs in each category (Fig. 10-3):

    A. _____

    B. _____

    C. _____

18. What is unique about the ribs in category *A* in the previous question?

    _____.

19. What is unique about the ribs in category *C* in the previous question?

    _____.

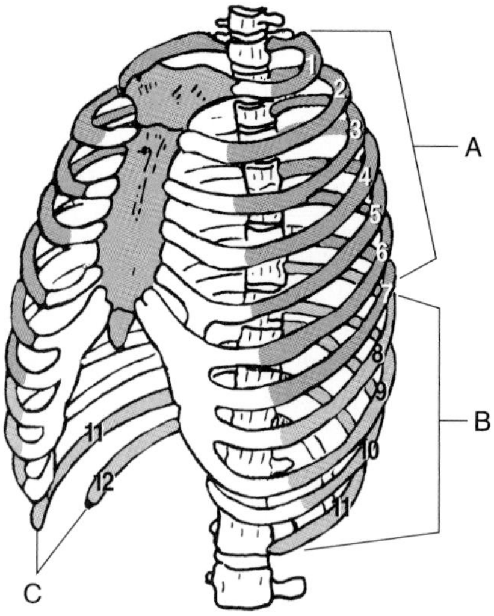

Fig. 10-3. Rib groups.

20. Identify the labeled parts of this posterior view of a typical rib (Fig. 10-4):

    A. _____

    B. _____

    C. _____

    D. _____

    E. _____

    F. _____

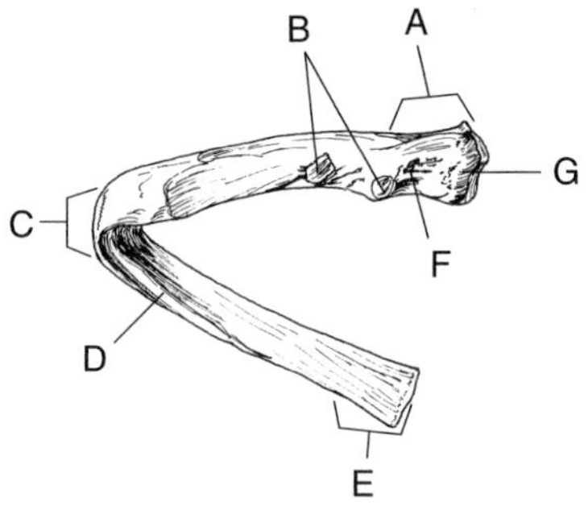

PART II: Radiographic Positioning

Fig. 10-4. Posterior view of a typical rib.

REVIEW EXERCISE B: Positioning of the Ribs and Sternum (see textbook pp. 339-350)

1. True/False: It is virtually impossible to visualize the sternum with a direct PA or anteroposterior (AP) projection.

2. True/False: A large, "deep-chested" (hypersthenic) patient requires more obliquity for a frontal view of the sternum as compared with a "thin chested" (asthenic) patient.

3. How much obliquity should be used for the oblique position of the sternum for a large, "deep chested" patient?

   _____.

4. List the ideal ranges (high or low) for the following exposure factors as they apply to an oblique position of the sternum.

   A. Kilovoltage peak range: _____

   B. Milliamperage: _____

   C. Exposure time: _____

5. What is the advantage of performing a breathing technique for radiography of the sternum?

    _____.

6. What is the primary reason that a source-image-receptor distance (SID) of less than 40 inches (100 cm) should not

    be used for sternum radiography? _____.

7. What other imaging option is available to study the sternum if routine RAO and lateral radiographs do not provide

    sufficient information? _____.

8. Circle the preferred positioning factor to demonstrate an injury to the ribs found **below** the diaphragm:

    A. General body position (erect/recumbent): _____

    B. Breathing instructions (inspiration/expiration): _____

    C. Recommended kilovoltage peak range: _____

9. An injury to the region of the eighth or ninth ribs would require the _____ (above or below)
    diaphragm technique.

10. To properly elongate and visualize the axillary aspect of the ribs, the patient's spine needs to be rotated

    _____ (toward or away) from the area of interest.

11. Which projections (AP or PA and anterior or posterior oblique) should be performed for an injury to the **anterior**

    aspect of the ribs? _____.

12. Which two rib projections should be performed for an injury to the **right posterior** ribs?

    _____.

13. How can the site of injury be marked for a rib series? _____

    _____.

14. If the physician suspects a pneumothorax or hemothorax has occurred as a result of a rib fracture, which additional
    radiographic projection(s) should be performed in addition to the routine rib projections?

    _____.

15. A flail chest is defined as a:

    A. Patient with an asthenic body habitus

    C. Patient with a chronic obstructivepulomonary
        disease (COPD; e.g., emphysema)

    B. Patient with pulmonary injury caused
        by blunt trauma to two or more ribs

    D. Patient with cardiac injury caused by blunt trauma

16. Osteolytic metastases of the ribs produce the following radiographic appearance:

    A. Irregular bony margins

    C. Sharp lucent lines through the ribs

    B. Increased bony density of the ribs

    D. Smooth, lucent "holes" in the rib

17. True/False: Magnetic resonance imaging (MRI) provides a more diagnostic image of rib metastases as compared with a nuclear medicine scan.

18. True/False: Patients can develop osteomyelitis as a postoperative complication following open heart surgery.

19. Which is preferred for a study of the sternum—RAO or left anterior oblique (LAO)

    _____.

    Why? _____.

20. Where is the central ray centered for the oblique and lateral projections of the sternum?

    _____.

21. What other position can be performed if the patient cannot assume a prone position for the RAO sternum?

    _____.

22. What is the recommended SID for a lateral projection of the sternum?

    _____.

    Why? _____.

23. Which of the following criteria apply to a radiograph for an evaluation of the oblique sternum?

    A.   The entire sternum should be adjacent to the spine and adjacent to the heart shadow.

    B.   The entire sternum should overlay the heart shadow and be adjacent to the spine.

    C.   The left sternoclavicular joint should be adjacent to the spinal column.

    D.   The second rib should lie directly over the manubrium of the sternum.

24. Where is the central ray centered for a PA projection of the sternoclavicular joints?

    A.   Level of T7   C.   At the vertebra prominens

    B.   Level of T2-3   D.   Level of xiphoid process

25. What type of breathing instructions should be given to the patient for a PA projection of the sternoclavicular joints?

    A.   Suspend respiration on inspiration.   C.   Suspended breathing is not necessary.

    B.   Use a breathing technique.

26. How much obliquity is recommended for an anterior oblique of the sternoclavicular joints?

    _____.

27. Which specific oblique position best demonstrates the **left** sternoclavicular joint next to the spine?

    _____.

28. Where is the central ray centered for an AP projection of the ribs for an injury located above the diaphragm?

    _____.

29. Which two specific oblique positions can be used to demonstrate the **left** axillary portion of the ribs?

    _____.

30. Which two specific projections or positions should be performed for an injury to the right anterior ribs?

_____.

31. How many degrees of rotation are needed for a routine oblique projection of the ribs? _____ .

32. Both the patient thyroid dose and the breast dose for a correctly collimated PA sternoclavicular (S-C) joint projection

are in the _____ range.

   A. 1 to 5 mrad   C. 300 to 400 mrad

   B. 25 to 100 mrad D. 500 to 1000 mrad

33. True/False: The thyroid dose for an anterior oblique rib projection is only about 5% of what it would be for a posterior oblique rib projection.

34. True/False: The breast dose for an anterior oblique rib projection is only about 5% of what it would be for a posterior oblique rib projection.

35. True/False: The amount of gonadal dose given for rib projections is less than 1 mrad.

REVIEW EXERCISE C: Problem Solving for Technical and Positioning Errors (see textbook pp. 339-350)

1. A radiograph of an RAO sternum reveals that part of the sternum is superimposed over the thoracic spine. Which

   specific positioning error is visible on this radiograph? _____

2. A radiograph of an RAO sternum reveals that the sternum is difficult to visualize because of excessive density. The following factors were used for this image: 75 kVp, 25 mA, 3-second exposure, 40 inch (100 cm) SID, Bucky, and 100-speed screens. Which one of these factors should be modified during the repeat exposure to produce a more

   diagnostic image? _____

3. A radiograph of an RAO sternum reveals that the sternum is poorly visualized because of excessive lung markings superimposed over the sternum. The following factors were used for this image: 65 kVp, 50 mA, 1-second exposure, 40 inch (100 cm) SID, Bucky, and 100-speed screens. Which of these factors can be altered to increase the visibility of the sternum? _____

4. A radiograph of a lateral projection of the sternum reveals that the patient's breasts are obscuring the sternum. What can be done to minimize the breast artifact over the sternum?

_____.

5. Repeat PA projections of the sternoclavicular joints do not clearly demonstrate them. What other imaging modality may produce a more diagnostic image of these joints?

_____.

6. **Situation.** A patient with trauma to the sternum and the left sternoclavicular joint region enters the emergency room. In addition to the sternum routine, the emergency room physician also asks for a specific projection to better demonstrate the left sternoclavicular joint. Describe the positioning routine, including the breathing instructions, that you would use. (HINT: Three projections are required.)

_____

_____.

7. A radiograph of the upper ribs demonstrates that the diaphragm is superimposed over the eighth ribs, which is in the area of interest. The following factors were used for the initial exposure: 65 kVp, 400 mA, 1/40 second, 400-speed screens, grid, suspended respiration on expiration, erect position, 40 inch (102 cm) SID. Which one of these factors can be modified to increase the visibility of the area of interest?

   _____.

8. **Situation:** A patient enters the emergency room on a backboard after being involved in a motor vehicle accident. Because of the condition of the patient, the emergency room physician orders a portable study of the sternum in the emergency room. Which two projections of the sternum would be most diagnostic yet minimize movement of the patient? (See Chapter 19 in the textbook for a demonstration.)

   _____.

8. **Situation:** A patient with trauma to the right upper anterior ribs enters the emergency room. Which positioning routine of the ribs should be performed? (Include general body position, breathing instructions, and specific projections or positions performed. Patient is able to sit in erect position.)

   _____.

10. **Situation:** A patient with trauma to the left lower anterior ribs enters the emergency room. Which positioning routine of the ribs should be performed? (Include general body position, breathing instructions, and specific positions performed.)

   _____.

REVIEW EXERCISE D: Critique Radiographs of the Bony Thorax (see textbook p. 352)

The following questions relate to the radiographs found at the end of Chapter 10 of the textbook. Evaluate these radiographs for the radiographic criteria categories *(1 through 5)* that follow. Describe the corrections needed to improve the overall image. The major, or "repeatable," errors are specific errors that indicate the need for a repeat exposure, regardless of the nature of the other errors.

A. Ribs above diaphragm (Fig. C10-43)

NOTE: This radiograph was included to keep you alert and present a challenge even to the most advanced student or technologist. To critique and evaluate this may require more information about this patient than was presented in the textbook. This patient came to the radiology department from the county morgue to be radiographed and the cause of death determined. This was a reported drowning victim whose body had been in the water for several days. Note the air in the lungs, which may suggest the cause of death was not drowning. No specific critique questions and answers are included for this unique radiograph; continue to the following radiograph.

B. Oblique sternum (Fig. C10-44)

   1. Structures shown: _____

   2. Part positioning: _____

   3. Collimation and central ray: _____

   4. Exposure criteria: _____

   5. Markers: _____

   Repeatable error(s): _____

C. **Ribs below diaphragm (Fig. C10-45)**

  1. Structures shown: _____

  2. Part positioning: _____

  3. Collimation and central ray: _____

  4. Exposure criteria: _____

  5. Markers: _____

  Repeatable error(s): _____

D. **Lateral sternum (Fig. C10-46)**

  1. Structures shown: _____

  2. Part positioning: _____

  3. Collimation and central ray: _____

  4. Exposure criteria: _____

  5. Markers: _____

  Repeatable error(s): _____

PART III: Laboratory Activities (see textbook pp. 286-303)

You must gain experience in positioning each part of the sternum and ribs before performing the following exams on actual patients. You can get experience in positioning and radiographic evaluation of these projections by performing exercises using radiographic phantoms and practicing on other students (although you will not be taking actual exposures).

The following suggested activities assume that your teaching institution has an energized lab and radiographic phantoms. If not, perform Laboratory Exercises B and C, the radiographic evaluation and the physical positioning exercises. (Check off each step and projection as you complete it.)

LABORATORY EXERCISE A: Energized Laboratory

  1. Using the chest radiographic phantom, produce radiographs of the following basic routines:

  _____ RAO sternum

  _____ PA sternoclavicular joints

  _____ AP (PA) ribs,

  _____ AP (PA) ribs, above and below diaphragm

  _____ Lateral sternum

  _____ RAO (LAO) sternoclavicular joints

  _____ Posterior and anterior oblique ribs, above diaphragm

  _____ Horizontal beam lateral sternum

LABORATORY EXERCISE B: Radiographic Evaluation

1. Evaluate and critique the radiographs produced during the previous experiments, additional radiographs provided by your instructor, or both. Evaluate each radiograph for the following points. (Check off when completed.):

    _____ Evaluate the completeness of the study. (Are all of the pertinent anatomic structures included on the radiograph?)

    _____ Evaluate for positioning or centering errors (e.g., rotation, off centering).

    _____ Evaluate for correct exposure factors and possible motion. (Are the density and contrast of the images acceptable?)

    _____ Determine whether markers and an acceptable degree of collimation and/or area shielding are visible on the images.

LABORATORY EXERCISE C: Physical Positioning

On another person, simulate performing all basic and special projections of the sternum and ribs as follows. (Check off each when completed satisfactorily.) Include the following six steps as described in the textbook.

Step 1. Appropriate size and type of film holder with correct markers
Step 2. Correct central ray placement and centering of part to central ray and/or film
Step 3. Accurate collimation
Step 4. Area shielding of patient where advisable
Step 5. Use of proper immobilizing devices when needed
Step 6. Approximate correct exposure factors, breathing instructions where applicable, and "making" exposure

Projections	Step 1	Step 2	Step 3	Step 4	Step 5	Step 6
• RAO sternum	_____	_____	_____	_____	_____	_____
• Erect lateral sternum	_____	_____	_____	_____	_____	_____
• Recumbent left posterior oblique (LPO) sternum	_____	_____	_____	_____	_____	_____
• Horizontal beam lateral sternum	_____	_____	_____	_____	_____	_____
• PA sternoclavicular joints	_____	_____	_____	_____	_____	_____
• Oblique sternoclavicular joints	_____	_____	_____	_____	_____	_____
• Rib routine for injury to right upper anterior ribs	_____	_____	_____	_____	_____	_____
• Rib routine for injury to left lower posterior ribs	_____	_____	_____	_____	_____	_____

*Optional exercise if the school or hospital has
a tomography unit:*

Projections	Step 1	Step 2	Step 3	Step 4	Step 5	Step 6
• *Frontal tomogram of the sternum*	_____	_____	_____	_____	_____	_____

ANSWERS TO REVIEW EXERCISES

Review Exercise A: Anatomy of the Bony Thorax, Sternum, and Ribs

1. A. Sternum
   B. Thoracic vertebra
   C. 12 pairs of ribs
2. A. Jugular (suprasternal) notch
   B. Facet for sternoclavicular joint
   C. Facet for first rib
   D. Manubrium
   E. Sternal angle
   F. Xiphoid process
   G. Costocartilage of seventh rib (last of "true" ribs)
   H. Tenth rib
   I. Costocartilage of second rib
   J. Clavicle
3. A. Corpus
   B. Gladiolus
4. 40
5. 6 inches (15 cm)
6. A. T9 or 10
   B. T4-5
7. Sternoclavicular joint
8. Costocartilage
9. True ribs connect to the sternum by their own costocartilage. False ribs are connected to the sternum via the costocartilage of the seventh rib.
10. True
11. False (called the sternal end)
12. D (tubercle)
13. A. Artery
    B. Vein
    C. Nerve
14. A. Posterior vertebral ends
    B. 3 to 5 inches (7.5 to 12.5 cm)
    C. First (anterior sternal end)
    D. Eighth or ninth
    E. 11
15. 1. B
    2. A
    3. B
    4. A
    5. A
    6. A
16. Synovial
17. A. True ribs, 1 through 7
    B. False ribs, 8 through 12
    C. Floating ribs, 11 through 12
18. Each rib attaches to the sternum by its own costocartilage.
19. They do not connect to anything anteriorly (thus the term "floating" ribs).
20. A. Vertebral end (posterior)
    B. Tubercles (for articulation with vertebrae)
    C. Angle portion of rib
    D. Costal groove
    E. Sternal end (anterior)
    F. Neck
    G. Head

Review Exercise B: Positioning of the Bony Thorax, Sternum, and Ribs

1. True
2. False (less obliquity)
3. Approximately 15°
4. A. Low (60 to 70)
   B. Low
   C. High (3 to 4 seconds) with breathing technique
5. It blurs lung markings and ribs, which improves the visibility of the sternum.
6. Increase in patient dose, especially skin dose
7. Computed tomography (CT) or nuclear medicine
8. A. Recumbent
   B. Expiration
   C. Medium (75 to 85)
9. Above
10. Away from
11. Posteroanterior (PA) and anterior obliques (Placing the area of interest closest to the image receptor [IR] is one recommended routine.)
12. Anteroposterior (AP) and right posterior oblique (RPO) (to shift spine away from area of interest)
13. By taping small, metallic "BB" over the site of the injury
14. Erect PA and lateral chest
15. B
16. A
17. False
18. True
19. Right anterior oblique (RAO); it places the sternum over the heart to provide a uniform background for added visibility of the sternum.
20. Mid sternum (midway between jugular notch and xiphoid)
21. Left posterior oblique (LPO) (oblique supine position)
22. 60 to 72 inches (152 to 183 cm); reduces magnification created by the long object-image receptor distance (OID)
23. B (entire sternum over heart shadow adjacent to spine)
24. B (level of T2-3)
25. A (suspend on inspiration)
26. 15°
27. LAO
28. 3 to 4 inches (8 to 10 cm) below the jugular notch, level of T7
29. RAO or LPO elongates the left axillary ribs (and shifts the spine away from the injury site).
30. PA and LAO (to shift spine away from injury site)
31. 45°
32. A (1 to 5 mrad)
33. False (only about one third, or 33%)
34. True (NOTE: A greater difference in breast dose exists for posterior versus anterior rib projections than for thyroid doses because of the more anterior surface placement of the breasts compared with the thyroid.)
35. True. The gonadal dose is so low that it is not listed on the dose charts for rib projections.

Review Exercise C: Problem-Solving for Technical and Positioning Errors

1. Underrotation or obliquity of the patient
2. Use a lower kilovoltage peak to 65 for higher contrast and to prevent overpenetration of the sternum.
3. Increase the exposure time (and lower the milliamperage) to allow for greater blurring of the lung markings.
4. Have the patient bring the breasts to the side; hold them in this position with a wide bandage.
5. CT
6. 15° to 20° RAO sternum with breathing technique; lateral sternum on inspiration; and 15° to 20° left anterior oblique (LAO) of sternoclavicular joint with suspended inspiration
7. Suspend respiration during inspiration to move the diaphragms below the eighth ribs.
8. LPO and horizontal beam lateral projections (may use 15° to 20° mediolateral central angle if patient cannot be in oblique position)
9. Erect PA and LAO (or RPO) position with suspended **inspiration**
10. Recumbent PA (or AP if the patient cannot assume prone position) and LPO (or RAO) positions with suspended **expiration**

Review Exercise D: Critique Radiographs of the Bony Thorax

A. Ribs above diaphragm (Fig. C10-43)
See explanation on p. 222.

B. Oblique sternum (Fig. C10-44)
1. All pertinent anatomic structures included
2. Sternum overobliqued; sternum away from the spine and rotated beyond heart shadow and distorted (NOTE: Because of additional patient dose, some departments may choose not to repeat this projection because the outline of the sternum is visible.)
3. Collimation not completely evident; central ray centering and IR placement correct
4. Acceptable exposure factors and processing
5. No evidence of anatomic side marker
Repeatable errors: criteria 2

B. Ribs below diaphragm (Fig. C10-45)
1. Right lower ribs cut off; only lower three pair of ribs demonstrated, indicating diaphragm is too low from poor expiration
2. No elevation of diaphragm; need to take exposure during expiration with the patient in a recumbent position to raise the diaphragm to the highest level
3. No evidence of collimation; acceptable central ray centering, but cassette should have been placed crosswise to prevent lateral margins of ribs from being cut off
4. Acceptable exposure factors and processing
5. Anatomic side marker evident but placed a little low and almost off the radiograph
Repeatable errors: criteria 1 and 3

D. Lateral sternum (Fig. C10-46)
1. Lower aspect of sternum cut off
2. Acceptable part positioning
3. No evidence of collimation; central ray centering and IR placement too high, causing lower sternum to be cut off
4. Acceptable exposure factors
5. No evidence of markers
Repeatable errors: criteria 1 and 3

SELF-TEST

My Score = _____%

This self-test should be taken only after completing all of the readings, review exercises, and laboratory activities for a particular section. The purpose of this test is not only to provide a good learning exercise but also to serve as a strong indicator of what your final evaluation grade will cover. It is strongly suggested that if you do not get at least a 90% to 95% grade on each self-test, you should review those areas in which you missed questions before going to your instructor for the final evaluation exam for this chapter. (There are 61 questions or blanks—each is worth 1.6 points.)

1. List the three parts of the sternum:

   A. _____

   B. _____

   C. _____

2. What is the most distal aspect of the sternum? _____.

3. What is the name of the palpable junction between the manubrium and body of the sternum?

   _____.

4. Which one of the following terms is another name for the body of the sternum?

   A. Shaft   C. Gladiolus

   B. Diaphysis   D. Sternal process

5. What distinguishes a true rib from a false rib?

   A. A true rib attaches directly to the sternum with it own costocartilage.

   B. A true rib possesses a costovertebral and a costotransverse joint.

   C. A false rib does not possess a head.

   D. A false rib is primarily composed of cartilage.

6. What distinguishes a floating rib from a false rib?

   A. A floating rib is found only at the T1, T10, and T11 levels.

   B. A floating rib does not possess a head.

   C. A floating rib has no costal groove.

   D. A floating rib does not possess costocartilage.

7. The fifth rib is an example of a _____ (true rib or false rib).

8. Which part of the sternum do the second ribs articulate?

   A. Midbody   C. Middle manubrium

   B. Upper manubrium   D. Sternal angle

9. Which of the structures below is found in the costal groove of each rib?

   A. Nerve   C. Vein

   B. Artery   D. All of the above

10. Match the following joints with the correct type of movement:

   _____ 1. Sternoclavicular   A. Plane (gliding)–diarthrodial

   _____ 2. Costovertebral joint   B. Immovable—synarthrodial

   _____ 3. First sternocostal joint

   _____ 4. Eighth interchondral joint

   _____ 5. Third costochondral union

11. Identify the structures labeled on the following radiographs of the sternum (Figs. 10-5 and 10-6).

Fig. 10-5

A. _____

B. _____ (joint)

C. _____

D. _____

E. _____

F. _____

G. _____

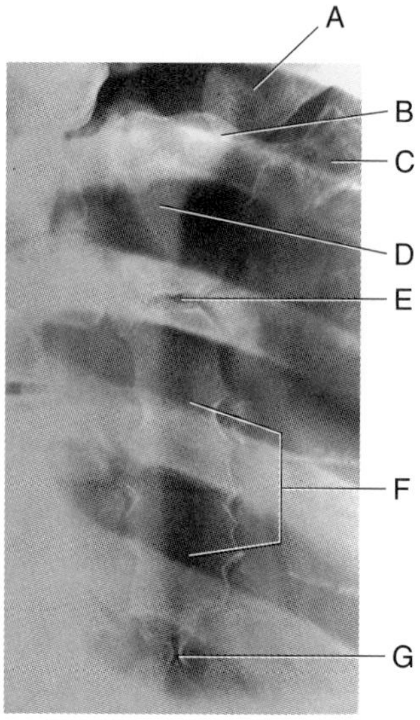

Fig. 10-5. The sternum (A through G).

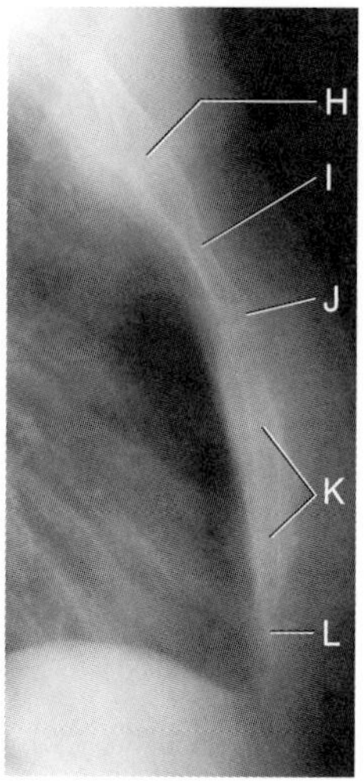

Fig. 10-6. The sternum (H through L).

Fig. 10-6

H. _____

I. _____

J. _____

K. _____

L. _____

12. List the correct positioning considerations for a study of the ribs above the diaphragm:

A. Breathing instructions: _____

B. Kilovoltage peak range: _____

C. General body position: _____

13. What is the minimum source-image distance (SID) for radiography of the sternum? (This is a radiation safety rule.)

_____.

14. Which one of the following breathing instructions should be employed for a right anterior oblique (RAO) position of the sternum?

    A. Suspended inspiration   C. Suspended expiration

    B. Breathing technique   D. Valsalva maneuver

15. List the two factors to be considered when determining which specific projections to include in the rib routine as described in the textbook.

    A. _____ .

    B. _____ .

16. Which two possible chest conditions may result from a rib injury requiring a posteroanterior (PA) and lateral chest projections to be included with the rib routine?

    A. _____   B. _____

17. A. What is the average degree of obliquity for an RAO position of the sternum?

    _____ .

    B. Does an asthenic patient require a little more or a little less obliquity than a hypersthenic patient?

    _____ .

18. For which of the following conditions of the bony thorax are nuclear medicine bone scans *not* normally performed?

    A. Patients with possible fractures   C. Patients with history of multiple myeloma

    B. Patients with osteoporosis   D. Patients with osteomyelitis

19. Pathology of the sternum is most commonly due to:

    A. Metastases   C. Infection

    B. Osteoporosis   D. Blunt trauma

20. What is the average breast dose range for: (A) a posterior oblique rib projection _____ and

    (B) an anterior oblique rib projection _____ ?

21. What other position could be used for the sternum if the patient cannot assume the RAO position?

    A. Left anterior oblique (LAO)   C. Left posterior oblique (LPO)

    B. Right posterior oblique (RPO)   D. Left lateral decubitus

22. How should the arms be positioned for a lateral projection of the sternum?

    A. Raised over the head   C. Depressed by holding 5 to 10 lb in each hand

    B. Drawn back   D. Extended in front of the thorax

23. Which radiographic sign can be evaluated to determine whether rotation is present on a PA projection of the sternoclavicular (SC) joints? _____ .

24. How much obliquity is required for the anterior oblique projection of the sternoclavicular joints?

    _____ .

25. Where is the central ray centered for an AP projection of the ribs below the diaphragm?

_____.

26. What range of kilovoltage peak should be used for ribs above the diaphragm?

A. 55 to 65 kVp   C. 80 to 90 kVp

B. 65 to 75 kVp   D. 90 to 100 kVp

27. Which one of the following positions or projections will best demonstrate the right axillary ribs?

A. LAO   C. RAO

B. LPO   D. PA

28. A radiograph of an RAO projection of the sternum reveals that the width of the sternum is foreshortened and the sternum is shifted away from the spine and out of the heart shadow. The patient has a large "barrel" chest. The technologist performed the RAO with 20° to 25° of obliquity and used a breathing technique. Which positioning error led to this radiographic outcome?

_____.

29. A radiograph of a lateral sternum reveals that anterior ribs are superimposed over the sternum. Which specific positioning error led to this radiographic outcome?

_____.

30. **Situation:** A patient with an injury to the **right lower posterior ribs** enters the emergency room. List the positioning routine that would be used for this patient. Include breathing instructions.

A. Positions performed: _____.

B. Breathing instructions: _____.

31. **Situation:** A patient with an injury to the left, upper, anterior ribs enters the emergency room. List the positioning routine that would be used for this patient and include positions used and breathing instructions.

A. Positions performed: _____.

B. Breathing instructions: _____.

32. **Situation:** A routine chest study reveals a possible lesion near the left sternoclavicular joint. A PA projection of the sternoclavicular joints is taken, but the area of interest is superimposed over the spine. What specific position can be

used to better demonstrate this region? _____.

33. True/False: The automatic exposure control (AEC) system is recommended for sternum and rib routines if the center chamber is utilized.

34. True/False: A breathing technique is recommended for studies of the sternoclavicular joints.

35. For the following critique questions, refer to the oblique sternum radiograph in Fig. C10-44 in your textbook.

   A. Which positioning error(s) are visible on this radiograph? More than one answer may be selected.

   (a) All essential anatomic structures are not demonstrated.

   (b) Central ray is centered incorrectly.

   (c) Collimation is not evident.

   (d) Exposure factors are incorrect.

   (e) No anatomic marker is visible on the radiograph.

   (f) Excessive obliquity of the sternum is evident.

   (g) Insufficient obliquity of the sternum is evident.

   B. Which of the previous criteria are considered "repeatable errors?" _____

   C. Which of the following modifications must be made during the repeat exposure? More than one answer may be selected.

   (a) Center central ray to middle aspect of sternum.

   (b) Increase collimation.

   (c) Decrease exposure factors.

   (d) Increase exposure factors.

   (e) Place anatomic side marker on IR before exposure.

   (f) Decrease obliquity of body.

   (g) Increase obliquity of body.

CHAPTER 11

Cranium

CHAPTER OBJECTIVES

After you have completed **all** the activities in this chapter, you will be able to:

_____ 1. List the eight cranial bones and describe their features, related structures, location, and function.

_____ 2. Using drawings and/or radiographs, identify specific structures of the eight cranial bones.

_____ 3. Define specific terminology, reference points, positioning lines, and topographic landmarks of the cranium

_____ 4. Identify specific radiographic and topographic landmarks of the cranium.

_____ 5. List the location, joint classification, and related terminology for the sutures and joints of the cranium and facial bones.

_____ 6. List the differences among the three shape and size (morphology) classifications of the skull and their implications to radiography of the cranium.

_____ 7. Identify alternative imaging modalities that best demonstrate specific conditions or disease processes of the cranium and brain.

_____ 8. Match specific pathologic indications of the cranium to the correct definition or statements.

_____ 9. Identify the correct size and type of film holder and central ray location, direction, and angle for basic and special projections of the cranium.

_____ 10. Identify which structures are best seen with specific projections of the cranium.

_____ 11. List the patient dose ranges for skin, midline, and thyroid for each basic and special projection of the cranium.

_____ 12. Identify the difference in dose ranges for the thyroid region for frontal projections (anteroposterior [AP]) compared with posteroanterior (PA) projections of the cranium (such as PA axial or PA Caldwell versus AP axial projections).

_____ 13. Given various hypothetical situations, identify the correct modification of a position and/or exposure factors to improve the radiographic image.

POSITIONING AND FILM CRITIQUE

_____ 1. Using a peer, position for basic and special projections of the cranium.

_____ 2. Using a cranial radiographic phantom, produce satisfactory radiographs of specific positions (if equipment is available).

_____ 3. Critique and evaluate cranial radiographs based on the four divisions of radiographic criteria: (1) structures shown, (2) position, (3) collimation and central ray, and (4) exposure criteria.

_____ 4. Distinguish between acceptable and unacceptable cranial radiographs based on exposure factors, motion, collimation, positioning, or other errors.

Learning Exercises

The following review exercises should be completed only after careful study of the associated pages in the textbook as indicated by each exercise.

   After completing each of these individual exercises, check your answers with the answer sheets that follow before continuing to the next exercise.

PART I: Radiographic Anatomy

REVIEW EXERCISE A: Anatomy of the Cranium (see textbook pp. 354-361)

1. Fill in the total number of bones:

   A. Cranium _____   B. Facial bones _____

2. List the four cranial bones that form the calvarium (skull cap):

   A. _____   C. _____

   B. _____   D. _____

3. List the four cranial bones that form the floor of the cranium:

   A. _____   C. _____

   B. _____   D. _____

4. Identify the cranial bones labeled on the drawings (Figs. 11-1 and 11-2). (All eight cranial bones, including each paired bone, are visible in at least one of the following drawings.)

   A. _____

   B. _____

   C. _____

   D. _____

   E. _____

   F. _____

   G. _____

   H. _____

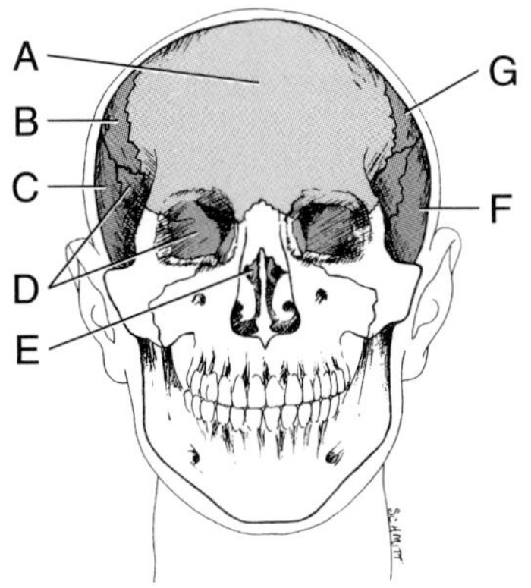

Fig. 11-1 Frontal view.

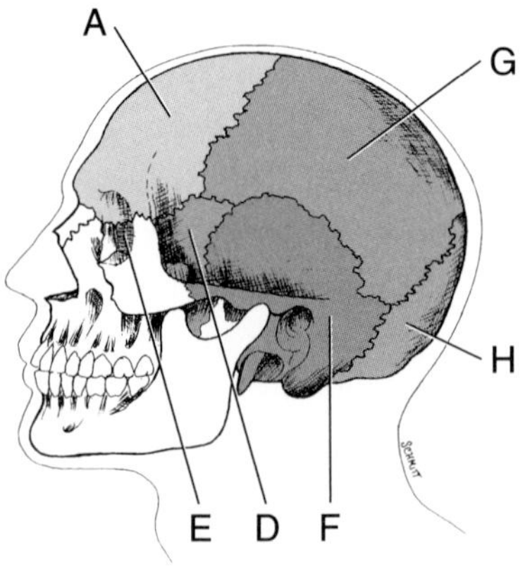

Fig. 11-2 Lateral view.

5. Identify all eight cranial bones on the two superior-view
    drawings (Figs. 11-3 and 11-4).

    A. _____

    B. _____

    C. _____

    D. _____

    E. _____

    F. _____

    G. _____

    H. _____

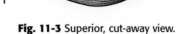
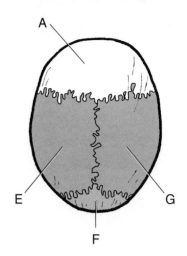

Fig. 11-3 Superior, cut-away view.   **Fig. 11-4** Superior view.

6. Identify the labeled parts on the three views of the ethmoid bone (Figs. 11-5 and 11-6).

    A. _____

    B. _____

    C. _____

    D. _____

    E. _____

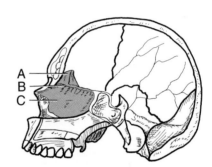

Fig. 11-5 Medial sectional view.

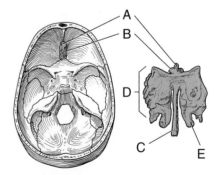

Fig. 11-6 Superior *(left)* and coronal sectional *(right)* views.

7. The small horizontal plate of the ethmoid seen in the above drawings is called the _____.

8. The vertical plate of the ethmoid bone forming the upper portion of the bony nasal septum is the

    _____.

9. Identify the labeled parts on the four views of the sphenoid (Figs. 11-7 through 11-10). Most of the parts are identified on more than one drawing:

A. _____

B. _____

C. _____

D. _____

E. _____

F. _____

G. _____

Foramina:

H. _____

I. _____

J. _____

K. _____

L. _____

M. _____

N. _____

O. _____

P. _____

Q. _____

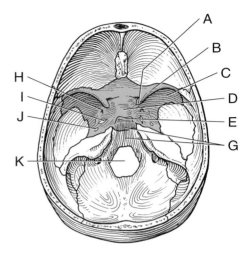

Fig. 11-7 Sphenoid, superior view.

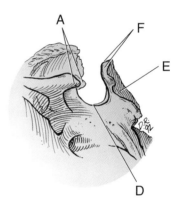

Fig. 11-8 Sphenoid, lateral view.

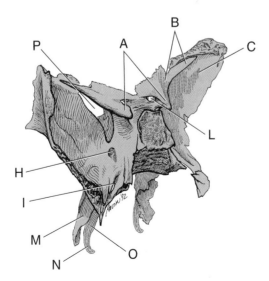

Fig. 11-9 Sphenoid, superior view.

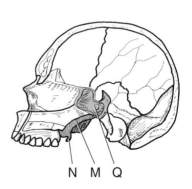

Fig. 11-10 Sphenoid, medial sectional view.

10. A structure found in the middle of the sphenoid bone that surrounds the pituitary gland is the _____.

11. The posterior aspect of the sella turcica is called the _____.

12. Which structure of the sphenoid bone allows for the passage of the optic nerve and is the actual opening into the orbit?

   _____

13. Which structures of the sphenoid bone help form part of the lateral walls of the nasal cavities?

   _____

14. Which radiographic cranial position best demonstrates the sella turcica? _____

15. Which aspect of the frontal bone forms the superior aspect of the orbit? _____

16. Identify the four major sutures and the six associated asterions and fontanels labeled on these drawings of an adult cranium and an infant cranium (Figs. 11-11 to 11-14):

Sutures:

A. _____

B. _____

C. _____

D. _____

Asterions:

E. _____

F. _____

G. Right and left _____

H. Right and left _____

Fontanels: *Associated adult asterion:*

I. _____ (_____)

J. _____ (_____)

K. Right and left _____ (_____)

L. Right and left _____ (_____)

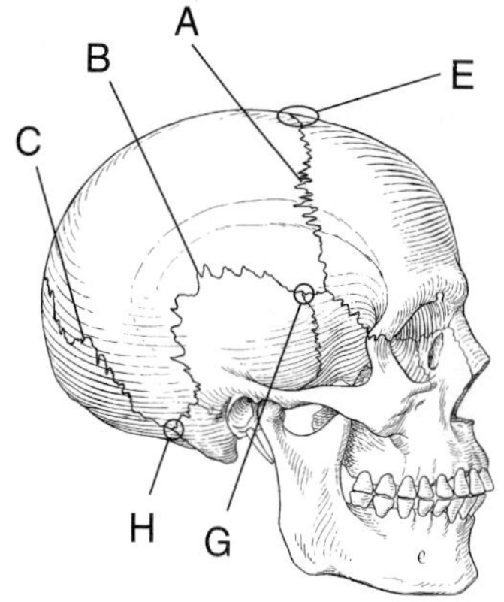

Fig. 11-11 Adult cranium, lateral view.

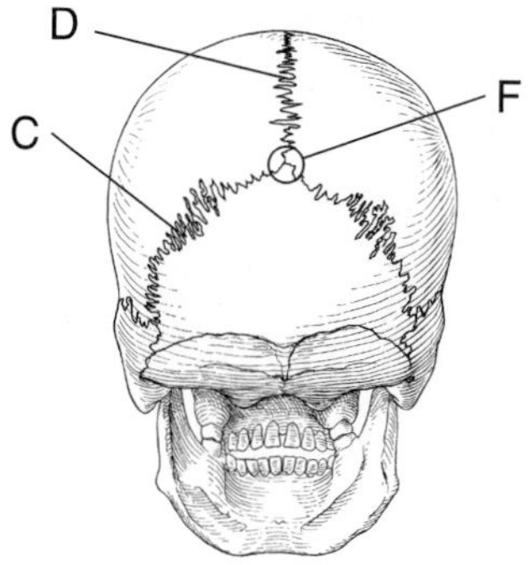

Fig. 11-12 Posterior view.

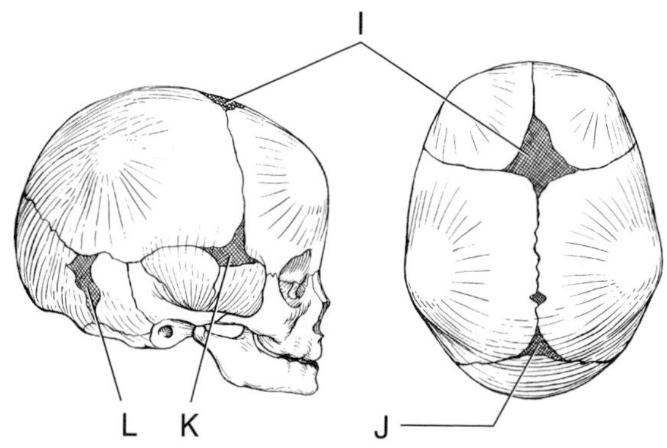

Fig. 11-13 Infant cranium, lateral view.   **Fig. 11-14** Infant cranium, superior view.

17. Cranial sutures are classified as being _____ joints.

18. Small irregular bones that sometimes develop in adult skull sutures are called _____ or

_____ bones and are most frequently found in the _____ suture.

19. Which term and initials describes the superior rim of the orbit? _____

20. What is the name of the notch that separates the orbital plates from each other? _____

21. Which cranial bones form the upper lateral walls of the calvarium? _____

22. Which cranial bone contains the foramen magnum? _____

23. A small prominence located on the squamous portion of the occipital bone is called the

_____.

24. What is the name of the oval processes found on the occipital bone that help form the occipito-atlantal joint?

_____

25. List the three aspects of the temporal bones:

A. _____   B. _____   C. _____

26. True/False: The mastoid portion of the temporal bone is the densest of the three aspects of the temporal bone.

27. Which external landmark corresponds with the level of the petrous ridge? _____

28. Which opening in the temporal bone serves as a passageway for nerves of hearing and equilibrium?

29. Identify the following cranial structures labeled on Figs. 11-15 and 11-16:

Fig. 11-15

A. _____

B. _____

C. _____ (suture)

D. _____ (suture)

E. _____

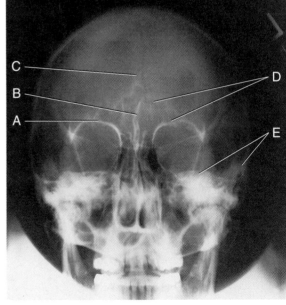

Fig. 11-15 Cranial structures, posteroanterior (PA) Caldwell projection.

Fig. 11-16

A. _____

B. _____

C. _____

D. _____ (suture)

E. _____

F. _____

G. _____

H. _____

I. _____

J. _____ (suture)

K. _____

L. _____

M. _____

N. _____

O. _____

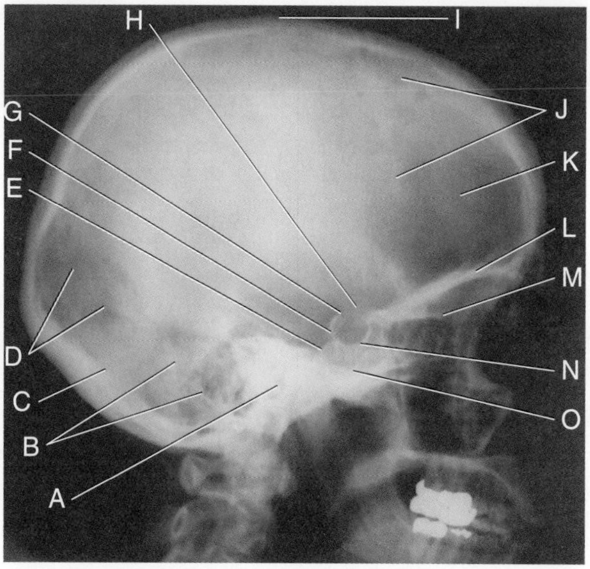

Fig. 11-16 Cranial structures, lateral projection.

PART II: Radiographic Positioning

REVIEW EXERCISE B: Skull Morphology, Topography, and Positioning of the Cranium (see textbook pp. 362-377)

1. List the three classifications of the skull and match them with the correct shape description listed on the right:

   CLASSIFICATION   *SHAPE DESCRIPTION*

   A. _____   a. Width is less than 75% of length

   B. _____   b. Width is 80% or more than length

   C. _____   c. Width is between 75% and 80% of length

2. Central ray angles and degree of rotation stated for basic skull positions are based on the

   _____ (average) skull, which has an angle between the midsagittal plane and the long axis

   of the petrous bone of _____°.

3. The long, narrow-shaped skull has an angle between the midsagittal plane and the long axis of the petrous bone of

   approximately _____°.

4. True/False: Two other terms for the orbitomeatal line (OML) are Reid's base line and the anthropologic base line.

5. There is a _____° difference between the orbitomeatal and infraorbitomeatal lines and _____° between the orbito-meatal and glabellomeatal lines.

6. Match the following cranial landmarks and positioning lines with the correct definition (use each choice only once):

_____ 1. Lateral junction of the eyelid   A. TEA

_____ 2. Posterior angle of the jaw   B. Supraorbital groove

_____ 3. A line between the infraorbital margin and external acoustic meatus (EAM)   C. Interpupillary line

_____ 4. The most prominent point of the external occipital protuberance   D. Nasion

_____ 5. A line between the glabella and alveolar process of the maxilla   E. Gonion

_____ 6. A line between the mental point and EAM   F. Tragus

_____ 7. A depression at the bridge of the nose   G. Outer canthus

_____ 8. The small cartilaginous flap covering the ear opening   H. Glabelloalveolar line

_____ 9. Corresponds to the highest level of the facial bone mass   I. OML

_____ 10. A line between the mid-lateral orbital margin and the EAM   J. Infraorbitomeatal line (IOML)

_____ 11. The center point of the EAM   K. Mentomeatal line

_____ 12. A positioning line that is primarily used for the modified Waters projection   L. Lips-meatal line

_____ 13. A line used in positioning to ensure that the skull is in a true lateral position   M. Glabella

_____ 14. Corresponds to the level of the petrous ridge   N. Inion

_____ 15. A smooth, slightly depressed area between the eyebrows   O. Auricular point

7. What is the average kilovoltage peak range for skull radiography? _____

8. True/False: According to HEW report 76-8031, the patient receives no detectable gonadal exposure during skull radiography when accurate collimation is used.

9. True/False: The anteroposterior (AP) axial (Towne) skull results in about 10 times more dose to the thyroid than a posteroanterior (PA) axial (Haas) projection.

10. The thyroid dose for a SMV projection of the skull is in the _____ range (which is the highest thyroid dose of any skull projection).

A. 10 to 50 mrad   C. 200 to 300 mrad

B. 50 to 100 mrad   D. 500 to 600 mrad

11. List the five most common errors made during skull radiography:

A. _____   C. _____   E. _____

B. _____   D. _____

12. Of the five causes listed in the previous question, which two are the most common?

    A. _____   B. _____

13. True/False: Adults with osteoporosis may require a 25% to 30% reduction in milliamperage seconds during skull projections.

14. Which one of the following imaging modalities is the most common neuroimaging procedure performed for the cranium?

    A. Computed tomography (CT)   C. Magnetic resonance imaging (MRI)

    B. Ultrasound   D. Nuclear medicine

15. Which of the following imaging modalities is usually performed on neonates with a possible intracranial hemorrhage?

    A. CT   C. MRI

    B. Ultrasound   D. Nuclear medicine

16. Which of the following imaging modalities is most commonly performed to evaluate patients for Alzheimer's disease?

    A. CT   C. MRI

    B. Ultrasound   D. Nuclear medicine

17. Match the following pathologic indications to the correct definition or statement (use each choice only once):

    _____ A. Fracture that may produce an air-fluid level in the sphenoid sinus   1. Osteoblastic neoplasm

    _____ B. Destructive lesion with irregular margins   2. Pituitary adenoma

    _____ C. Also called a "ping pong" fracture   3. Basal skull fracture

    _____ D. Proliferative bony lesion of increased density   4. Paget's disease

    _____ E. A tumor that may produce erosion of the dorsum sellae   5. Osteolytic neoplasm

    _____ F. Also known as *osteitis deformans*   6. Depressed skull fracture

    _____ G. A bone tumor that originates in the bone marrow   7. Multiple myeloma

18. Which one of the following pathologic indications may require an increase in manual exposure factors?

    A. Paget's disease   C. Multiple myeloma

    B. Metastatic neoplasm   D. Basal skull fracture

19. Which cranial bone is best demonstrated with an AP axial (Towne method) projection of the skull?

    _____

20. When using a 30° caudad angle for the AP axial (Towne) projection of the skull, which positioning line should be perpendicular to the image receptor?

    A. OML   C. GAL

    B. IOML   D. AML

21. A properly positioned AP axial (Towne) projection should place the dorsum sellae into the middle aspect of the:

    A. Orbits   C. Foramen magnum

    B. Clivus   D. Anterior arch of C1

22. A lack of symmetry of the petrous ridges indicates which of the following problems with a radiograph of an AP axial projection:

    A. Tilt   C. Flexion or extension

    B. Central ray angle   D. Rotation

23. If the patient cannot flex the head adequately for the AP axial (Towne) projection, the technologist could place the

    _____ perpendicular to the image receptor and angle the central ray _____ ° caudad.

24. What evidence on an AP axial (Towne) radiograph indicates whether the correct central ray angle and correct head

    flexion were used? _____

25. What central ray angle should be used for the PA axial (Haas method) projection for the cranium?

    _____

26. Where is the central ray centered for a lateral projection of the skull? _____

27. Which specific positioning error is present if the mandibular rami are *not* superimposed on a lateral skull radiograph?

    A. Tilt   C. Overflexion of head and neck

    B. Rotation   D. Incorrect central ray angle

28. Where will the petrous ridges be projected with a 15° PA axial (Caldwell) projection of the cranium?

    _____

29. Which specific positioning error is present if the petrous ridges are projected **higher** in the orbits than expected for

    a 15° PA axial projection? _____

30. Which projection of the cranium produces an image of the frontal bone with little or no distortion?

    _____

31. With a possible trauma patient, what must be determined before performing the submentovertex (SMV) projection

    of the skull? _____

32. Where is the central ray centered for a lateral projection of the sella turcica? _____

33. Which skull positioning line is placed parallel to the plane of the IR for the SMV projection?

    A. OML   C. AML

    B. IOML   D. GML

34. Which one of the following AP axial projections best visualizes the anterior clinoids and projects the dorsum sella just above the foramen magnum?

    A. 30° caudal to IOML   C. 30° caudal to OML

    B. 37° caudal to IOML   D. 45° caudal to OML

35. Which one of the following projections best demonstrate the sella turcica in profile?

  A. AP axial   C. 15° PA axial

  B. SMV   D. Lateral

36. Which one of the following projections best demonstrates the foramen rotundum?

  A. SMV   C. 30° PA axial

  B. 25° to 30° AP axial   D. Lateral

37. Which one of the following projections best demonstrates the clivus?

  A. AP axial   C. Lateral

  B. 15° PA   D. SMV

REVIEW EXERCISE C: Problem Solving for Technical and Positioning Errors (see textbook pp. 362-377)

  1. A radiograph of an AP axial projection of the cranium reveals that the right petrous ridge is wider than the left side. Which **specific** positioning error is present on this radiograph?

  _____

  2. A radiograph of a 15° PA axial projection of the cranium indicates that the petrous ridges are projected at the inferior orbital margin. Which positioning error(s) led to this radiographic outcome?

  _____

  _____

  3. A radiograph of a 15° PA axial (Caldwell) projection indicates that distance between the midlateral borders of the orbit and lateral margin of the skull is not equal. Which positioning error led to this radiographic outcome?

  _____

  4. A radiograph of an SMV projection of the skull reveals that the mandibular condyles are within the petrous bone. Which specific positioning error led to this problem?

  _____

  5. A radiograph of a lateral projection of the skull reveals that the orbital plates are not superimposed (one orbital plate is slightly superior to the other). Which specific positioning error led to this radiographic outcome?

  _____

  6. A lateral skull radiograph demonstrates one mandibular ramus about 0.5 cm more anterior than the other. Which positioning error occurred?

  _____

  7. An AP axial (Towne) radiograph demonstrates the dorsum sellae projected above or superior to, rather than within, the foramen magnum. Which positioning error occurred?

  _____

  8. **Situation:** A patient comes to the radiology department with a possible tumor of the pituitary gland. Which projection of the cranium best demonstrates any bony involvement of the sella turcica?

  _____

9. **Situation:** A patient with a possible linear fracture of the right parietal bone enters the emergency room. Which single projection of the skull best demonstrates this fracture?

    _____

10. **Situation:** A patient comes to the radiology department for a skull series, but the patient cannot assume the correct position for either version of the AP axial Towne projection because of a very short neck and severe spinal kyphosis. What can the technologist do to demonstrate the occipital bone?

    _____

11. **Situation:** A patient with a possible basal skull fracture enters the emergency room. Which specific position may provide radiographic evidence of this fracture?

    _____

12. **Situation:** A neonate has a clinical history of craniosynostosis. Because of the age of the patient, the physician does not order a radiographic procedure of the cranium. What other imaging modality can be performed to evaluate the patient for this condition?

    _____

REVIEW EXERCISE D: Critique Radiographs of the Cranium (see textbook p. 378)

The following questions relate to the radiographs found at the end of Chapter 11 of the textbook. Evaluate these radiographs for the radiographic criteria categories (*1* through *5*) that follow. Describe the corrections needed to improve the overall image. The major, or "repeatable," errors are specific errors that indicate the need for a repeat exposure, regardless of the nature of the other errors.

A. **Lateral skull: 4-year-old (Fig. C11-62)**

    1. Structures shown: _____

    2. Part positioning: _____

    3. Collimation and central ray: _____

    4. Exposure criteria: _____

    5. Markers: _____

    Repeatable error(s): _____

B. **Lateral skull: 54 year-old, traumatic injury (Fig. C11-63)**

    1. Structures shown: _____

    2. Part positioning: _____

    3. Collimation and central ray: _____

    4. Exposure criteria: _____

    5. Markers: _____

    Repeatable error(s): _____

C. AP axial: Towne skull (Fig. C11-64)

1. Structures shown: _____

2. Part positioning: _____

3. Collimation and central ray: _____

4. Exposure criteria: _____

5. Markers: _____

    Repeatable error(s): _____

D. AP or PA skull (Fig. C11-65)

How can you determine whether this was a PA or an AP projection? _____

_____

1. Structures shown: _____

2. Part positioning: _____

3. Collimation and central ray: _____

4. Exposure criteria: _____

5. Markers: _____

    Repeatable error(s): _____

E. AP or PA skull (Fig. C11-66)

Is this an AP or a PA skull? Compare with Fig. C11-65, and look at size of the orbits. _____

_____

1. Structures shown: _____

2. Part positioning: _____

3. Collimation and central ray: _____

4. Exposure criteria: _____

5. Markers: _____

    Repeatable error(s): _____

PART III: Laboratory Exercises (see textbook pp. 370-377)

You must gain experience in positioning each part of the cranium before performing the following exams on actual patients. You can get experience in positioning and radiographic evaluation of these projections by performing exercises using radiographic phantoms and practicing on other students (although you will not be taking actual exposures).

    The following suggested activities assume that your teaching institution has an energized lab and radiographic phantoms. If not, perform Laboratory Exercises B and C, the radiographic evaluation and the physical positioning exercises. (Check off each step and projection as you complete it.)

LABORATORY EXERCISE A: Energized Laboratory

1. Using the skull radiographic phantom, produce radiographs of the following basic routines:

   _____ 15° PA axial skull   _____ PA axial (Haas)   _____ AP axial sella turcica

   _____ Lateral skull   _____ SMV   _____ Lateral sella turcica

   _____ AP axial skull

LABORATORY EXERCISE B

1. Evaluate and critique the radiographs produced during the previous experiments, additional radiographs provided by your instructor, or both. Evaluate each radiograph for the following points. (Check off when completed.):

   _____ Evaluate the completeness of the study. (Are all of the pertinent anatomic structures included on the radiograph?)

   _____ Evaluate for positioning or centering errors (e.g., rotation, off centering).

   _____ Evaluate for correct exposure factors and possible motion. (Are the density and contrast of the images acceptable?)

   _____ Determine whether markers and an acceptable degree of collimation and/or area shielding are visible on the images.

LABORATORY EXERCISE C: Physical Positioning

On another person, simulate performing all basic and special projections of the sternum and ribs as follows. (Check off each when completed satisfactorily.) Include the following six steps as described in the textbook.

   Step 1. Appropriate size and type of film holder with correct markers
   Step 2. Correct central ray placement and centering of part to central ray and/or film
   Step 3. Accurate collimation
   Step 4. Area shielding of patient where advisable
   Step 5. Use of proper immobilizing devices when needed
   Step 6. Approximate correct exposure factors, breathing instructions where applicable, and "making" exposure

Projections	Step 1	Step 2	Step 3	Step 4	Step 5	Step 6
Skull series: basic						
• AP axial (Towne)	____	____	____	____	____	____
• Lateral skull	____	____	____	____	____	____
• PA 15° axial (Caldwell)	____	____	____	____	____	____
Skull series: special						
• PA axial (Haas)	____	____	____	____	____	____
• SMV	____	____	____	____	____	____
Sella turcica: basic						
• Lateral	____	____	____	____	____	____
• AP axial (Towne)	____	____	____	____	____	____

ANSWERS TO REVIEW EXERCISES

Review Exercise A: Anatomy of the Cranium

1. A. 8
   B. 14
2. A. Frontal
   B. Right parietal
   C. Left parietal
   D. Occipital
3. A. Right temporal
   B. Left temporal
   C. Sphenoid
   D. Ethmoid
4. A. Frontal
   B. Right parietal
   C. Right temporal
   D. Sphenoid
   E. Ethmoid
   F. Left temporal
   G. Left parietal
   H. Occipital
5. A. Frontal
   B. Ethmoid
   C. Sphenoid
   D. Left temporal
   E. Left parietal
   F. Occipital
   G. Right parietal
   H. Right temporal
6. A. Crista galli
   B. Cribriform plate
   C. Perpendicular plate
   D. Lateral labyrinth (mass)
   E. Middle nasal conchae (turbinate)
7. Cribriform plate
8. Perpendicular plate
9. A. Anterior clinoid processes
   B. Lesser wing
   C. Greater wing
   D. Sella turcica
   E. Dorsum sellae
   F. Posterior clinoid process
   G. Clivis
   H. Foramen rotundum
   I. Foramen ovale
   J. Foramen spinosum
   K. Jugular foramen
   L. Optic foramen
   M. Lateral pterygoid process (plate)
   N. Pterygoid hamulus
   O. Medial pterygoid process (plate)
   P. Superior orbital fissure
   Q. Body of sphenoid (sinus)
10. Sella turcica
11. Dorsum sellae
12. Optic foramen
13. Medial and lateral pterygoid processes
14. Lateral

15. Orbital or horizontal portion
16. A. Coronal
    B. Squamosal
    C. Lambdoidal
    D. Sagittal
    E. Bregma
    F. Lambda
    G. Pterion
    H. Asterion
    I. Anterior (bregma)
    J. Posterior (lambda)
    K. Sphenoid (pterion)
    L. Mastoid (asterion)
17. Fibrous or synarthrodial
18. Sutural or Wormian, lambdoidal
19. Supraorbital margin, or SOM
20. Ethmoidal notch
21. Right and left parietals
22. Occipital
23. External occipital protuberance, or inion
24. Occipital condyles, or lateral condylar portions
25. A. Squamous
    B. Mastoid
    C. Petrous
26. False (petrous portion)
27. Top of the ear attachment, or TEA
28. Internal acoustic meatus
29. *Fig. 11-15*
    A. Supraorbital margins of right orbit
    B. Crista galli of ethmoid
    C. Sagittal suture-posterior skull
    D. Lambdoidal suture-posterior skull
    E. Petrous ridge
    Fig. 11-16
    A. External acoustic meatus (EAM)
    B. Mastoid portion of temporal bone
    C. Occipital bone
    D. Lambdoidal suture
    E. Clivus
    F. Dorsum sellae
    G. Posterior clinoid processes
    H. Anterior clinoid processes
    I. Vertex of skull
    J. Coronal suture
    K. Frontal bone
    L. Orbital plates of frontal bone
    M. Cribform plate
    N. Sella turcica
    O. Body of sphenoid bone: sphenoid sinus

Review Exercise B: Skull Morphology, Topography, and Positioning of the Cranium

1. A. Mesocephalic (c)
   B. Brachycephalic (b)

   C. Dolichocephalic (a)
2. Mesocephalic, 47
3. ±40
4. False (Two other terms for the *infraorbitomeatal* line)
5. 7° to 8°, 7° to 8° (same degrees of difference)
6. 1. G
   2. E
   3. J
   4. N
   5. H
   6. K
   7. D
   8. F
   9. B
   10. I
   11. O
   12. L
   13. C
   14. A
   15. M
7. 75 to 85 kVp
8. True
9. True
10. C. (200 to 300 mrad)
11. A. Rotation
    B. Tilt
    C. Excessive flexion
    D. Excessive extension
    E. Incorrect central ray angulation
12. A. Rotation
    B. Tilt
13. True
14. A. Computed tomography (CT)
15. B. Ultrasound
16. D. Nuclear medicine
17. A. 3
    B. 5
    C. 6
    D. 1
    E. 2
    F. 4
    G. 7
18. A. Paget's disease
19. Occipital
20. A. Orbitomeatal line (OML)
21. C. Foramen magnum
22. D. Rotation
23. Infraorbitomeatal line (IOML), 37
24. Dorsum sellae and posterior clinoids should be projected into the foramen magnum.
25. 25° cephalad
26. 2 inches (5 cm) above the EAM
27. B. Rotation
28. In the lower one third of the orbits
29. Excessive flexion or insufficient central ray angle
30. 0° posteroanterior (PA)

31. Rule out any possible cervical fractures or subluxation.
32. ½ inch (2 cm) anterior and ½ inch (2 cm) superior to EAM
33. B. IOML
34. A. 30° caudal to IOML
35. D. Lateral
36. C. 30° PA axial
37. C. Lateral

Review Exercise C: Problem-Solving for Technical and Positioning Errors

1. Rotation of skull present; rotation of skull toward left
2. Excessive extension or excessive caudad central ray angle—projects the petrous ridges lower than expected (should be in the lower third of the orbit)
3. Rotation of the skull
4. Insufficient extension of the skull, or central ray was not perpendicular to IOML
5. Skull tilt
6. Skull rotation
7. Central ray angled less than 37° to the IOML, or less than 30° to the OML (would be caused by 30° angle to IOML)
8. Collimated, lateral projection of the sella turcica
9. Right lateral projection of the skull
10. Should perform the PA axial projection or Haas method
11. Horizontal beam lateral position—will demonstrate a possible air-fluid level in the sphenoid sinus
12. Ultrasound—a noninvasive means of evaluating the newborn's cranium

Review Exercise D: Critique Radiographs

A. Lateral skull: 4-year-old (Fig. C11-62)
   1. Foreign bodies (earrings) obscuring essential anatomic structures
   2. Correct part positioning, but patient's hand seen supporting mandible; can use positioning sponge if needed to support skull
   3. No evidence of collimation; correct central ray and film placement
   4. Appears underexposed on this printed copy (may be a repeatable error if actual radiograph also appears this light)
   5. No evidence of anatomic side marker
   Repeatable errors: criteria 1 and possibly 4

B. Lateral skull: 54-year-old, traumatic injury (Fig. C11-63)
   1. Vertex of the skull just slightly cut off (may be repeatable error because of proximity to the site of trauma)
   2. Tilted and rotated skull (separation of the orbital plates from the tilt, and separation of the greater wings of the sphenoid, the rami of the mandible, and the EAMs—all indicating rotation)
   3. No evidence of collimation; slightly high central ray centering if the photo borders are also the collimation borders, which would add to the tilt appearance
   4. Acceptable exposure factors
   5. No evidence of anatomic side marker
   Repeatable errors: criteria 1and 2

C. AP axial: Towne skull (C11-64)
   1. Entire occipital bone and foramen magnum demonstrated
   2. Correct part positioning
   3. No evidence of collimation; overangled central ray; anterior arch of C1 projected into the foramen magnum rather than the dorsum sellae
   4. Acceptable but slightly underexposed exposure factors

   5. No evidence of anatomic side marker
   Repeatable errors: criteria 3

D. AP or PA skull (Fig. C11-65)
AP projection, as indicated by the large size of the orbits, which was caused by magnification from increased object-image distance (OID) (can compare with radiograph that follows)
   1. All pertinent anatomic structures demonstrated but with some foreshortening of frontal bone
   2. Petrous ridges not in the lower third of orbits; position requires more flexion or less central ray angle as an AP; skull slightly rotated (note distance between orbits and lateral margins of skull)
   3. No evidence of collimation; less central ray angle needed (see previous answer) (can compare with correctly angled central ray on PA radiograph in Fig. C11-66)
   4. Acceptable exposure factors
   5. No evidence of anatomic side marker
   Repeatable errors: criteria 2 and 3

E. AP or PA skull (Fig. C11-66)
PA 15° Caldwell projection
   1. All pertinent anatomic structures not demonstrated; patient ID marker and side marker obscuring skull
   2. Correct part positioning
   3. Evidence of collimation (circular cone); size of cassette too small for the skull; correct central ray placement and angle (petrous ridges in lower third of orbit)
   4. Acceptable exposure factors
   5. Evidence of anatomic side marker, but it is placed over skull; patient ID marker is over upper right cranium (both repeatable errors.)
   Repeatable errors: criteria 1 and 5

SELF-TEST

My Score = _____%

This self-test should be taken only after completing all of the readings, review exercises, and laboratory activities for a particular section. The purpose of this test is not only to provide a good learning exercise but also to serve as a strong indicator of what your final unit evaluation grade will cover. It is strongly suggested that if you do not get at least a 90% to 95% grade on each self-test, you should review those areas in which you missed questions before going to your instructor for the final unit evaluation exam.

1. Which one of the following bones is *not* part of the floor of the cranium?

    A. Temporal   B. Ethmoid   C. Occipital   D. Sphenoid

2. Which aspect of the frontal bone is thin walled and forms the forehead?

    A. Orbital   B. Horizontal   C. Squamous   D. Superciliary margin

3. Which four cranial bones articulate with the frontal bone?

    A. _____   C. _____

    B. _____   D. _____

4. Which structures are found at the widest aspect of the skull? _____

5. What is the name of a prominent landmark (or "bump") found on the external surface of the occipital bone?

    _____

6. List the number of individual bones that articulate with the following cranial bones:

    A. Parietal bone _____

    B. Occipital bone _____

    C. Temporal bone _____

    D. Sphenoid _____

    E. Ethmoid _____

7. What is the thickest and densest structure in the cranium? _____

8. True/False: The hypophysis is another term for the pituitary gland.

9. True/False: The sphenoid bone articulates with all the other cranial bones.

10. The shallow depression just posterior to the base of the dorsum sellae and anterior to the foramen magnum is the:

    _____.

11. What is the name of the paired collections of bone found inferior to the cribriform plate that contain numerous air

    cells and help form the lateral walls of the nasal cavity? _____

12. Which small section of bone is located superior to the cribriform plate? _____

13. What is the formal term for the left sphenoid fontanel in the adult? _____

14. What is the name of the cranial suture formed by the inferior junction of the parietals to the temporal bones?

_____

15. What are the two terms for the small, irregular bones found in the adult skull sutures?

_____

16. Match the following structures to their related cranial bone:

_____ 1. Pterygoid hamulus   A. Occipital

_____ 2. Anterior clinoid processes   B. Frontal

_____ 3. Glabella   C. Sphenoid

_____ 4. Foramen ovale   D. Ethmoid

_____ 5. Perpendicular plate   E. Temporal

_____ 6. Superior nasal conchae   F. Parietal

_____ 7. Foramen magnum

_____ 8. Cribriform plate

_____ 9. Zygomatic process

_____ 10. Lateral condylar portions

_____ 11. Superciliary arch

_____ 12. External acoustic meatus (EAM)

_____ 13. Inion

_____ 14. Sella turcica

_____ 15. Petrous ridge

17. Identify the following cranial structures labeled on the following radiographs (Figs. 11-17 and 11-18).

Fig. 11-17:

STRUCTURE   **BONE(S)**

A. _____

B. _____

C. _____

D. _____ (suture)

E. _____

F. _____

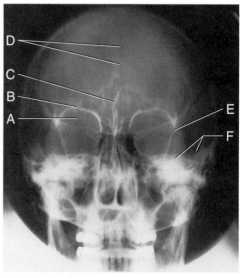

Fig. 11-17 PA Caldwell cranium.

Fig. 11-18:

G. _____

H. _____

I. _____

J. _____

K. _____

L. _____

M. _____

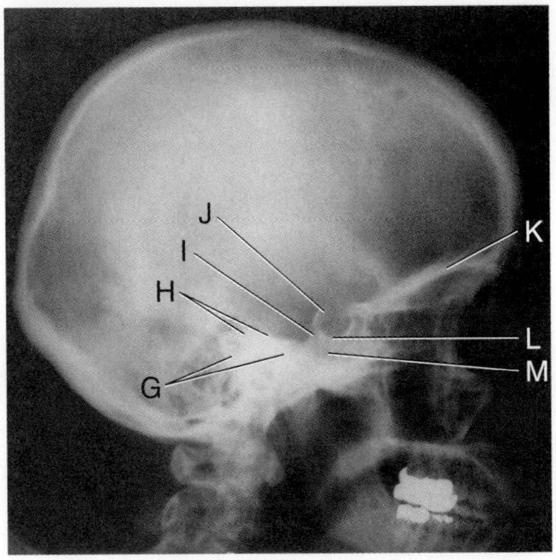

Fig. 11-18 Lateral cranium.

18. Which one of the following skull classifications applies to a skull with an angle of 54° between the midsagittal plane and the long axis of the petrous bone?

    A. Mesocephalic   C. Brachycephalic

    B. Dolichocephalic   D. None of the above

19. Which of the above classifications is considered the average-shape skull? _____

20. Identify the labeled landmarks and positioning lines used in skull and facial bone positioning as shown in Fig. 11-19 (including abbreviations):

    A. _____

    B. _____

    C. _____

    D. _____

    E. _____

    F. _____

    G. _____

    H. _____

    I. _____

    J. _____

    K. _____

    L. _____

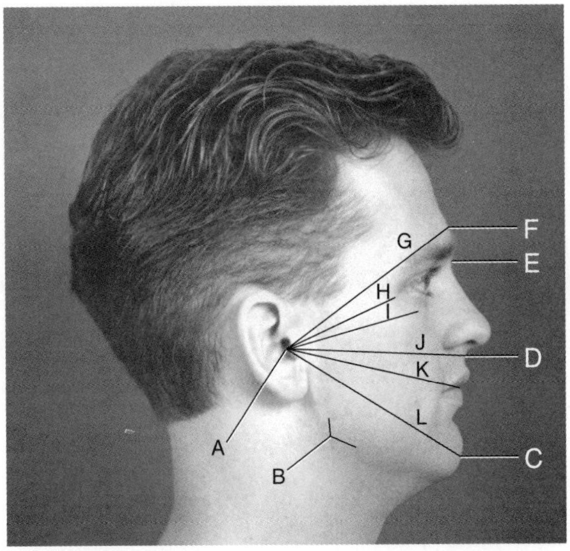

Fig. 11-19 Skull and facial bone landmarks and positioning lines

21. The center point of structure *A* as used for the positioning lines in the previous question is called the

_____.

22. Which one of the following terms is defined as the large cartilaginous aspect of the external ear?

    A. Pinna   C. Glabella

    B. Tragus   D. Acanthion

23. Reid's base line is also more commonly referred to as:

    A. GML   C. OML

    B. IOML   D. GAL

24. How much of a difference in degrees is there between the OML and IOML?

    A. 10°   C. 3°

    B. 7° to 8°   D. None. They represent the same positioning line.

25. Which one of the following positioning errors almost always results in a repeat exposure of a cranial position?

    A. Rotation   C. Slight flexion

    B. Incorrect central ray placement   D. None of the above

26. Match the following pathologic indications to the correct definition or statement (use each choice only once):

    _____ A. Bone tumor originating in the bone marrow   1. Linear fracture

    _____ B. Fracture evident by sphenoid sinus effusion   2. Paget's disease

    _____ C. Condition that begins with bony destruction followed by bony repair   3. Depressed fracture

    _____ D. Destructive lesion with irregular margins   4. Osteolytic neoplasm

    _____ E. Fracture of the skull with jagged or irregular lucent line   5. Multiple myeloma

    _____ F. Tangential view may be helpful to determine extent or degree of this fracture   6. Basal fracture

27. Which one of the following pathologic indications may require a decrease in manual exposure factors?

    A. Pituitary adenoma   C. Paget's disease

    B. Linear skull fracture   D. Multiple myeloma

28. Which one of the following imaging modalities may be used to examine a possible cranial bleed caused by trauma?

    A. Computed tomography (CT)   C. Ultrasound

    B. Magnetic resonance imaging (MRI)   D. Nuclear medicine

29. Which one of the following imaging modalities provides an excellent distinction between normal and abnormal brain tissue?

    A. CT   C. Ultrasound

    B. MRI   D. Nuclear medicine

30. Which two projections of the cranium project the dorsum sellae within the foramen magnum?

    A. _____

    B. _____

31.   A.   What central ray angle is used for the anteroposterior (AP) axial projection (Towne method) with the IOML

      perpendicular to the image receptor? _____

      B.   What is the central ray angle for this same projection with a perpendicular OML?_____

32.   Where is the central ray centered for a lateral projection of the cranium? _____

33.   To prevent tilting of the skull for the lateral projection of the cranium, the _____ line is
      placed perpendicular to the image receptor.

34.   Where should the petrous ridges be located, on the image, for a well-positioned, 30° caudad, posteroanterior (PA)

      axial (alternate PA Caldwell) projection? _____

35.   Where is the central ray centered for a submentovertex (SMV) projection of the skull?

      _____

36.   A.   How much is the central ray angled to the IOML for an AP axial projection of the sella turcica when the poste-

      rior clinoid processes are of primary interest? _____

      B.   How much is the central ray angled to the IOML when the anterior clinoid processes are of primary interest?

      _____

37.   A radiograph of an AP axial projection for the cranium reveals that the dorsum sellae is projected just above rather
      than into the foramen magnum. What must be modified during the repeat exposure to correct this problem?

      _____

38.   A radiograph of a lateral projection of the cranium reveals that the mandibular rami are *not* superimposed. What
      type of positioning error is present on this radiograph?

      _____

39.   A radiograph of a 15° caudad PA axial projection of the cranium reveals that the petrous ridges are at the level of
      the supraorbital margin. Without changing the central ray angle, how must the head position be modified during the
      repeat exposure to produce a more acceptable image?

      _____

      _____

40.   **Situation:** A patient with a possible basilar skull fracture enters the emergency room. The physician wants a projec-
      tion to demonstrate a possible sphenoid sinus effusion. Which projection of the cranium would be best for this situa-
      tion?

      _____

41.   **Situation:** The same patient in the previous situation also requires a frontal projection of the skull. The physician
      wants the projection to demonstrate the frontal bone and place the petrous ridges in the lower one third of the orbits,
      but it has not been determined whether the patient's cervical spine has been fracture so the patient can't be moved
      from a supine position. What should the technologist do to obtain this image?

      _____

42. **Situation:** A patient comes to the radiology department for a skull series. Because of the size of his shoulders, he is unable to flex his neck sufficiently to place the OML perpendicular to the IR for the AP axial projection. His head cannot be raised due to possible cervical trauma. What other options does the technologist have to obtain an acceptable AP axial projection?

_____

_____

43. For the following critique questions, refer to the radiograph of the lateral skull shown in Fig. C11-63 (p. 378) of your textbook.

   A. Which positioning error(s) are visible on this radiograph? More than one answer may be selected.

      (a) All essential anatomic structures are not demonstrated.

      (b) Central ray is centered incorrectly.

      (c) Collimation is not evident.

      (d) Exposure factors are incorrect.

      (e) No anatomic marker is visible on the radiograph.

      (f) Tilt of skull is evident.

      (g) Rotation of skull is evident.

      (h) Excessive flexion and extension are evident.

   B. Which of the previous criteria are considered "repeatable errors?"

   C. Which of the following modifications must be made during the repeat exposure? More than one answer may be selected.

      (a) Increase collimation.

      (b) Center central ray correctly.

      (c) Decrease exposure factors.

      (d) Increase exposure factors.

      (e) Place anatomic marker on image receptor before exposure.

      (f) Adjust skull to place midsagittal plane parallel to plane of image receptor to eliminate rotation and tilt.

      (g) Adjust skull to eliminate excessive flexion and extension.

44. For the following critique questions, refer to the radiograph of the Caldwell position shown in Fig. C11-65 (p. 378) of your textbook.

   A. Which positioning error(s) are visible on this radiograph? More than one answer may be selected.

      (a) All essential anatomic structures are not demonstrated.

      (b) Central ray is centered incorrectly.

      (c) Collimation is not evident.

      (d) Exposure factors are incorrect.

      (e) No anatomic marker is visible on the radiograph.

      (f) Central ray is angled insufficiently.

      (g) No anatomic marker is visible on the radiograph.

      (h) Tilt of skull is evident.

      (i) Rotation of skull is evident.

B. Which of the previous criteria are considered "repeatable errors?" (Petrous ridges should be in the lower third of the orbits.)

C. Which of the following modifications must be made during the repeat exposure? More than one answer may be selected.

   (a) Increase collimation.

   (b) Center central ray correctly.

   (c) Decrease exposure factors.

   (d) Increase exposure factors.

   (e) Place anatomic marker on image receptor before exposure.

   (f) Align midsagittal plane perpendicular to the image receptor to eliminate rotation and tilt.

   (g) Decrease central ray angle or increase flexion.

   (h) Increase central ray angle or increase extension.

Facial Bones

After you have completed **all** the activities of this chapter, you will be able to:

_____ 1. List the specific features, characteristics, location, and functions of the fourteen facial bones.

_____ 2. List the seven cranial and facial bones that make up the bony orbit.

_____ 3. Using drawings and/or radiographs, identify specific structures of the facial bone region.

_____ 4. Explain the advantages of performing facial bone projections erect.

_____ 5. Identify alternative imaging modalities that best demonstrate specific facial bone pathology.

_____ 6. Identify specific types of fractures of the facial bone region.

_____ 7. Identify basic and special projections of the facial bones and list the correct size of image receptor, central ray location, direction, and angulation of the central ray for each projection.

_____ 8. List which structures are best seen with basic and special projections of the facial bones.

_____ 9. Identify the basic operational and positioning considerations when performing a mandible study using the Panorex unit.

_____ 10. List patient dose ranges for skin, midline, and thyroid doses for specific projections of the facial bones.

_____ 11. Given various hypothetical situations, identify the correct modification of a position and/or exposure factors to improve the radiographic image.

_____ 12. Given radiographs of specific facial projections/positions, identify specific errors in positioning and exposure factors.

POSITIONING AND FILM CRITIQUE

_____ 1. Using a peer, position for basic and special projections of the facial bones.

_____ 2. Using a cranial radiographic phantom, produce satisfactory radiographs of specific positions (if equipment is available).

_____ 3. Critique and evaluate facial bone radiographs based on the four divisions of radiographic criteria: (1) Structures shown, (2) position, (3) collimation, and CR (4) exposure criteria.

_____ 4. Distinguish between acceptable and unacceptable cranial radiographs resulting from exposure factors, motion, collimation, positioning, or other errors.

Learning Exercises

The following review exercises should be completed only after careful study of the associated pages in the textbook as indicated by each exercise.

    After completing each of these individual exercises, check your answers with the answer sheets that follow before continuing to the next exercise.

PART I: Radiographic Anatomy

REVIEW EXERCISE A : Radiographic Anatomy of the Facial Bones (see textbook pp. 360-368)

1. Which of the following bones is not a facial bone?

    A. Middle nasal conchae   C. Lacrimal bone

    B. Vomer   D. Mandible

2. What is the largest immovable bone of the face? _____

3. List the four processes of the maxilla:

    A. _____   C. _____

    B. _____   D. _____

4. Which one of the above mentioned processes is considered most superior? _____

5. Which soft-tissue landmark is found at the base of the anterior nasal spine? _____

6. Which facial bones form the posterior aspect of the hard palate? _____

7. Which two cranial bones articulate with the maxilla? _____

8. Which facial bones are sometimes called the "cheek bones"? _____

9. Which of the following bones does not articulate with the zygomatic bone?

    A. Temporal   C. Frontal

    B. Maxilla   D. Sphenoid

10. Which facial bone is associated with the tear ducts? _____

11. The purpose of the _____ is to divide the nasal cavity into compartments and circulate air coming into the nasal cavities. (Include both terms for these bones.)

12. True/False: The majority of the nose is formed by the right and left nasal bones.

13. A deviated nasal septum is most likely to occur at the junction between _____

    and _____ .

14. Match the following mandibular terms to the correct definition (use each choice only once):

      _____ A. Gonion   1. Vertical portion of mandible

      _____ B. Mandibular notch   2. The chin

      _____ C. Body   3. Mandibular angle

      _____ D. Condyloid process   4. The point of union between both halves of the mandible

      _____ E. Coronoid process   5. Bony process located anterior to mandibular notch

      _____ F. Ramus   6. Horizontal portion of mandible

      _____ G. Mentum   7. Posterior process of upper ramus

      _____ H. Symphysis menti   8. "U"- shaped notch

15. Identify the labeled facial bones visible on Figs. 12-1 and 12-2.

Paired bones:

A. _____

B. _____

C. _____

D. _____

E. _____

Single bone:

F. _____

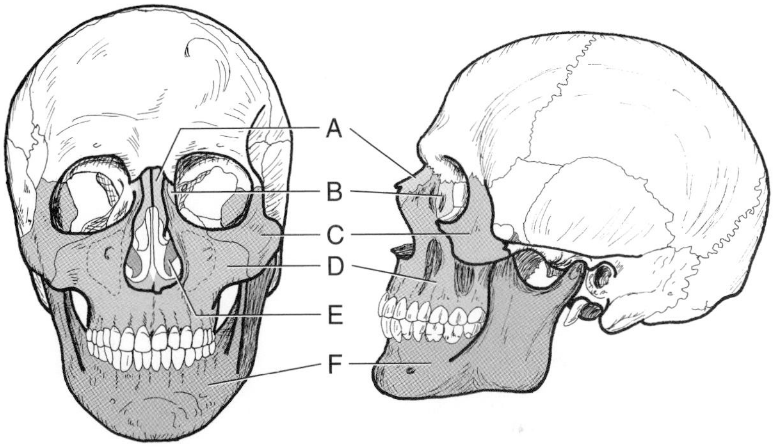

Fig. 12-1 Frontal view.   **Fig. 12-2** Side view.

16. The one single facial bone and the one pair of facial bones not visible from the exterior and not demonstrated on the above drawings are the _____ and _____ , respectively. (These are demonstrated on special view drawings in the following questions.)

17. Identify the labeled structures and the facial bones of which they are a part on this inferior surface view of the maxillae (Fig. 12-3).

           Structure   *Bone(s)*

A. _____ (_____)

B. _____ (_____)

C. _____ (_____)

D. _____ (_____)

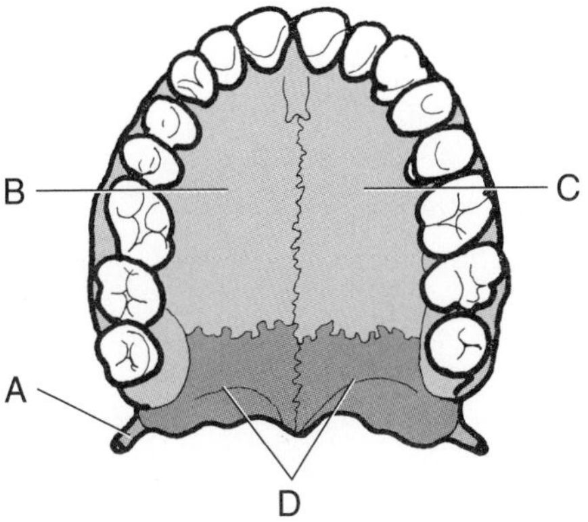

Fig. 12-3 Inferior surface view of the maxillae.

18. List the three structures that form the nasal septum as shown on Fig. 12-4:

    A. _____

    B. _____

    C. _____

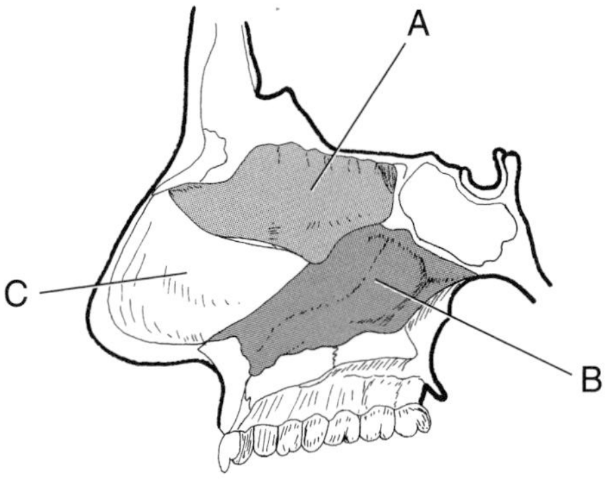

Fig. 12-4 Nasal septum.

19. Identify the parts of the mandible and skull as labeled on Figs. 12-5 and 12-6.

    A. _____

    B. _____

    C. _____

    D. _____

    E. _____

    F. _____

    G. _____

    H. _____

    I. _____

    J. _____

    K. (Cranial bone) _____

    L. (Joint) _____

    M. (Key landmark) _____

    N. (Landmark) _____

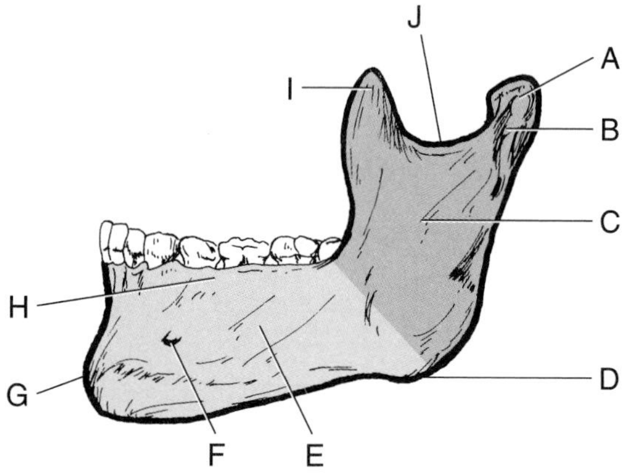

Fig. 12-5 Mandible.

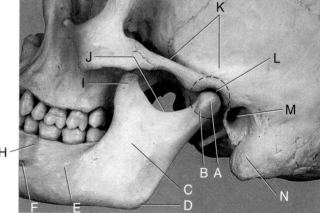

Fig. 12-6 Lateral skull and mandible.

20. Identify the seven bones that form the orbit and indicate whether they are cranial or facial bones (Fig. 12-7).

A. _____ (_____)

B. _____ (_____)

C. _____ (_____)

D. _____ (_____)

E. _____ (_____)

F. _____ (_____)

G. _____ (_____)

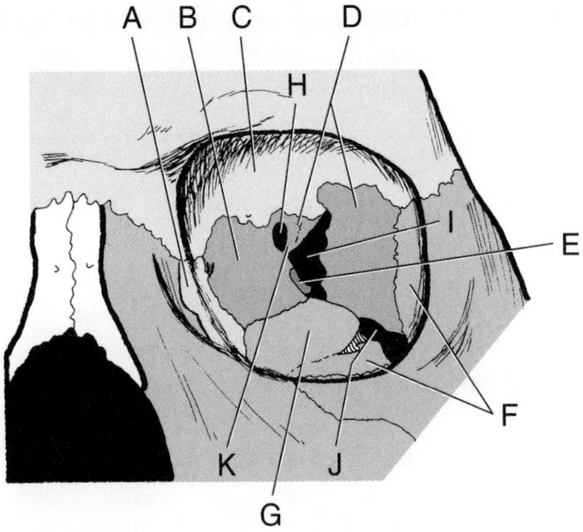

Fig. 12-7 Slightly oblique frontal view of orbit, **A-K.**

21. Identify the three foramina contained within the orbits as labeled on Fig. 12-7.

H. _____

I. _____

J. _____

Small section of bone:

K. _____

22. From anterior to posterior, the cone-shaped orbits project upward at an angle of _____ degrees and toward the

midsagittal plane at an angle of _____ degrees.

PART II: Radiographic Positioning

REVIEW EXERCISE B: Positioning of the Facial Bones, Nasal Bones, Zygomatic Arches, and Optic Foramina and Orbits (see textbook pp. 390-403)

1. True/False: Facial bone studies should be performed recumbent whenever possible.

2. True/False: A horizontal beam lateral position should be taken for the geriatric patient unable to assume the erect position.

3. True/False: An increase in milliamperage seconds of 25% to 30% may be required for the geriatric patient with advanced osteoporosis.

4. True/False: Radiography of the facial bones has decreased because of increased use of CT and MRI.

5. True/False: Nuclear medicine is not used in diagnosing occult facial bone fractures.

6. True/False: MRI is an excellent imaging modality for the detection of small metal foreign bodies in the eye.

7. What is the name of the fracture that results from a direct blow to the orbit and leads to a disruption of the inferior

orbital margin? _____

8. A "free-floating" zygomatic bone is the result of a _____ type fracture.

9. What is the major disadvantage of performing a straight PA projection for facial bones, with no CR angulation or neck extension, as compared with other PA facial bone projections?

   _____

10. Where is the CR centered for a lateral position for facial bones?

    A. Outer canthus   C. Zygoma

    B. Acanthion   D. Nasion

11. What is the proper name method for the parietoacanthial projection of the facial bones? _____

12. Which structures are best seen with a parietoacanthial projection?

    _____

13. What CR angle must be used to project the petrous ridges below the orbital floor with the PA axial (Caldwell method) projection?

    _____

    A. None. CR is perpendicular.   C. 20°

    B. 30°   D. 45°

14. Which structures specifically are visualized better on the modified parietoacanthial (Waters) projection as compared

    with the basic Waters projection? _____

15. Give two reasons why projections of the facial bones are performed PA rather than AP when possible?

    A. _____   B. _____

16. What are three technical differences between the lateral projection of the cranium as compared with the lateral for the facial bones? (Disregard anatomy visualized and image receptor size.)

    A. _____

    B. _____

    C. _____

17. The parietoacanthial (Waters) projection for the facial bones will have the _____ line per-

    pendicular to the image receptor, which places the OML at a _____ angle to the tabletop and image receptor.

18. Where does the CR exit for a parietoacanthial (Waters) projection of the facial bones?

    _____

19. Where does the CR exit for a 15° PA axial (Caldwell) projection for facial bones?

    _____

20. The modified parietoacanthial (modified Waters) projection requires that the _____ line is

    perpendicular to the image receptor, which places the OML at a _____ angle to the tabletop and image receptor.

21. True/False: Lateral projections for nasal bones generally are taken bilaterally for comparison.

22. True/False: The tangential projection for a unilateral zygomatic arch requires that the skull be rotated and tilted 15° **away from** the affected side.

23. True/False: Both oblique inferosuperior (tangential) projections for the zygomatic arch generally are taken for comparison.

24. True/False: The gonadal and/or thyroid dose for all facial bone projections is NDC (no discernible contribution).

25. For a PA Waters projection, the petrous ridges should be projected directly below the _____

    and projected into the lower half of the maxillary sinuses or below the _____ in a modified

    Waters projection.

26. For the superoinferior projection of the nasal bones, the image receptor is placed perpendicular to the

    _____ line (include both full name and abbreviations).

27. Which specific facial bone structures (other than the mandible) are best demonstrated with the submentovertex (SMV)

    projection if correct exposure factors are used (soft tissue technique)?_____

28. Where is the CR centered for an AP axial projection for zygomatic arches?

    _____

29. List the proper name and the common descriptive names used for the parieto-orbital projection for optic foramen.

    A. _____   B. _____

30. The three aspects of the face that should be in contact with the head unit or tabletop when beginning positioning for

    the parieto-orbital projection are the (A) _____, _____, and

    _____. The final angle between the midsagittal plane and the film should be (B)

    _____ with the (C) _____ line perpendicular to the film. This places

    the optic foramen in the (D) _____ quadrant of the orbit.

31. Match the following facial bone projection that **best** matches with the "structures best seen" (use each choice only once):

    _____ 1. Floor of orbits (blowout fractures)   A. Lateral (nasal bones)

    _____ 2. Optic foramen   B. Parietoacanthial projection

    _____ 3. View of single zygomatic arch   C. Parieto-orbital projection

    _____ 4. Profile image of nasal bones and nasal septum D. Submentovertex projection

    _____ 5. Bilateral zygomatic arches   E. Modified Waters method

    _____ 6. Inferior orbital rim, maxillae, nasal septum, F. Oblique inferosuperior projection
             nasal spine, zygomatic bone and arches

REVIEW EXERCISE C: Positioning of the Mandible and Temporomandibular joints (TMJ)(see textbook pp. 404-412)

1. Which projection for the mandible results in a thyroid dose that is four or five times greater than the thyroid dose for any other projection described in this chapter? _____

2. Which projection of the mandible will project the opposite half of the mandible away from the side of interest?

   _____

3. What must be done to prevent the ramus of the mandible from being superimposed over the cervical spine with an axiolateral projection of the mandible? _____

4. How much skull rotation toward the image receptor is required with an axiolateral projection for demonstrating the following:

   A. Body of the mandible _____

   B. Mentum region _____

   C. Ramus region _____

   D. General survey of the mandible _____

   E. What CR angle is needed for all of these projections? _____

5. What specific positioning error has been committed if both sides of the mandible are largely superimposed with an axiolateral projection?

   _____

6. Where should the CR exit for a **PA axial** projection of the mandible? _____

7. Which skull line is placed perpendicular to the image receptor for a PA or PA axial projection of the mandible?

   _____

8. True/False: For a true frontal view of the mandibular body (if this is the area of interest), the AML should be perpendicular to the image receptor.

9. True/False: The CR should be angled 20 to 25° caudad for the PA axial projection of the mandible.

10. Which aspect of the mandible is best visualized with an AP axial projection? _____

11. What CR angle is required for the AP axial projection of the mandible if the OML is placed perpendicular to the image receptor? (A) _____ If the IOML is perpendicular, what CR angle is needed? (B)

    _____

12. Describe where the CR is centered, and where it will pass through, for an AP axial projection of the mandible.

    _____

13. Which projection of the mandible will demonstrate the entire mandible, including the coronoid and condyloid processes?

_____

14. Which imaging system provides a single, frontal perspective of the entire mandible? _____

15. What provides the inherent collimation during a Panorex procedure? _____

16. For a Panorex of the mandible, the _____ line is adjusted to be parallel to the floor.

17. What type of image receptor must be used with Panorex? _____

18. True/False: The modified Law method provides a bilateral and functional study of the TMJs.

19. True/False: The mandibular condyles move anteriorly as the mouth is opened.

20. Which projection of the TMJs requires that the skull be kept in a true lateral position?

    A. Modified Law   C. Axiolateral oblique projection

    B. Schuller   D. Modified Towne

21. The axiolateral (Schuller method) projection described for the TMJs requires a CR angle of _____ degrees

    _____ (caudad or cephalad).

22. The axiolateral oblique projection of the TMJs is commonly referred to as the (A) _____

    method, which requires a (B) _____ degree head rotation from lateral and a (C) _____ degree caudad CR angle.

23. Which projection best visualizes the condyloid processes and the temporomandibular fossae?

_____

24. Aligning the _____ plane perpendicular to the IR will prevent rotation of either a PA or AP axial mandible.

REVIEW EXERCISE D: Problem Solving for Technical and Positioning Errors (see textbook pp. 390-412)

1. A radiograph of a lateral projection of the facial bones reveals that the mandibular rami are not superimposed. What positioning error led to this radiographic outcome?

_____

2. A radiograph of a parietoacanthial (Waters) projection reveals that the petrous ridges are projected within the maxillary sinuses. Is this an acceptable image? If not, what must be done to improve the image during the repeat exposure?

_____

3. A radiograph of a parietoacanthial (Waters) projection reveals that the distance between the lateral margins of the orbits and the lateral aspect of the skull is not equal. What type of positioning led to this radiographic outcome?

_____

4. A radiograph of a 30° PA axial projection of the facial bones reveals that the petrous ridges are projected at the level of the inferior orbital margins. Is this an acceptable image for this projection? If not, what must be done to improve the quality of the image during the repeat exposure?

_____

5. A radiograph of a superoinferior projection of the nasal bones reveals that the glabella is superimposed over the nasal bones. What positioning error led to this radiographic outcome, and how can it be corrected?

_____

_____

6. A lateral radiograph of the facial bones demonstrates that the gonions (angles) of the mandible are not superimposed; one is about 1 cm superior to the other. How would this be corrected on a repeat exposure?

_____

7. A radiograph of a parieto-orbital (Rhese) projection reveals that the optic foramen is incorrectly located in the upper outer quadrant of the orbit. What must be done to correct this problem during the repeat exposure?

_____

_____

8. A radiograph of an axiolateral projection of the mandible reveals that the body of the mandible is severely foreshortened. The body of the mandible was the area of interest. What positioning error led to this radiographic outcome?

_____

_____

9. **Situation:** A patient with a possible fracture of the nasal bones enters the emergency room. The physician is concerned about deviation of the bony nasal septum along with possible nasal bones fracture. What radiographic routine would be best for this situation?

_____

_____

_____

10. **Situation:** A patient with a possible blowout fracture of the right orbit enters the emergency room. In addition to the basic facial bone routine, what additional single projection would best demonstrate this type of injury?

_____

11. **Situation:** A patient with a possible fracture of the left zygomatic arch enters the emergency room. Neither the AP axial nor the submentovertex projection demonstrate this side well. The radiologist is indecisive as to whether this zygomatic arch is fractured. What other projections can the technologist provide to better define this area?

_____

12. **Situation:** As part of a study of the zygomatic arches, the technologist attempts to perform the SMV position. Because of the size of the patient's shoulders, he is unable to flex the neck adequately to place the IOML parallel to the image receptor. What other options does the technologist have to produce an acceptable SMV projection?

_____

REVIEW EXERCISE E: Critique Radiographs of the Facial Bones (see textbook p. 413)

The following questions relate to the radiographs found at the end of Chapter 12 of the textbook. Evaluate these radiographs for positioning accuracy as well as exposure factors, collimation, and correct use of anatomical markers. Describe the corrections needed to improve the overall image. The major, or "repeatable," error(s) are specific errors that indicate the need for a repeat exposure, regardless of the nature or degree of the other errors. Answers to each critique are given at the end of the laboratory activity exercise.

A. PA Waters (Fig. C12-107)
Description of possible error:

1. Structures shown: _____

2. Part positioning: _____

3. Collimation and central ray: _____

4. Exposure criteria: _____

5. Markers: _____

Repeatable error(s): _____

B. SMV mandible (Fig. C12-108)
Description of possible error:

1. Structures shown: _____

2. Part positioning: _____

3. Collimation and central ray: _____

4. Exposure criteria: _____

5. Markers: _____

Repeatable error(s): _____

C. Optic Foramina, Rhese Method (Fig. C12-109)
Description of possible error:

1. Structures shown: _____

2. Part positioning: _____

3. Collimation and central ray: _____

4. Exposure criteria: _____

5. Markers: _____

Repeatable error(s): _____

D. Optic Foramina, Rhese Method (Fig. C12-110)
Description of possible error:

1. Structures shown: _____

2. Part positioning: _____

3. Collimation and central ray: _____

4. Exposure criteria: _____

5. Markers: _____

Repeatable error(s): _____

E. Lateral Facial Bones (Fig. C12-111)
Description of possible error:

1. Structures shown: _____

2. Part positioning: _____

3. Collimation and central ray: _____

4. Exposure criteria: _____

5. Markers: _____

Repeatable error(s): _____

PART III: Laboratory Exercises (see textbook pp. 394-412)

You must gain experience in positioning each part of the facial bones before performing the following exams on actual patients. You can get experience in positioning and radiographic evaluation of these projections by performing exercises using radiographic phantoms and practicing on other students (although you will not be taking actual exposures).

The following suggested activities assume that your teaching institution has an energized lab and radiographic phantoms. If not, perform Laboratory Exercises B and C, the radiographic evaluation, and the physical positioning activities. (Check off each step and projection as you complete it.)

LABORATORY EXERCISE A: Energized Laboratory

1. Using the skull radiographic phantom, produce radiographs of the following basic routines:

Facial bones	*Zygomatic arches*	*Temporomandibular joints*
_____ Parietoacanthial (Waters)	_____ Submentovertex (SMV)	_____ Modified Law
_____ Modified Waters	_____ Oblique tangential	_____ Schuller method
_____ Lateral	_____ AP axial	_____ AP axial
_____ 15° PA axial (Caldwell)	*Mandible*	*Optic foramina*
Nasal bones	_____ Axiolateral	_____ Parieto-orbital (Rhese)
_____ Lateral	_____ PA	
_____ Superoinferior (tangential)	_____ AP axial	
_____ SMV		

LABORATORY EXERCISE B: Radiographic Evaluation

1. Evaluate and critique the radiographs produced during the previous experiments, additional radiographs provided by your instructor, or both. Evaluate each radiograph for the following points. (Check off when completed.):

    _____ Evaluate the completeness of the study. (Are all pertinent anatomic structures included on the radiograph?)

    _____ Evaluate for positioning or centering errors (e.g., rotation, off centering).

    _____ Evaluate for correct exposure factors and possible motion. (Are the density and contrast of the images acceptable?)

    _____ Determine whether markers and an acceptable degree of collimation and/or area shielding are visible on the images.

LABORATORY EXERCISE C: Physical Positioning

On another person, simulate performing all basic and special projections of the facial bones as follows. (Check off each when completed satisfactorily.) Include the following six steps as described in the textbook.

Step 1. Appropriate size and type of film holder with correct markers
Step 2. Correct CR placement and centering of part to CR and/or film
Step 3. Accurate collimation
Step 4. Area shielding of patient where advisable
Step 5. Use of proper immobilizing devices when needed
Step 6. Approximate correct exposure factors, breathing instructions where applicable, and "making" exposure

Projections	Step 1	Step 2	Step 3	Step 4	Step 5	Step 6
Facial bones						
• Parietoacanthial (Waters)	____	____	____	____	____	____
• Modified parietoacanthial	____	____	____	____	____	____
• Lateral facial bones	____	____	____	____	____	____
• 15° PA axial (Caldwell)	____	____	____	____	____	____
Nasal bones						
• Laterals	____	____	____	____	____	____
• Superoinferior nasal bones	____	____	____	____	____	____
Zygomatic arches						
• Submentovertex (SMV)	____	____	____	____	____	____
• Oblique tangential	____	____	____	____	____	____
• AP axial	____	____	____	____	____	____
Optic foramina						
• Parieto-orbital (Rhese)	____	____	____	____	____	____
Mandible						
• PA	____	____	____	____	____	____
• AP axial	____	____	____	____	____	____
• Axiolateral (general survey)	____	____	____	____	____	____
Temporomandibular joints						
• Modified Law	____	____	____	____	____	____
• Schuller method	____	____	____	____	____	____
• AP axial	____	____	____	____	____	____

Answers to Review Exercises

Review Exercise A: Anatomy of the Facial Bones

1. A. Middle nasal conchae
2. Maxilla
3. A. Frontal process
   B. Zygomatic process
   C. Alveolar process
   D. Palatine process
4. Frontal process
5. Acanthion
6. Horizontal portion of the palatine bones
7. Frontal and ethmoid
8. Zygomatic or malar bones
9. D. Sphenoid
10. Lacrimal bones
11. Conchae or turbinates
12. False, most of nose is made up of cartilage
13. Septal cartilage, vomer, pushed laterally to one side
14. A. 3
    B. 8
    C. 6
    D. 7
    E. 5
    F. 1
    G. 2
    H. 4
15. A. Nasal bones
    B. Lacrimal bones
    C. Zygomatic bones
    D. Maxillary bones
    E. Inferior nasal conchae
    F. Mandible
16. Vomer and palatine bones
17. A. Pterygoid hamulus, sphenoid
    B. Right palatine process, left maxilla
    C. Left palatine process, left maxilla
    D. Horizontal portions, right and left palatine bones
18. A. Perpendicular plate of ethmoid
    B. Vomer
    C. Septal cartilage
19. A. Condyle
    B. Neck
    C. Ramus
    D. Gonion or mandibular angle
    E. Body
    F. Mental foramen
    G. Mentum or mental protuberance
    H. Alveolar process
    I. Coronoid process
    J. Mandibular notch
    K. Temporal bone
    L. Temporomandibular joint (TMJ)
    M. External auditory meatus (EAM)
    N. Mastoid process

20. A. Lacrimal-facial
    B. Ethmoid-cranial
    C. Frontal-cranial
    D. Sphenoid-cranial
    E. Palatine-facial
    F. Zygomatic-facial
    G. Maxilla-facial
21. H. Optic foramen
    I. Superior orbital fissure
    J. Inferior orbital fissure
    K. Sphenoid strut
22. 30, 37

Review Exercise B: Positioning of the Facial Bones

1. False (should be performed erect for possible fluid levels)
2. True
3. False (decrease of 25%-30%)
4. True
5. False (is used for this)
6. False (strong magnets in MRI prohibit this)
7. Blowout fracture
8. Tripod
9. Dense petrous pyramids superimpose the orbits obscuring facial bone structures
10. C. Zygoma
11. Waters method
12. Orbits including infraorbital rims, bony nasal septum, maxillae, zygomatic bones and arches
13. B. 30°
14. Orbital rims and orbital floors
15. A. Reduces OID of facial bones
    B. Reduces exposure to anterior facial bones and neck structures such as thyroid glands
16. A. Facial bone lateral projections are unilateral: cranial laterals are bilateral
    B. IR is placed lengthwise for facial bones but crosswise for the cranium
    C. CR is centered to the zygoma for facial bones and 2 inches (5 cm) above the EAM for the cranium
17. Mentomeatal, 37
18. Acanthion
19. Nasion
20. Lips—meatal, 55°
21. True
22. False (toward the affected side)
23. True
24. False (thyroid gland dose is significant for 5 MV and HP axial projections)
25. Maxillary sinuses, Inferior orbital rims
26. Glabelloalveolar (GAL)
27. Zygomatic arches

28. 1 inch (2.5 cm) superior to glabella to pass through mid arches
29. A. Rhese method
    B. Three-point landing
30. A. Cheek, nose, and chin
    B. 53°
    C. Acanthiomeatal
    D. Lower outer
31. 1-E
    2-C
    3-F
    4-A
    5-D
    6-B

Review Exercise C: Positioning of the Mandible and Temporomandibular Joints (TMJ)

1. Submentovertex (SMV)
2. Axiolateral
3. Extend the chin
4. A. 30°
   B. 45°
   C. 0°, true lateral
   D. 10-15°
   E. 25° cephalad
5. Insufficient cephalic CR angle
6. Acanthion—at lips for PA projection
7. Orbitomeatal OML
8. True
9. False (cephalad)
10. Condyloid process
11. (A) 35-40° caudad
    (B) 42-47°
12. Glabella, to pass through midway between EAM and angle of mandible
13. Submentovertex—SMV projection
14. Panoramic tomography—Panorex
15. Narrow, vertical slit diaphragm
16. Infraorbitomeatal –IOML
17. Curved, nongrid cassette
18. True
19. True
20. B. Schuller
21. 25-30, caudad
22. A. Modified Law,
    B. 15
    C. 15
23. Modified Towne with 40° caudad angle—see Note on page 406 in textbook
24. Midsagittal

Review Exercise D: Problem Solving for Technical and Positioning Errors

1. Rotation of the head
2. No. The petrous ridges should be projected just below the maxillary

sinuses. The patient's head needs to be extended more.

3. Rotation of the head

4. Yes, this image meets the evaluation criteria for a 30° PA axial projection.

5. Excessive flexion of the head and neck or incorrect CR angle will project the glabella into the nasal bones. The CR must be aligned with the glabelloalveolar line.

6. The head was tilted. Ensure that the IPL is perpendicular to the film.

7. Increase extension of the head and neck. The AML should be placed perpendicular to the film to ensure that the optic foramen is open and is projected into the lower outer quadrant of the orbit (head rotation is correct).

8. Insufficient rotation of the head toward the IR. The head should be rotated 30° toward the IR to prevent foreshortening of the body.

9. PA Waters and R and L laterals. The PA Waters or the optional PA axial would demonstrate any possible septal deviation. The lateral projections would demonstrate any possible fracture of the nasal bones or anterior nasal spine. (The superoinferior projection would provide an axial perspective but is considered an optional projection in most departments and not part of the routine unless specifically requested.)

10. Modified parietoacanthial (Modified Waters) projection

11. Perform the oblique inferosuperior (tangential) projections. These projections are most ideal to demonstrate a depressed fracture of the zygomatic arch. (Bilateral projections are generally taken for comparison.)

12. Angle CR as to place it perpendicular to the IOML. If possible, angle image receptor to maintain a perpendicular relationship between the CR and image receptor.

Review Exercise E: Critique Radiographs of the Facial Bones

A. PA Waters (C12-107)
1. Pertinent anatomy is all included but not well demonstrated due to positioning and exposure errors.
2. Skull is underextended. This led to the petrous ridges being projected into the lower maxillary sinuses. Also, skull appears to be rotated.
3. Collimation is not evident. CR and film placement appears correct.
4. Facial bone region appears to be overexposed with very poor contrast.
5. Anatomical side marker is not evident.

Repeatable error (s): Criteria 2 and 4

B. SMV mandible (C12-108)
1. Pertinent anatomy is included but not well demonstrated due to positioning error.
2. Skull is underextended and/or CR angle is incorrect. (IOML was not parallel to film and not perpendicular to CR.) Mandible is foreshortened and rami projected into temporal bone.
3. Collimation is not evident. CR centering and film placement is correct.
4. Image appears to be slightly underexposed.
5. Anatomical side marker is not evident.

Repeatable error (s): Criterion 2 (possibly 4)

C. Optic foramina, Rhese method (C12-109)
1. Optic foramen is included but is slightly distorted.
2. Skull is rotated excessively toward a PA. (The skull is rotated more than 53° from the lateral position. This led to the optic foramen being projected into the mid lower aspect of the orbit.)

3. Collimation is not evident. CR and film placement are correct.
4. Exposure factors are acceptable.
5. Anatomical side marker is not evident.

Repeatable error (s): Criterion 2 (The foramen is well demonstrated, and this may not be a repeatable error by itself.)

D. Optic foramina, Rhese method (C12-110)
1. Optic foramen is distorted and totally obscured.
2. Skull appears to be overextended. (The AML was not perpendicular.) This projects the optic foramina into the infraorbital rim structure. Skull also appears to be underrotated, toward a lateral position. (If the skull is rotated less than 53° from the lateral position, the optic foramen will be projected into the lateral margin of the orbit.)
3. Collimation is evident and appears satisfactory. CR and film placement are correct.
4. Exposure factors are acceptable.
5. Anatomical side marker is not evident.

Repeatable error (s): Criteria 1 and 2

E. Lateral facial bones (C12-111)
1. Very distal end of mandible is cut off. Probably would not justify repeat exposure unless this was a specific area of interest.
2. Skull is rotated. (Note the separation of rami of mandible, greater wings of sphenoid and orbits).
3. Collimation is evident and acceptable (except for cut-off of lower tip of mandible). CR and film placement are acceptable.
4. Exposure factors appear to be satisfactory.
5. Anatomical side marker is not evident.

Repeatable error (s): Criterion 2 (possibly 1)

SELF-TEST

My Score = _____%

Directions: This self-test should be taken only after completing **all** of the readings, review exercises, and laboratory activities for a particular section. The purpose of this test is not only to provide a good learning exercise but also to serve as a strong indicator of what your final evaluation grade will be. It is strongly suggested that if you do not get at least a 90% to 95% grade on each self-test, you should review those areas in which you missed questions before going to your instructor for the final evaluation exam for this chapter. (There are a total of 54 questions or blanks—each is worth 1.9 points.)

1. The majority of the hard palate is formed by:

   A. Maxilla   C. Zygomatic bone

   B. Palatine bones   D. Mandible

2. Which of the following is not an aspect of the maxilla?

   A. Frontal process   C. Zygomatic process

   B. Body   D. Ramus

3. Match the following statements/characteristics to the correct facial bone (use each choice only once):

   _____ A. Mandible   1. Contains four processes

   _____ B. Lacrimal bones   2. Forms lower, outer aspect of orbit

   _____ C. Palatine bones   3. Lie just anterior and medial to the frontal process of maxilla

   _____ D. Inferior nasal conchae   4. Unpaired bone in the adult

   _____ E. Nasal bones   5. Located anteriorly in medial aspect of orbit

   _____ F. Maxilla   6. Help to mix air drawn into nasal cavity

   _____ G. Zygomatic bone   7. Possesses a vertical and horizontal portion

4. Identify the seven (cranial and facial) bones that form the bony orbit (Fig. 12-8).

   A. _____

   B. _____

   C. _____

   D. _____

   E. _____

   F. _____

   G. _____

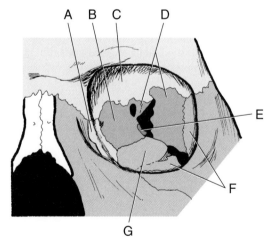

Fig. 12-8 Slightly oblique frontal view of orbit, **A-G.**

5. True/False: Facial bone studies should be performed erect whenever possible.

6. True/False: A LeForte fracture produces a "free-floating" zygomatic bone.

7. Which frontal projection of the facial bones will best visualize the region of the maxilla and orbits?

_____

8. For possible cranial trauma, which single projection of the facial bones will best demonstrate any possible air/fluid levels in the sinuses if the patient can't stand or sit erect?

_____

9. Which body plane is placed parallel to the film with a true lateral projection of the facial bones?

_____

10. A. What is the angle between the OML and plane of image receptor with a parietoacanthial (Waters) projection?

_____

   B. This will place the _____ perpendicular to the IR.

11. The CR is centered to exit at the level of the _____ for a well-positioned parietoacanthial projection.
   A. Nasion   C. Inner canthus
   B. Glabella   D. Acanthion

12. The CR is centered to exit at the level of the _____ for a well-positioned 15° PA axial projection of the facial bones.
   A. Nasion   C. Mid orbits
   B. Glabella   D. Acanthion

13. Where are the petrous ridges projected for a modified parietoacanthial projection?

_____

14. True/False: The lateral projection of the nasal bones should be performed using a small focal spot, detail screens, and close collimation.

15. True/False: The CR should be angled as needed to be parallel to the glabellomeatal line (GML) for the superoinferior projection of the nasal bones.

16. Which positioning line is placed perpendicular to the image receptor for a modified parietoacanthial projection?

_____

17. Where is the CR centered for a lateral projection of the nasal bones?

_____

18. Which positioning line, if placed parallel to the image receptor, will ensure adequate extension of the head for the submentovertex projection for zygomatic arches?

_____

19. How much tilt and rotation are required for the oblique inferosuperior (tangential) projection for zygomatic

   arches? _____

20. How much CR angle is required for the AP axial projection for the zygomatic arches if the IOML is placed perpendicular to the IR? (Hint: the same as for an AP axial skull.) _____

21. The proper name method for the "three-point landing" projection for the optic foramen is the

_____.

22. Where should the optic foramen be located with a well positioned parieto-orbital projection?

_____

23. What type of CR angulation should be used for an axiolateral projection of the mandible?

_____

24. Which one of the following factors will prevent superimposition of the ramus upon the cervical spine for the axiolateral mandible projection?

   A. Angle CR 10 to 15° cephalad   C. Extend chin slightly

   B. Have patient open mouth during exposure   D. Rotate head toward film

25. How much skull rotation toward the image receptor is required for the axiolateral projection for the mentum?

   A. 10 to 15°   C. 45°

   B. 30°   D. None; keep skull in true lateral position

26. How much CR angulation should be used for a PA axial projection of the mandible?

   A. None   C. 20 to 25° cephalad

   B. 10 to 15° cephalad   D. 5° cephalad

27. What structures are better defined when increasing CR angulation from 35 to 40° caudad with the AP axial projection for mandible?

_____

28. Where is the CR centered for a submentovertex (SMV) projection of the mandible?

_____

29. The thyroid dose range for the submentovertex (SMV) projection of the mandible is:

   A. 10-50 mrad   C. 200-300 mrad

   B. 50-100 mrad   D. 400-500 mrad

30. During a Panorex procedure, it is important to keep the _____ positioning line parallel to the floor.

   A. OML   C. IOML

   B. AML   D. GAL

31. What type of CR angulation is utilized for the AP axial projection of the TMJs with the OML perpendicular to the image receptor? _____

32. True/False: The modified Law method requires a tube angulation of 25°.

33. True/False: The Schuller method requires that the skull is placed in a true lateral position.

34. True/False: A grid is not required for the oblique inferosuperior (tangential) projection for zygomatic arches.

35. A radiograph of a 15° PA projection of the facial bones reveals that the petrous ridges are projected at the level of the mid orbital rims. What specific positioning error or what CR angling error led to this radiographic outcome?

   _____

36. Which positioning line should be perpendicular to the image receptor for the Rhese method projections for optic foramina?

   A. Acanthomeatal (AML)   C. Infraorbitomeatal (IOML)

   B. Mentomeatal (MML)   D. Glabellomeatal (GML)

37. A radiograph of a submentovertex projection of the mandibular condyles reveals that the arches are superimposed over the petrous pyramids. What adjustment to this position is needed to avoid this problem during the repeat exposure?

   _____

   _____

38. **Situation:** A patient with severe facial bone injuries comes into the emergency room. The patient is in a cervical collar and cannot be moved. What type of positioning routine should be performed for this situation?

   _____

   _____

39. A superoinferior, tangential projection for the nasal bones was taken with the following factors: 8 x 10 inches (18 x 24 cm) image receptor crosswise, detail screen table-top, 75 kVp, 3 mAs, 40 inches (102 cm) SID. The resultant radiograph was unsatisfactory. What factors should be changed for the repeat exposure?

   _____

40. **Situation:** A patient with possible facial fractures, including a possible "blowout" fracture to the right orbit, was brought from the emergency room to the radiology department. What special facial bone projection should be included with the basic facial bone routine of a lateral, parietoacanthial (Waters) and PA axial (Caldwell)?

   _____

   _____

CHAPTER 13

Paranasal Sinuses, Mastoids, and Temporal Bones

CHAPTER OBJECTIVES

After you have completed **all** the activities of this chapter, you will be able to:

_____ 1. List the location, function, and characteristics of the four groups of paranasal sinuses.

_____ 2. Using drawings and radiographs, identify specific paranasal sinuses.

_____ 3. List the three main portions of the temporal bones.

_____ 4. Identify specific structures of the external, middle, and internal ear.

_____ 5. Using drawings, identify the three divisions of the ear and the structures found in each division.

_____ 6. Using radiographs, identify specific structures of the temporal bone.

_____ 7. Match specific pathologic indications of the paranasal sinuses and temporal bone to the correct definition.

_____ 8. Identify which radiographic projection and/or procedure best demonstrates a specific pathologic indication.

_____ 9. List the dose ranges for patient skin dose and midline dose for each projection of the sinuses, mastoids, and temporal bones.

_____ 10. Identify basic and special projections of the paranasal sinuses and temporal bones and list the correct size and type of image receptor, central ray location, direction, and angulation for each position.

_____ 11. Given various hypothetical situations, identify the correct modification of a position and/or exposure factors to improve the radiographic image.

_____ 12. Given radiographs of specific paranasal sinus and temporal bone projections, identify positioning and exposure factors errors.

POSITIONING AND FILM CRITIQUE

_____ 1. Using a peer, position for basic projections of the paranasal sinuses and temporal bone.

_____ 2. Using appropriate radiographic phantom, produce satisfactory radiographs of specific positions (if equipment is available).

_____ 3. Critique and evaluate paranasal sinus and temporal bone radiographs based on the four divisions of radiographic criteria: (1) structures shown, (2) position, (3) collimation and CR, and (4) exposure criteria.

_____ 4. Distinguish between acceptable and unacceptable spine radiographs due to exposure factors, motion, collimation, positioning, or other errors.

Learning Exercises

The following review exercises should be completed only after careful study of the associated pages in the textbook as indicated by each exercise.

   After completing each of these individual exercises, check your answers against the answer sheets that follow before continuing to the next exercise.

PART I: Radiographic Positioning

REVIEW EXERCISE A: Radiographic Anatomy of the Paranasal Sinuses, Mastoids, and Temporal Bones (see textbook pp. 416-423)

1. What is the older term for the maxillary sinuses? _____.

2. An infection of the teeth may travel upward and involve the _____ sinus.

3. Specifically, where are the frontal sinuses located? _____.

4. The frontal sinuses rarely become aerated before the age of _____.

5. Which aspect of the ethmoid bone contains the ethmoid sinuses? _____.

6. The drainage pathways for the paranasal sinuses are called the:

    A. Uncinate process   C. Paranasal meatus

    B. Osteomeatal complex   D. Lateral masses

7. Which sinus will be projected through the open mouth with a PA axial transoral projection? _____.

8. Identify the sinuses, structures, or bones labeled on Fig. 13-1:

    A. _____

    B. _____

    C. _____

    D. _____

    E. _____

    F. _____

    G. _____

    H. _____

    I. _____

    J. _____

    K. _____

    L. _____

    M. _____

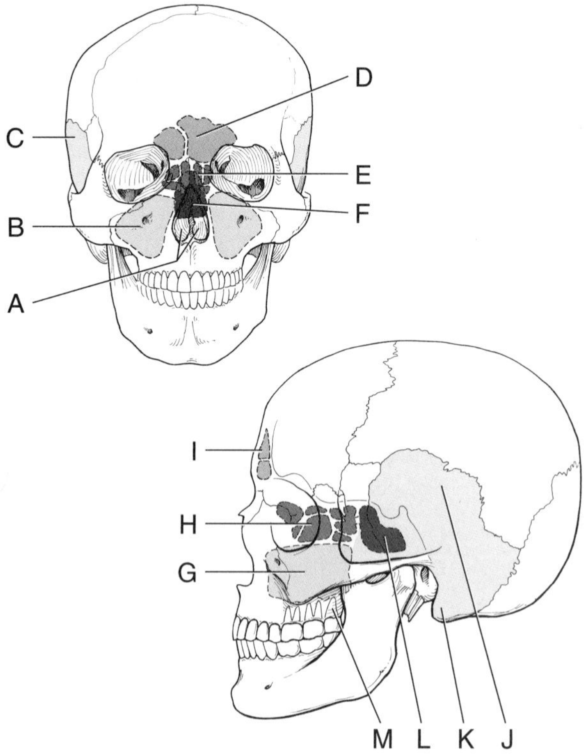

Fig. 13-1. Frontal and lateral views.

9. Identify the following paranasal sinuses labeled on Fig. 13-2 and 13-3:

Fig. 13-2

A. _____

B. _____

C. _____

D. _____

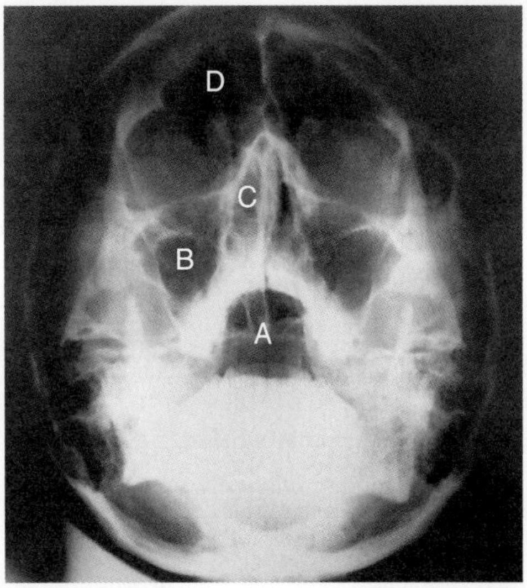

Fig. 13-2. Paranasal sinuses. PA axial transoral projection.

Fig. 13-3

E. _____

F. _____

G. _____

H. _____

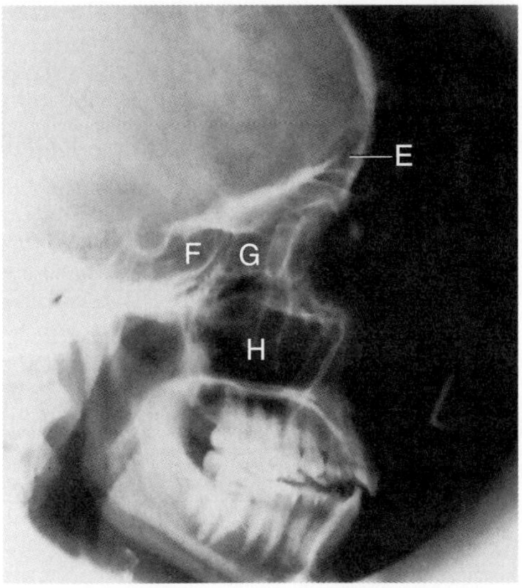

Fig. 13-3. Paranasal sinuses. Lateral projection

10. List the three aspects of the temporal bone:

A. _____ B. _____ C. _____

11. Which aspect of the temporal bone is considered the most dense? _____.

12. Which structure makes up the cartilaginous, external ear? _____.

13. On average, how long is the external acoustic meatus (EAM)? _____.

14. Which small membrane marks the beginning of the middle ear? _____.

15. What is the collective term for the small bones of the middle ear? _____.

16. Which structure allows for communication between the nasopharynx and middle ear? _____.

17. What is the major function of this structure (question #16)? _____.

18. Which structure serves as an opening between the mastoid portion of the temporal bone and the middle ear?

    _____.

19. What is the name of the thin plate of bone that separates the mastoid air cells from the brain? _____.

20. Which one of the auditory ossicles pick up sound vibrations from the tympanic membrane?

    _____.

21. Which one of the auditory ossicles is considered to be the smallest? _____.

22. Which one of the auditory ossicles resembles a premolar tooth? _____.

23. What is the name of the small membrane that connects the middle to the inner ear? _____.

24. Which two sensory functions occur within the inner ear?

    A. _____   B. _____

25. What is the name of the small membrane that will move outward to transmit impulses to the auditory nerve, thus

    creating the sense of hearing? _____.

26. True/False: The cochlea is a closed system relating to the sense of hearing.

27. Identify the structures labeled on Fig. 13-4:

    A. _____

    B. _____

    C. _____

    D. _____

    E. _____

    F. _____

    G. _____

    H. _____

    I. _____

    J. _____

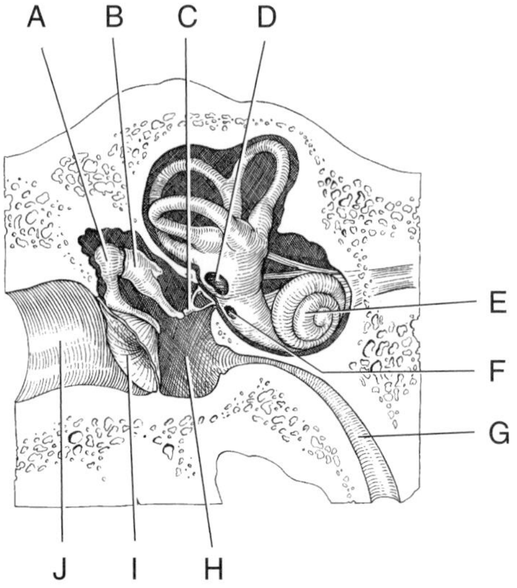

Fig. 13-4. Structures of the middle and external ear.

PART II: Radiographic Positioning

REVIEW EXERCISE B: Positioning of the Paranasal Sinuses, Mastoids, and Temporal Bones
(see textbook pp. 424-439)

1. What kVp range should be used for sinus radiography? _____.

2. To demonstrate any possible air or fluid levels within the sinuses, it is important to:

   A. _____

   B. _____

3. Why are the auricles taped forward for certain lateral projections of the temporal bone?

   _____.

4. True/False: Temporal bone studies require that both sides be radiographed for comparison purposes.

5. True/False: Ultrasound of the maxillary sinuses to rule out sinusitis is feasible.

6. True/False: Magnetic resonance imaging is the preferred modality to study soft tissue changes and masses within the sinuses.

7. Match the following pathologic indications for the paranasal sinuses and temporal bone to the correct definition or statement (use each choice only once):

   _____ A. Sinusitis   1. Bacterial infection of the mastoid process

   _____ B. Otosclerosis   2. Infection of the bone and marrow, secondary to sinusitis

   _____ C. Mastoiditis   3. Hereditary disease involving excessive bone formation of middle and inner ear

   _____ D. Acoustic neuroma   4. Benign, cystlike mass or tumor of the middle ear

   _____ E. Secondary osteomyelitis 5. This condition may be chronic or acute

   _____ F. Cholesteatoma   6. Benign tumor of the auditory nerve sheath

8. Which one of the following radiographic appearances pertains to an acoustic neuroma?

   A. Expansion of the internal acoustic canal   C. Increased density in the sinus

   B. Bone destruction within the middle ear   D. Sinus mucosal thickening

9. Which one of the following imaging modalities will best demonstrate otosclerosis?

   A. MRI   C. Conventional radiography

   B. CT   D. Ultrasound

10. List the four most commonly performed basic or routine projections for paranasal sinuses:

    A. _____   C. _____

    B. _____   D. _____

11. Which single projection for a paranasal sinus routine provides an image of all four sinus groups?

    _____.

12. If the patient cannot stand for the lateral projection of the paranasal sinuses, it should be taken:

    _____.

13. Which paranasal sinuses are best demonstrated with a PA (Caldwell) projection? _____.

14. To avoid angling the CR for the erect PA Caldwell sinus projection, the head should be adjusted so the OML is

_____ degrees from horizontal.

15. A.   Which paranasal sinuses are best demonstrated with a parietoacanthial (Water) projection?

_____.

    B.   The orbitomeatal line (OML) forms a _____ degree angle with the film with this projection.

16. Which positioning line is placed perpendicular to the image receptor for a parietoacanthial projection?

_____.

17. Where are the petrous ridges located on a well-positioned parietoacanthial projection?

_____.

18. Which paranasal sinuses are demonstrated with a submentovertex (SMV) projection of the paranasal sinuses?

_____.

19. Where should the CR exit for both the PA parietoacanthial (Waters) and the PA transoral (open-mouth Waters)

projection? _____.

20. What is the one major difference in positioning between the parietoacanthial and PA axial transoral projections?

_____.

21. Which sinuses are projected thorough the oral cavity with the PA axial transoral projection?

_____.

22. Which two projections of the mastoid routine presented in the textbook provide a relative lateral perspective of the mastoid air cells?

    A.   _____   B.   _____

23. Which positioning line should be perpendicular to the image receptor to prevent incorrect tilting of the skull for the

axiolateral oblique (Modified Law) projection? _____.

24. The axiolateral oblique (Modified Law) projection of the mastoids requires a _____ degree caudad CR angle and a

_____ degree rotation of the skull toward the image receptor.

25. A.   What is the proper name (method) for the posterior profile projection for mastoids? _____.

    B.   The petrous pyramid should be _____ (parallel or perpendicular) to the IR with this posterior profile projection for the mastoids.

    C.   For this projection the head is rotated _____ degrees and the CR angled _____ degrees

         _____, (caudad or cephalad) which visualizes the _____ (upside or downside) mastoids.

26. Which of the following projections provides a comparative, bilateral view of both right and left mastoids with a single exposure?

    A. Posterior profile   C. AP axial

    B. Axiolateral oblique   D. Anterior profile

27. What CR angulation should be utilized for the axiolateral (Schuller) method for mastoids?

    A. 15° caudad   C. Perpendicular beam

    B. 12° cephalad   D. 25 to 30° caudad

28. Where is the CR centered for an anterior profile (Arcelin method) projection of the mastoids?

    _____.

29. Which projection of the mastoids provides an "end-on" perspective of the downside petrous bone?

    _____.

30. Match the following projections with the anatomy best seen (use each choice only once):

    PROJECTION   *ANATOMY*

    _____ 1. Lateral sinus   A. Profile image of upside mastoids

    _____ 2. Parietoacanthial   B. Sphenoid sinus in oral cavity

    _____ 3. PA Caldwell   C. End-on view of downside mastoids

    _____ 4. Modified Law   D. Inferior view of sphenoid sinus

    _____ 5. PA transoral   E. Bilateral view of petrous bones

    _____ 6. Mayer method   F. All four paranasal sinuses

    _____ 7. SMV for sinuses   G. Best view of maxillary sinuses

    _____ 8. Arcelin method   H. Lateral view of downside mastoid air cells

    _____ 9. AP axial (Towne)   I. Best view of frontal and ethmoid sinuses

REVIEW EXERCISE C: Problem Solving for Technical and Positioning Errors (see textbook: pp. 428-439)

1. A radiograph of a PA (Caldwell) projection for sinuses reveals that the petrous ridges are projected into the lower half of the orbits and over the ethmoid sinuses. The technologist used a horizontal beam for the projection. Also, the skull was positioned to place the OML at a 15° angle from the horizontal plane. What positioning modification is needed to correct this problem during the repeat exposure?

    _____.

2. A radiograph of a parietoacanthial projection reveals that the distance between the midsagittal plane and the outer orbital margin are not equal. What positioning error is present on this radiograph?

    _____.

3. A radiograph of a submentovertex projection for sinuses reveals that the distance between the mandibular condyles and lateral border of the skull are not equal. What positioning error is present on this radiograph?

   _____.

4. A radiograph of a PA transoral projection reveals that the sphenoid sinus is superimposed over the upper teeth and the nasal cavity. How must the initial position be modified to avoid this problem during the repeat exposure?

   _____.

5. A radiograph of an axiolateral oblique (modified Law) projection for mastoids reveals that the external ear has cast a shadow over the mastoid air cells. What can be done to avoid this problem during the repeat exposure?

   _____.

6. A radiograph of an AP axial projection for mastoids reveals the petrous ridges are not symmetrical. What specific positioning error is present on this radiograph?

   _____.

7. A radiograph of a Stenvers method for mastoids reveals that the petrous bone appears to be foreshortened. The patient's skull was classified as being dolichocephalic. What must be done to create a better profile image of the

   mastoids? _____.

   _____.

   _____.

8. A radiograph of a parietoacanthial projection reveals that the petrous ridges are projected just below the maxillary sinuses. What positioning error (if any) is present?

   _____.

9. **Situation:** A patient with a clinical history of sinusitis comes to the radiology department for a sinuses study evaluation. The patient is quadriplegic and can't be placed erect. Which single projection demonstrates any air-fluid levels present in the sinuses?

   _____.

10. **Situation:** A patient comes to the radiology department to rule out a possible polyp within the sphenoid sinus. What routine and/or special projections would provide the best overall assessment of the sinuses for this patient?

    _____.

    _____.

11. **Situation:** A patient comes to the radiology department for a mastoid series. He cannot lie prone on the table or stand erect. Which projections of the mastoids could be performed on this patient?

    _____.

    _____.

12. **Situation:** A patient with a clinical history of acoustic neuroma comes to the radiology department. Which imaging modality (modalities) is recommended for this type of pathology?

    _____.

REVIEW EXERCISE D: Critique Radiographs of the Paranasal Sinuses, Mastoids, and Temporal Bones
(see textbook p. 440)

The following questions relate to the radiographs found at the end of Chapter 13 of the textbook. Evaluate these radiographs for positioning accuracy as well as exposure factors, collimation, and correct use of anatomical markers. Describe the corrections needed to improve the overall image. The major, or "repeatable," error(s) imply that these specific errors require a repeat exposure be taken regardless of the nature or degree of the other errors. Answers to each critique are given at the end of the laboratory activities.

A. **Parietoacanthial transoral (open-mouth Waters) (Fig. C13-66)**
Description of possible error:

1. Structures shown: _____

2. Part positioning: _____

3. Collimation and central ray: _____

4. Exposure criteria: _____

5. Markers: _____

Repeatable error(s): _____

B. **Parietoacanthial (Waters) (Fig. C13-67)**
Description of possible error:

1. Structures shown: _____

2. Part positioning: _____

3. Collimation and central ray: _____

4. Exposure criteria: _____

5. Markers: _____

Repeatable error(s): _____

C. **Submentovertex (SMV) (Fig. C13-68)**
Description of possible error:

1. Structures shown: _____

2. Part positioning: _____

3. Collimation and central ray: _____

4. Exposure criteria: _____

5. Markers: _____

Repeatable error(s): _____

D. Submentovertex (SMV) (Fig. C13-69)
   Description of possible error:

   1.   Structures shown: _____

   2.   Part positioning: _____

   3.   Collimation and central ray: _____

   4.   Exposure criteria: _____

   5.   Markers: _____

   Repeatable error(s): _____

PART III: Laboratory Exercises (see textbook pp. 424-439)

You must gain experience in positioning each part of the paranasal sinuses, mastoids, and temporal bone before performing these exams on actual patients. You can get experience in positioning and radiographic evaluation of these projections by performing exercises using radiographic phantoms and practicing on other students (although you will not be taking actual exposures).

   The following suggested activities assume that your teaching institution has an energized lab and radiographic phantoms. If not, perform Laboratory Exercises B and C, the radiographic evaluation, and the physical positioning exercises. (Check off each step as you complete it.)

LABORATORY EXERCISE A: Energized Laboratory

   1.   Using the skull radiographic phantom, produce radiographs of the following basic routines:

Sinuses	*Temporal Bone*
_____ Parietoacanthial (Waters)	_____ AP sacrum
_____ Lateral	_____ Posterior profile (Stenvers)
_____ PA	_____ Anterior profile (Arcelin)
_____ Submentovertex (SMV)	_____ AP axial (Towne)
	_____ AP axiolateral oblique (Mayer)

LABORATORY EXERCISE B: Radiographic Evaluation

   1.   Evaluate and critique the radiographs produced during the previous experiments, additional radiographs provided by your instructor, or both. Evaluate each radiograph for the following points. (Check off when completed.):

   _____ Evaluate the completeness of the study. (Are all of the pertinent anatomic structures included on the radiograph?)

   _____ Evaluate for positioning or centering errors (e.g., rotation, off centering).

   _____ Evaluate for correct exposure factors and possible motion.

   _____ (Are the density and contrast of the images acceptable?)

   _____ Determine whether markers and an acceptable degree of collimation and/or area shielding are visible on the images.

LABORATORY EXERCISE C: Physical Positioning

On another person, simulate performing all basic and special projections of the paranasal sinuses, mastoids, and temporal bone as follows. (Check off each when completed satisfactorily.) Include the following six steps as described in the textbook.

Step 1. Appropriate size and type of film holder with correct markers
Step 2. Correct central ray placement and centering of part to central ray and/or film
Step 3. Accurate collimation
Step 4. Area shielding of patient where advisable
Step 5. Use of proper immobilizing devices when needed
Step 6. Approximate correct exposure factors, breathing instructions where applicable, and "making" exposure

	Step 1	Step 2	Step 3	Step 4	Step 5	Step 6
Sinus projections						
• Parietoacanthial (Waters)	___	___	___	___	___	___
• Lateral	___	___	___	___	___	___
• PA	___	___	___	___	___	___
• Submentovertex (SMV)	___	___	___	___	___	___
• Parietoacanthial transoral (open-mouth Waters)	___	___	___	___	___	___
Temporal bone projections						
• Axiolateral oblique (modified Law)	___	___	___	___	___	___
• Axiolateral (Schuller)	___	___	___	___	___	___
• Posterior profile (Stenvers)	___	___	___	___	___	___
• Anterior profile (Arcelin)	___	___	___	___	___	___
• AP axial (Towne)	___	___	___	___	___	___
• AP axiolateral oblique (Mayer)	___	___	___	___	___	___

ANSWERS TO REVIEW EXERCISES

Review Exercise A: Anatomy of the Paranasal Sinuses, Mastoids, and Temporal Bones

1. Antrum of Highmore
2. Maxillary
3. Between the inner and outer tables of the skull, posterior to the glabella
4. Before 6 years old
5. Lateral masses or labyrinths
6. B. Osteomeatal complex
7. Sphenoid sinus
8. A. Nasal cavity (fossae)
   B. Maxillary sinuses
   C. Right temporal bone (squamous portion)
   D. Frontal sinuses
   E. Ethmoid sinuses
   F. Sphenoid sinuses
   G. Maxillary sinuses
   H. Ethmoid sinuses
   I. Frontal sinuses
   J. Squamous portion of left temporal bone
   K. Mastoid portion of left temporal bone
   L. Sphenoid sinus
   M. Roots of upper teeth (alveolar process
   Fig. 13-2
9. A. Sphenoid sinus
   B. Maxillary sinuses
   C. Ethmoid sinuses
   D. Frontal sinus
   Fig. 13-3
   E. Frontal sinuses
   F. Sphenoid sinus
   G. Ethmoid sinuses
   H. Maxillary sinuses
10. A. Squamous
    B. Mastoid
    C. Petrous
11. Petrous portion
12. Auricle or pinna
13. 1 inch or 2.5 cm
14. Tympanic membrane (eardrum)
15. Auditory ossicles
16. Eustachian or auditory tube
17. To equalize the atmospheric pressure within the middle ear
18. Aditus
19. Tegmen tympani
20. Malleus
21. Stapes
22. Incus
23. Oval or vestibular window
24. A. Hearing
    B. Equilibrium
25. Round or cochlear window
26. True
27. A. Malleus
    B. Incus
    C. Stapes
    D. Oval window
    E. Cochlea
    F. Round window
    G. Eustachian tube
    H. Tympanic cavity
    I. Tympanic membrane
    J. External acoustic meatus (EAM) or canal

Review Exercise B: Positioning of the Paranasal Sinuses, Mastoids, and Temporal Bones

1. 70-80 kVp
2. A. Perform positions erect when possible
   B. Use horizontal x-ray beam
3. Prevent shadows from the cartilaginous ear superimposing the mastoid air cells
4. True
5. True
6. True
7. A. 5
   B. 3
   C. 1
   D. 6
   E. 2
   F. 4
8. A. Expansion of the internal acoustic canal
9. B. CT
10. A. Lateral
    B. PA Caldwell
    C. Parietoacanthial (Waters)
    D. Submentovertex (SMV)
11. Lateral
12. Cross-table with horizontal x-ray beam
13. Frontal and anterior ethmoid
14. 15
15. A. Maxillary
    B. 37
16. Mentomeatal (MML)
17. Just below the maxillary sinuses
18. Sphenoid, ethmoid, and maxillary sinuses
19. At the acanthion
20. The mouth is open with the PA transoral projection
21. Sphenoid sinuses
22. A. Axiolateral oblique (modified Law) projection
    B. Axiolateral oblique (Schuller) projection
23. Interpupillary
24. 15, 15
25. A. Stenvers
    B. Parallel
    C. 45, 12, cephalad, downside
26. C. AP axial

27. D. 25-30° caudad
28. 1 in. (2.5 cm) anterior and 3/4 in. (2 cm) superior to elevated EAM
29. AP axial oblique (Mayer and Owen) projection
30. 1. F, 2. G, 3. I, 4. H, 5. B, 6. C, 7. D, 8. A, 9. E

Review Exercise C: Problem Solving for Technical and Positioning Errors

1. The head and neck need to be extended more to project the petrous ridges below the ethmoid sinuses.
2. Rotation of the head
3. Tilt of the head
4. Increase extension of the head and neck to project the entire sphenoid sinus through the oral cavity.
5. Tape the patient's auricle forward to prevent it from superimposing the mastoids.
6. Rotation of the head
7. A dolichocephalic skull requires more rotation of the skull as compared with an average-shaped skull (mesocephalic). The 45° rotation for the Stenvers needs to be increased to at least 50° for the dolichocephalic skull.
8. None. The petrous ridges should be below the floors of the maxillary sinuses on a well-positioned parietoacanthial projection.
9. The most diagnostic projection is the horizontal beam lateral projection to demonstrate any air/fluid levels.
10. The PA transoral special projection in addition to the routine four sinuses projection series (the lateral, PA Caldwell, parietoacanthial, and SMV).
11. AP axial (Towne) and anterior profile oblique (Arcelin) and axiolateral oblique (Mayer or Owen) projections could be performed without turning the patient from the supine position.
12. MRI or CT

Review Exercise D: Critique Radiographs of the Paranasal Sinuses, Mastoids, and Temporal Bones

A. Parietoacanthial transoral (open-mouth Waters) (C13-66)
   1. Sphenoid and maxillary sinuses not well demonstrated. Petrous ridges are projected into lower

aspect of maxillary sinuses. The base of skull is superimposed over sphenoid sinus.

2. Skull is underextended, leading to errors previously described. (Chin not elevated sufficiently.)

3. Collimation is not centered to film. CR is centered too low (inferior) according to circular collimation on top, but this is not a repeatable error by itself. Film appears centered high, not aligned with CR.

4. Exposure factors are acceptable.

5. Anatomical side marker is not evident.
   Repeatable errors:
   Criteria 1 and 2

B. Parietoacanthial (Waters) (C13-67)

1. Maxillary sinuses not well demonstrated. Petrous ridges are projected into lower aspect of maxillary sinuses. Artifacts appear to be either surgical clips and devices or external hair pins or clips.

2. Skull is underextended and severely rotated.

3. Collimation is not evident. CR centering and film placement are slightly low.

4. Exposure factors are acceptable.

5. Anatomical side marker is not evident.
   Repeatable errors:
   Criteria 1 and 2

C. Submentovertex (SMV) (C13-68)

1. Maxillary and ethmoid sinuses not well demonstrated and partially cut off. Mandible is superimposed over sinuses.

2. Skull is grossly underextended and tilted. (Also some rotation.)

3. Collimation would have been OK if centering would have been correct. CR centering is off laterally. This led to cut-off of the anatomy.

4. Exposure factors are acceptable.

5. Anatomical side marker is not evident.
   Repeatable errors: Criteria 1, 2, and 3 (CR centering)

D. Submentovertex (SMV) (C13-69)

1. Part of ethmoid and maxillary sinuses not well demonstrated due to superimposed mandible. Earrings were not removed.

2. Skull is underextended and slightly rotated to the right.

3. Collimation is acceptable. CR centering and film placement are acceptable but slightly anterior.

4. Exposure factors are acceptable for the sphenoid/ethmoid sinuses.

5. Anatomical side marker is not evident.
   Repeatable errors:
   Criteria 1 and 2

SELF-TEST

My Score = _____%

This self-test should be taken only after completing **all** of the readings, review exercises, and laboratory activities for a particular section. The purpose of this test is not only to provide a good learning exercise but also to serve as a strong indicator of what your final evaluation grade will be. It is strongly suggested that if you do not get at least a 90% to 95% grade on each self-test, you should review those areas in which you missed questions **before** going to your instructor for the final evaluation exam for this chapter. (There are a total of 58 questions or blanks—each is worth 1.7 points.)

1. On average, how many separate cavities make up the frontal sinus? _____.

2. True/False: All of the paranasal sinuses are contained within cranial bones except the maxillary sinuses.

3. True/False: All of the paranasal sinuses except the sphenoid communicate with the nasal cavity.

4. True/False: In general, all the paranasal sinuses are not fully developed until age 6 or 7.

5. True/False: The frontal sinuses are usually larger in men than in women.

6. Identify the labeled structures on Figs. 13-5, 13-6, and 13-7, which are radiographs of the paranasal sinuses:

A. _____   H. _____

B. _____   I. _____

C. _____   J. _____

D. _____   K. _____

E. _____   L. _____

F. _____   M. _____

G. _____

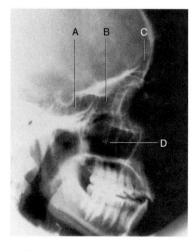

Fig. 13-5. Paranasal sinuses, A-D.

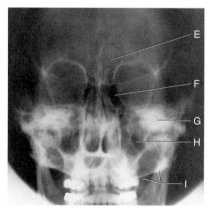

Fig. 13-6. Paranasal sinuses, E-I.

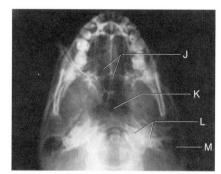

Fig. 13-7. Paranasal sinuses, J-M.

7. Which aspect of the ethmoid bone contains the ethmoid air cells? _____.

8. The sphenoid sinus lies directly inferior to the _____.

9. Which aspect of the temporal bone is considered to be thinnest? _____.

10. Which aspect of the temporal bone contains the organs of hearing and balance? _____.

11. The correct term for the eardrum is the _____.

12. Which one of the following middle ear structures is considered to be most lateral?

    A. Malleus   C. Stapes

    B. Incus   D. Oval window

13. Which structure helps equalize atmospheric pressure in the middle ear? _____.

14. What passes through the internal acoustic meatus? _____.

15. The aditus is an opening between the _____ and the _____ portion of the temporal bone.

16. An infection of the mastoid air cells, if untreated, can lead to a serious infection of the brain called

    _____.

17. Which auditory ossicle attaches to the oval window?

    A. Malleus   C. Stapes

    B. Incus   D. None

18. The internal ear is divided into the osseous or bony labyrinth and the _____ labyrinth.

19. List the three divisions of the bony labyrinth of the inner ear.

    A. _____   B. _____   C. _____

20. Identify the structures labeled on Fig. 13-8:

    A. _____

    B. _____

    C. _____

    D. _____

    E. _____

    F. _____

    G. _____

    H. _____

    I. _____

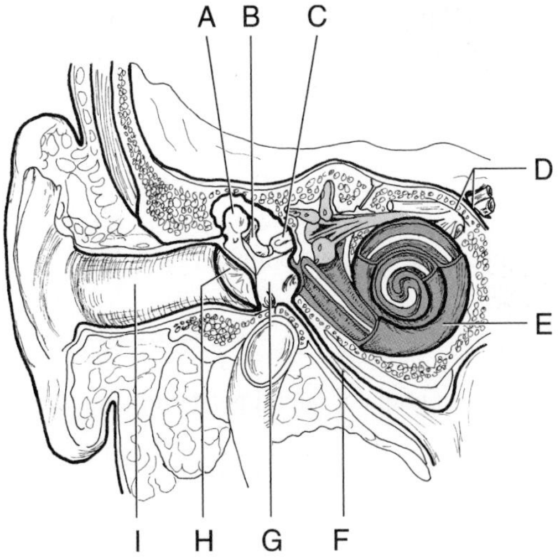

Fig. 13-8. Three divisions of the ear.

21. True/False: Ultrasound of the sphenoid sinus can be performed to rule out sinusitis.

22. A benign, cystlike mass of the middle ear is a/an:

    A. Acoustic neuroma   C. Cholesteatoma

    B. Osteomyelitis   D. Acoustic sarcoma

23. True/False: Otosclerosis is a hereditary disease.

24. Which one of the following imaging modalities would best demonstrate bony erosion of the maxillary sinus due to acute sinusitis?

    A. CT   C. Ultrasound

    B. MRI   D. Conventional radiography

25. The skin dose range for an AP axial (Towne) projection for either the mastoids and/or temporal bone is:

    A. 10-50 mrad   C. 300-400 mrad

    B. 100-200 mrad   D. Over 500 mrad

26. Where is the CR centered for a lateral projection of the paranasal sinuses? _____

27. Why should patients remain in an erect position for at least 5 minutes before sinus radiography?

    _____

28. Which projection is best for demonstrating the maxillary sinuses? _____

29. Why should a completely horizontal CR be utilized for the erect PA (Caldwell) projection rather than the usual 15°

    caudad angle? _____

30. A radiograph of an axiolateral (Schuller) projection of the mastoid air cells reveals that the opposite or "up-side" mastoid is projected on the mastoid of interest. What positioning error may have led to this radiographic outcome?

    _____

31. A radiograph of a submentovertex (SMV) projection of the sinuses reveals the mandible is superimposed over an aspect of the ethmoid and maxillary sinuses. What modification is needed to improve this image during the repeat exposure?

    _____

32. A radiograph of an AP axial (Towne) projection for mastoids reveals that the dorsum sellae is projected above the foramen magnum. Also, the petrous pyramids appear foreshortened. What modification is needed to correct the errors present on the initial radiograph?

    _____

33. A radiograph of lateral position for sinuses reveals that the greater wings of the sphenoid bone are not superim

    posed. What specific positioning error is present? _____

34. **Situation:** A patient comes to the radiology department for a mastoid series. The positioning routine includes a posterior profile (Stenvers) projection. Classification of the skull reveals that the patient has a brachycephalic skull. What specific degree of obliquity is needed for the posterior profile projection?

_____

_____

_____

35. **Situation:** A patient with a clinical history of secondary osteomyelitis comes to the radiology department. Which imaging modalities or procedures can be performed that will demonstrate the extent of damage to the sinuses?

_____

SELF-TEST ANSWERS

Chapter 1
Principles, Terminology, and Radiation Protection
Self-Test A: General, Systemic, and Skeletal Anatomy and Arthrology
1.
   - A. Integumentary
   - D. Osseous
2. C. 206
3. B. Circulatory
4. B. Urinary
5. D. Integumentary
6. B. Axial and appendicular
7. A. Spongy or cancellous
8. C. Nyaline or articular cartilage
9. D. Diploe
10. A. Diaphysis
11. C. Epiphyses
12. A. Fibrous
13. B. Cartilaginous
14. C. Distal tibiofibular joint
15.
   1. C
   2. A
   3. B
   4. D
   5. C
   6. A
   7. D
   8. C
16. D. Fibrous
17.
   1. E
   2. A
   3. F
   4. C
   5. B
   6. D
   7. B
   8. D

Self-Test B: Radiographic Terminology
1. C. Midcoronal
2. False
3. C. Sagittal plane
4.
   1. E
   2. I
   3. G
   4. J
   5. A
   6. K
   7. C
   8. H
   9. B
   10. F
   11. L
   12. D

5.
   1. L
   2. G
   3. F
   4. J
   5. A
   6. H
   7. D
   8. C
   9. B
   10. K
   11. I
   12. E
6. D. Projection
7. A. LAO
8. C. Ventral decubitus
9. D. Anteroposterior
10. A. Tangential

Self-Test C: Basic Imaging Principles
1. C. Kilovoltage peak
2. True
3. A. Density
4. B. milliamperage seconds
5. False
6. B. Decrease to 5 mAs
7. B. Kilovoltage peak
8. C. 110 kVp 2mAs
9. A. 60 kVp, 30 mAs
10. True
11. False
12. False
13. D. Shorten the exposure time
14. D. 0.3 mm focal spot and 40-inch SID
15. D. Distortion
16. C. 72-inch SID and 3-inch OID.
17. False

Self-Test D: Positioning Principles
1. False
2. False
3. D. None of the x-ray equipment manufactured after 1994
4. True
5.
   1. B
   2. B
   3. A
   4. A
   5. B
   6. A
   7. A
   8. B
   9. A
   10. A
6. C. Two
7. B. 10 × 12
8. C. 100

9. A. Iliac crest
10. B. Jugular notch
11. A. T-9/10.
12. D. Hypersthenic

Self-Test E: Digital Imaging
1. False
2. True
3. D. Bar code reader
4. A. Laser
5. C. 80%
6. False
7. False
8. True
9. True
10. False
11. C. Radiology information system
12. A. Set of communication standards among PACS
13. D. Teleradiology

Self-Test F: Radiation Protection
1. B. Gray
2. D. Roentgen
3. D. 5 rem or 50 mSv
4. A. 25 rem or 250 mSv
5. B. 0.1 rem or 1 mSv
6. D. 10 R/minute
7. A. 3 to 4 R/minute
8. A. Absorb lower energy x-rays
9. A. AP thoracic spine (7 × 17 collimation)
10. C. 50 to 90%
11. C. Shadow shield
12. False
13. True
14. True
15. False

Chapter 2
Chest
1.
   - A. 5. Sternum
   - B. 3. Thyroid-cartilage
   - C. 4. Scapula
   - D. 2. Larynx
   - E. 1. Clavicle
2. D. Vertebra prominens
3. C. Jugular notch
4. A. Right and left bronchi
5. B. Carina
6. D. Hilum
7. B. Alveoli
8. B. Hilar pleura
9. C. Hemothorax
10. A. Costophrenic angle
11. C. Epiglottis
12. D. Asthenic
13. D. 130 kVp, 600 mA, 1/60 sec, 72 in. SID

14.
  A. 8
  B. 10
  C. 1
  D. 5
  E. 4
  F. 11
  G. 9
  H. 13
  I. 7
  J. 3
  K. 6
  L. 12
  M. 2
15.
  A. Superior portion of left lung
  B. Jugular notch (superior margin of manubrium)
  C. Trachea
  D. Esophagus
16.
  A. Esophagus
  B. Descending aorta
  C. T4 vertebra
  D. Trachea
  E. Superior vena cava
  F. Ascending aorta
  G. Sternum
  H. Left lung region
17. A. Pigg-O-Stat
18. C. 65 kVp, short exposure time
19. A. To reduce patient dose
20. D. To reduce chest rotation
21. A. Remove scapulae from lung fields
22. C. 3 to 4 inches (8 to 10 cm) below jugular notch
23. True. CT is replacing bronchography to study the bronchial tree.
24. A. Atelectasis
25. C. Chylothorax
26. B. Pulmonary emboli
27. D. Tuberculosis
28. A. Be Reduced
29. C. Rotation into an LAO position
30. Yes, 10 ribs showing is acceptable. (Some healthy patients can inhale deeper and show 11 ribs.)
31. Yes. The costophrenic angles must be visualized on both the PA and lateral projections.
32. D. Raise upper limbs higher
33. No. This separation is acceptable and is caused by the divergent x-ray beam.
34. B. Perform AP semi-axial projection
35. C. Yes. Decrease exposure factors
36. A. Left lateral decubitus
37. B. 60 degrees LAO
38. D. Left lateral decubitis

39.
  A. (a), (c), (f) (slight rotation is evident)
  B. Criterion (a)
  C. (a), (f), (g)
40.
  A. (b), (c), (f)
  B. Criteria (b) and (f)
  C. (a), (d), (e)

Chapter 3
Abdomen
1. D. Peritioneum
2. C. Psoas muscles
3. A. Duodenum
4. C. Ileocecal valve
5.
  1. D
  2. H
  3. G
  4. F
  5. C
  6. A
  7. I
  8. B
  9. E
6. D. Kidney
7. C. Ureter
8. D. Gallbladder
9. D. Mesentery
10.
  A. RLQ
  B. RUQ
  C. LUQ
  D. LUQ
  E. RUQ
  F. LLQ
  G. RLQ
  H. RUQ and LUQ
  I. RUQ
11. A
12.
  1. A
  2. A
  3. B
  4. A
  5. B
  6. A
  7. C
  8. B
  9. C
  10. B
13. A. T9-10
14.
  1. E
  2. A
  3. G
  4. B
  5. C
  6. F
  7. D
15. B. Greater trochanter
16. A. Iliac crest
17. A. Short exposure time

18. D. Ascites
19. B. Ileus
20. A. Intussusception
21. D. Ulcerative colitis
22. C. Pneumoperitoneum
23. B. Diaphragm
24. B. Ascites
25. D. Ileus
26.
  A. Iliac crest
  B. Lumbar spine
  C. Psoas muscles
  D. Coccyx
  E. Symphysis pubis
  F. Obturator foramen
27.
  A. Liver
  B. Gallbladder
  C. Duodenum
  D. Stomach
  E. Splenic flexure of colon
  F. Pancreas
  G. Spleen
  H. Left kidney
  I. Abdominal aorta
  J. Inferior vena cava
28. B. 78 kVp, 600mA, 1/30 sec, grid, 40 in. SID
29. C. Rotation toward the right
30. A. Expiration
31. B. Use two cassettes placed crosswise
32. D. 5 minutes
33. B. Diaphragm
34. A. Left lateral decubitus
35. D. AP erect abdomen
36. B. Left lateral decubitus
37. C. Dorsal decubitus
38.
  A. True
  B. False (250 to 300 range)
  C. False (AP is about 35% greater than PA)
  D. True (testes are out of primary field)
39.
  A. (a), (b), (c), (g)
  B. Criteria (a) and (c)
  C. (b), (c), (g)
40.
  A. (a), (b)
  B. Criterion (a)
  C. (b)

Chapter 4
Upper Limb
1.
  A. A. 14
  B. B. 8
  C. B. 27
2.
  A. 7
  B. 4

C. 2
D. 5
E. 1
F. 6
3.
   A. 11
   B. 13
   C. 4
   D. 15
   E. 7
   F. 17
   G. 5
   H. 18
   I. 12
   J. 1
   K. 16
   L. 8
   M. 2
   N. 3
   O. 9
   P. 14
   Q. 6
   R. 10
4. C. Hamate
5. D. Trapezium
6. A. Scaphoid
7. D. Scaphoid and trapezium
8.
   A. 6
   B. 3
   C. 8
   D. 2
   E. 5
   F. 11
   G. 9
   H. 1
   I. 4
   J. 7
   K. 10
9. C. PA-Radial deviation
10. C. Scaphoid
11. A. PA-Ulnar deviation
12. B. Scaphoid
13. D. Ulna
14. A. Anterior aspect of distal
     humerus
15. C. Lateral and medial epicondyle
16. A. Medial aspect of coronoid
     process
17. A. Head of ulna
18.
   A. 4
   B. 3
   C. 2
   D. 1
   E. 4
19.
   A. 2
   B. 1
   C. 4
   D. 3
   E. 2
   F. 9

   G. 7
   H. 5
   I. 4
   J. 1
   K. 10
   L. 1
   M. 3
   N. 6
   O. 8
20.
   A. 5
   B. 3
   C. 8
   D. 7
   E. 11
   F. 1
   G. 2
   H. 4
   I. 10
   J. 9
   K. 6
21. True
22. False
23. B. Causes the proximal radius to
     cross over the ulna
24. A. Supinated
25. B. Pronated
26.
   A. 3
   B. 4
   C. 1
   D. 2
   E. 1
   F. 4
   G. 2
27. False
28. B. Parallel to long axis of the IR
29. D. Soft-tissue structures within
     certain synovial joints
30.
   1. F
   2. H
   3. G
   4. E
   5. B
   6. D
   7. A
   8. C
31. C. Gout
32. A. Affected PIP joint
33. D. All of the above
34. B. Third MP joint
35. A. Increased OID
36. C. Bennett's fracture
37. True
38. False
39. D
40. True
41. C. Decrease obliquity of hand
42. A. Rotate upper limb medially
43. C. Rotate wrist laterally 5 to 10°
44. A. Insufficient medial rotation

45. B. Place humerus/forearm in
     same horizontal plane
46. B. Wrist
47. C. Wrist
48. D. 68 to 70 kVp or 10 mAs
49. A. Coyle method
50.
   1. A. Lateral rotation
   A. (c), (e), (g)
   B. Criteria (e) and (g)
Note: Insufficient lateral rotation may
be considered a marginal repeatable
error by itself. But with no anatomical
marker visible, both of these errors
make it repeatable.
   C. (a), (e), (g)
51.
   1. B. Radial deviation
   A. (a), (b)
   B. Criteria (a) and (b)
   C. b

Chapter 5
Proximal Humerus and
Shoulder Girdle
1. D
2. C. Acromioclavicular
3. B. Medial angle
4. D. Coracoid process
5. False
6. A. Scapular spine
7. C. Acromion
8. B. Spheroidal
9.
   A. 3
   B. 11
   C. 5
   D. 8
   E. 12
   F. 10
   G. 7
   H. 2
   I. 9
   J. 4
   K. B. External
   L. 2
   M. 12
   N. 3
   O. 6
   P. 13
   Q. 1
   R. 8
   S. A. Inferosuperior axial
     projection—Lawrence
     method
10. A. Center and right AEC chambers
     activated
11. True
12. True
13. D. Nuclear medicine
14. A. Ultrasound

15.
1. D
2. E
3. C
4. F
5. G
6. A
7. B
16. D. Scapular Y or Neer method
17. A. Osteoarthritis
18. B. Rheumatoid arthritis
19. A. External rotation
20. C. 1 in (2.5 cm) inferior to coracoid process
21. C. Internal rotation
22. B. 25° medially
23. B. Use exaggerated, external rotation
24. A. 25° anterior and medial
25. D. Grashey method
26. C. 10 to 15
27. B. Reduced OID
28. A. Neer method
29. B. Transthoracic lateral
30. A. 10 to 15° caudad
31. C. Scapulohumeral dislocations
32. True
33. True
34.
1. B. (66 mrad)
2. C. (3 to 8 mrad)
3. C. (1 to 3 mrad)
4. B. (45 mrad)
5. A. (1005 mrad)
6. C. (10 mrad)
7. C. (1 mrad)
8. C. (0 mrad)
35. D. Rotate body more toward affected side
36. C. Garth method
37. A. Increase CR angulation
38. A. AC joint series—Non-weight and weight-bearing projections
39.
A. (b), (c), (e), (f)
B. Criteria (b), (e), (f)
C. (a), (b), (f)
40.
A. (a), (b), (d), (e)
B. Criteria (a), (b), (d), (e)
C. (a), (b), (d), (e)

Chapter 6
Lower Limb
1. B. Tail
2. False
3. A. Plantar surface near head of 1st metatarsal
4. D. Navicular
5. C. Intermediate
6. B. Subtalar joint
7. B. Tibial plafond
8. False (not the lateral aspect)

9.
1. D
2. G
3. B
4. F
5. A
6. E
7. C
10.
A. 3
B. 4
C. 5
D. 1
E. 2
F. C. AP ankle
11.
A. 7
B. 9
C. 4
D. 2
E. 3
F. 1
G. 8
H. 5
I. 10
J. 2
K. 6
12. A. Fig. 6-11
13. A. Affected MTP joint
14. B. 10 to 15° posterior
15. C. Tangential
16. D. 30 to 40°
17. D. Dorsoplantar projection
18. A. 10° posterior
19. C. AP oblique-medial rotation
20. D. Intercondylar tubercles
21. A. Intercondylar fossa
22. A. (5 to 7°)
23. True
24. B. Base
25. C. Cruciate
26. C. Menisci
27.
A. 3
B. 9
C. 6
D. 8
E. 1
F. 4
G. 2
H. 10
I. 5
J. 7
28. B. AP oblique-medial rotation
29.
A. 3
B. 5
C. 1
D. 6
E. 2
F. 3
G. 5
H. 1

I. 4
J. 7
30. B. Under rotation toward IR
31. True
32. C. Over rotation of knee toward IR
33. D. Osgood-Schlatter disease
34. D. Osteomalacia
35. A. Osteogenic sarcoma
36. B. Runner's knee
37. C. Base of third metatarsal
38. B. AP oblique (15-20° medial rotation)
39. D. Interepicondylar
40. B. Proximal tibiofibular
41. True
42. D. All of the above
43. D. Merchant
44. C. Requires overflexion of knee
45. B. Lateral rotation of lower limb
46. C. Increase central ray angle to 45°
47. A. Increase CR angulation to 40°
48. D. AP and horizontal beam lateral position
49.
A. (a), (d), (e), (g)
B. Criteria (a), (d), (e), (g)
C. (d), (e), (g)
50.
A. (a), (g), (c)
B. Criteria (a) (anterior tubercle is obscured), (g)
C. (a), (f)

Chapter 7
Proximal Femur and Pelvis
1.
A. Left hip bone
B. Right hip bone
C. Sacrum
D. Coccyx
2.
A. Ilium
B. Ischium
C. Pubis
3. D. All of the above
4. Obturator foramen
5. B. Lesser trochanter
6.
A. Body
B. Ramus
7. Brim of the pelvis
8.
1. B
2. A
3. A
4. B
5. A
6. B
7. B
9. Cephalopelvimetry

10.
  A. Greater trochanter
  B. Neck of femur
  C. Acetabulum
  D. Anterior superior iliac spine (ASIS)
  E. Crest of ilium
  F. Ischial spine
  G. Superior ramus of pubis
  H. Symphysis pubis
  I. Ischial tuberosity
  J. Female
  K. Neck of femur
  L. Lesser trochanter
  M. Greater trochanter
  N. Ischial tuberosity
  O. Axiolateral (inferior-superior) (Danelius-Miller method)
  P. Ala (wing) of left ilium
  Q. Body of left ilium
  R. Body of left pubis
  S. Ramus of left ischium
  T. Greater trochanter
  U. Lesser trochanter
  V. Neck of right femur
  W. AP bilateral frog-legs (modified Cleaves method)

11.
  1. M
  2. M
  3. F
  4. F
  5. F
  6. M

12. A. Ischial spines
13. Fovea capitis
14. C. Fractured proximal femur
15. D. Ankylosing spondylitis
16.
  1. F
  2. B
  3. A
  4. E
  5. D
  6. C

17. C. Limited view of the lesser trochanter in profile
18. B. 200 to 500
19. True
20. A. Bi-lateral frog-leg
21. D. 30-45° cephalad
22. True
23. False. (Midway between ASIS and symphysis pubis)
24. False. (Trauma projection)
25. Anterior oblique acetabulum Judet method
26. B. AP axial method
27. 1 inch (2.5 cm) medial from the upside ASIS
28. Less
29. Right (downside) joints

30. The AP axial outlet projection (Taylor method) will elongate the pubis and ischium and define this region more completely.
31. It is soft tissue from the unaffected thigh. This leg must be flexed and elevated high enough to keep it from superimposing the affected hip.
32. PA axial, CR 30 to 35 degrees caudad and 25 to 30 degrees right and left anterior oblique projections with patient semi-prone.
33. No. It is an acceptable image because the lesser trochanters should not be visible at all or only minimally on a well-positioned AP hip projection.
34. AP pelvis and bilateral "frog-leg"
35. B. Reverse central ray angle
36.
  A. (a), (e)
  B. (a), (e)
  C. (e), (f)
37.
  A. (a), (b), (f), (h)
  B. (a), (b), (f), (h)
  C. (b), (g), (h)

Chapter 8
Cervical and Thoracic Spine

1. Lower border of first lumbar (L1) vertebrae
2. Five
3. A. Thoracic; D. Sacral
4. True
5. Kyphosis
6. Scoliosis
7. Herniated nucleus pulposus (HNP)
8. Intervertebral foramina
9. Zygapophyseal joints
10. C. Nucleus pulposus
11. False (vertebral artery and vein)
12. False (C-Spine possesses bifid spinous processes)
13. 45
14. Transverse atlantal ligament
15. Zygapophyseal joint
16. Demifacets
17. C. T11; D. T12
18. A. Each have three foramina (one in each transverse process plus usual vertebral foramina).
  B. Spinous processes have bifid tip.
19. Presence of facets for articulation with ribs
20. Lateral
21.
  A. Anterior arch (with anterior tubercle), C1 (atlas)
  B. Dens (odontoid process), C2
  C. Transverse atlantal ligament, C2

  D. Transverse foramen, C1
  E. Superior facets (atlanto-occipital articulation), C1
  F. Posterior arch, C1
  G. Dens (odontoid process), C2
  H. Transverse process, C1
  I. Articular pillar (lateral mass), C2
  J. Right zygapophyseal joint, C2 to C3
  K. Bifid tip, spinous process, C4
  L. Vertebra prominens (spinous process), C7
  M. Superior articular process, T10
  N. Intervertebral disk space, T10 to T11
  O. Facet for costovertebral joint, T11
  P. Right zygapophyseal joint, T11 to T12
  Q. Right intervertebral foramen, T12 to L1
  R. Facet of inferior articular process, L2
  S. Lower thoracic (T10, 11, and 12) and upper lumbar (L1 and 2).
  T. Evident by facets for articulation with ribs on upper three but not on lower two. (Note also that the last two thoracic vertebrae do not have facets on transverse processes for costotransverse joints, characteristic of T11 and T12.)

22.
  A. Lateral mass (articular pillar), C1
  B. Zygapophyseal joint, C1 to C2
  C. Body, C2
  D. Spinous process (superimposed by body), C2
  E. Inferior articular process, C2
  F. Dens (odontoid process), C2
  G. Upper incisors (teeth)
23. Lateral
24. Left zygapophyseal joints (downside joints)
25. 1) B
  2) A
  3) C
  4) D
  5) F
  6) E
26. D. Nuclear medicine
27. B. Clay shoveler's fracture
28. A. Scoliosis and/or kyphosis
29. False. Most common at the L4 to L5 level
30.
  A. Close side collimation
  B. Use a lead blocker on table-top behind patient
31. AP open-mouth projection

32.
  A. 15 to 20 degrees cephalad
  B. 15 to 20 degrees caudad
  C. 15 to 20 degrees cephalad
33. B. LAO
34.
  A. Suspend respiration on full expiration
  B. Have patient hold 5 to 10 lb. in each hand.
35. Swimmer's, cervicothoracic lateral
36.
  A. Fuchs method
  B. Judd method
37. Tilt and/or rotation of the spine
38. Not keeping spine parallel to the film and/or not aligning the CR perpendicular to spine
39. Yes. (The technologist needs to assume there may be a fracture present. A horizontal beam cross-table lateral projection should be taken for all suspected trauma to the cervical spine. A physician must examine the radiograph and clear the patient for the remaining projections.)
40. AP open-mouth projection. Note that a horizontal beam lateral must be taken and cleared first.
41. C. 100 to 200 mrad
42. D. Four times greater
43. D. 900 to 1000 mrad
44. C. 10 to 15 times greater
45.
  A. (a), (c), (f)
  B. Criteria (a), (f)
  C. Criteria (a), (e), (f)
46.
  A. (a), (b), (c), (g)
  B. Criteria (a), (c), (g)
  C. Criteria (c), (d)

Chapter 9
Lumbar Spine, Sacrum, and Coccyx

1. C. Larger and more blunt
2. C. Promontory
3. B. 30
4. 45
5. C. Between superior and inferior articular processes
6.
  A. Left ala superior articular process
  B. Left ala of sacrum
  C. Pelvic (anterior) sacral foramina
  D. Apex of sacrum
  E. Right and left superior articular processes

  F. Sacral promontory (also seen on frontal view)
  G. Auricular surface (sacroiliac joint)
  H. Coccyx
  I. Apex of coccyx
  J. Horn (cornu) of coccyx
  K. Horn (cornu) of sacrum
  L. Median sacral crest
7.
  A. Spinous process
  B. Lamina
  C. Transverse process
  D. Pedicle (also shown on lateral view)
  E. Vertebral foramen
  F. Body (also shown on lateral view)
  G. Superior articular process
  H. Inferior articular process
  I. Region of articular facets (R and L sides superimposed as seen on a lateral view)
  J. Intervertebral notch or foramen
8. Large body and large blunt spinous process
9. Synovial, plane (gliding)
10.
  A. Superior articular process (ear)
  B. Transverse process (nose)
  C. Pedicle (eye)
  D. Inferior articular (leg)
  E. Pars interarticularis (neck)
  F. Zygapophyseal joint (between L-4/5)
11. Zygapophyseal
12. B. Lower costal margin
13. False (would obscure essential anatomy).
14. False (ovaries are slightly anterior, thus AP results in about 30% greater gonadal dose than PA).
15. Opens the intervertebral disk space by reducing the normal lumbar curvature of the spine.
16. False. The lead blocker should be used with digital imaging to prevent secondary scatter from reaching radiosensitive image receptor.
17. True
18. C. Compression fracture
19. B. Spina bifida
20. A. Ankylosing spondylitis
21. 1 to 1.5 in. (3 to 4 cm) above the iliac crest
22. Right, the upside joints
23. 50 degrees from plane of table
24. A patient with a wide pelvis and narrow thorax
25. B. 5 to 10°, caudad
26. A. 35°, cephalad

27. Level of ASIS at the midline of the body
28. True
29. AP (PA) projection, Ferguson method (with and without block under convex side of curve)
30. Hyperextension and hyperflexion lateral projection
31. Midway between the symphysis pubis and ASIS
32.
  A. Close collimation
  B. Use a lead blocker on table-top behind patient
33. To reduce gonadal dose
34. C. 1000 to 1500 mrad
35. Right rotation.
36. Decrease obliquity of the spine
37. Insufficient cephalad CR angulation
38. A lateral projection (may include a coned down spot AP/PA and lateral of the L3 region)
39. AP, lateral, L5-S1 spot lateral and right and left 30 degree obliques
40.
  A. (a), (b), (c), (e), (f)
  B. (a), (b), (f)
  C. (a), (b), (e), (f)

Chapter 10
Bony Thorax

1.
  A. Manubrium
  B. Body
  C. Xiphoid process
2. Xiphoid process
3. Sternal angle
4. C. Gladiolus
5. A. Attaches directly to sternum
6. D. Does not possess costocartilage
7. True rib
8. D. Sternal angle
9. D. All of the above
10.
  1. A
  2. A
  3. B
  4. A
  5. B
11.
  A. Left clavicle
  B. Left SC joint
  C. First rib (sternal end)
  D. Manubrium
  E. Sternal angle
  F. Body
  G. Xiphoid
  H. Jugular notch
  I. Manubrium
  J. Sternal angle

K. Body
L. Xiphoid
12.
  A. Suspended inspiration
  B. Low (65 to 75)
  C. Erect (if patient is able)
13. 40 in. (100 cm)
14. B. Breathing technique

15.
  A. Place the area of interest closest to film.
  B. Rotate the spine away from the area of interest.
16.
  A. Pneumothorax
  B. Hemothorax
17.
  A. 15 to 20 degrees
  B. More
18. C. Patients with history of multiple myeloma
19. D. Blunt trauma
20.
  A. 66 mrad (50 to 100 range)
  B. 3 mrad (2 to 5 range)
21. C. (LPO)
22. B. Drawn back
23. The SC joints are equal distance from the midline of spine
24. 15 degrees
25. Midway between the xiphoid process and lower rib cage
26. B. 65 to 75 kVp
27. A. LAO
28. Overobliquity of the sternum. A large-chested patient only requires approximately 15 degrees of rotation. Overobliquity will lead to foreshortening along the width of the sternum and will shift the sternum away from the spine.
29. Rotation of the upper body from a true lateral will cause the ribs to be superimposed over the sternum.
30.
  A. AP and RPO performed recumbent
  B. Suspend upon expiration
31.
  A. PA and RAO performed recumbent
  B. Expose upon inspiration
32. 15 to 20 degrees LAO (a RAO with less obliquity of only 15 degrees would also demonstrate the left SC joint region by aligning it next to the spinal column).
33. False. (AEC is generally not recommended for rib routines due to the

need for high-contrast, optimum detail exposures, which can generally be better achieved manually.)
34. False. Exposure is made with suspended respiration on inspiration.

35.
  A. (c), (e), (f)
  B. (f)
  C. (b), (c), (f)

Chapter 11
Cranium
1. C. Occipital
2. C. Squamous
3.
  A. Right parietal
  B. Left parietal
  C. Sphenoid
  D. Ethmoid
4. Parietal tubercles or eminences
5. External occipital protuberance or inion
6.
  A. 5
  B. 6
  C. 3
  D. 7
  E. 2
7. Petrous pyramids
8. True
9. True
10. Clivus
11. Lateral labyrinth or masses
12. Crista galli
13. Left pterion
14. Squamosal suture
15. Sutural or Wormian bones
16.
  1. C
  2. C
  3. B
  4. C
  5. D
  6. D
  7. A
  8. D
  9. E
  10. A
  11. B
  12. E
  13. A
  14. C
  15. E

17.
  A. Oribital plate, frontal
  B. Supraorbital margin (SOM), frontal

C. Crista galli, ethmoid
D. Sagittal suture, parietals
E. Midlateral orbital margin, zygoma
F. Petrous ridge, temporal
G. Petrous portion, temporal
H. Petrous ridge, temporal
I. Dorsum sellae, sphenoid
J. Posterior clinoid processes, sphenoid
K. Orbital roofs (plates), frontal
L. Sella turcica, sphenoid
M. Body (sphenoid sinus), sphenoid
18. C. Brachycephalic
19. A. Mesocephalic
20.
  A. External auditory meatus (EAM)
  B. Angle (gonion) of mandible
  C. Mental point (mentum)
  D. Acanthion
  E. Nasion
  F. Glabella
  G. Glabellomeatal line (GML)
  H. Orbitomeatal line (OML)
  I. Infraorbitomeatal line (IOML)
  J. Acanthomeatal line (AML)
  K. Lips-meatal line (LML)
  L. Mentomeatal line (MML)
21. Auricular point
22. A. Pinna
23. B. IOML
24. B. 7 to 8°
25. A. Rotation
26.
  A. 5
  B. 6
  C. 2
  D. 4
  E. 1
  F. 3
27. D. Multiple myeloma
28. A. CT
29. B. MRI
30.
  A. AP axial projection (Towne method)
  B. PA axial projection (Haas method)
31.
  A. 37 degrees caudad
  B. 30 degrees caudad
32. 2 in. (5 cm) superior to the EAM
33. Interpupillary
34. At level of, or slightly inferior to, the inferior orbital rim
35. ¾ in. (2 cm) anterior to the level of the EAMs, midway between the angles of the mandible

36.
  A. 37 degrees
  B. 30 degrees
37. Decrease caudad CR angle by about 7 degrees
38. Rotation
39. Increase extension of the skull to bring the OML perpendicular to the IR (this will project the petrous ridges into the lower one third of the orbits).
40. Horizontal beam lateral skull projection will demonstrate any possible air/fluid levels
41. Perform the AP projection with a 15 degree cephalad CR angle to the OML
42. Use the IOML instead of OML and angle CR an additional 7 degrees caudad for a total of 37 degrees.
43.
  A. (a), (b), (c), (e), (f), (g)
  B.
    Criteria (a), (*b), (c), (e), (f), (g) (*Note: CR appears to be slightly high. Not a major error, though.)
  C. (a), (b), (e), (f)
44.
  A. (c), (e), (g), (i)
  B. (*c), (e), (g), (i) (*Note: Petrous ridges should be in the lower 1/3 of orbits.)
  C. (a), (e), (f), (g)

Chapter 12
Facial Bones

1. A. Maxilla
2. D. Ramus
3.
  A. 4
  B. 5
  C. 7
  D. 6
  E. 3
  F. 1
  G. 2
4.
  A. Lacrimal
  B. Ethmoid
  C. Frontal
  D. Sphenoid
  E. Palatine
  F. Zygomatic
  G. Maxilla
5. True
6. False (The tripod fracture does this.)

7. Parietoacanthial (Waters) projection (dense petrous pyramids are projected below the maxillary sinuses)
8. Horizontal beam (cross-table) lateral projection
9. Midsagittal plane
10.
  A. 37 degrees
  B. Mentomeatal line (MML)
11. D. Acanthion
12. A. Nasion
13. Lower half of the maxillary sinuses
14. True
15. False (glabelloalveolar, GAL)
16. Lips-meatal line (LML)
17. 1/2 in. (1.25 cm) inferior to nasion
18. Infraorbitomeatal line (IOML)
19. 15 degrees rotation and 15 degrees tilt toward the affected side
20. 37 degrees caudad
21. Rhese method
22. Lower outer quadrant of the orbit
23. 25 degrees cephalad
24. C. Extend chin slightly
25. C. 45°
26. C. 20 to 25° cephalad
27. Temporomandibular fossae
28. 1½ in. (4 cm) inferior to mandibular symphysis (or midway between angles of mandible)
29. C. 200 to 300 mrad
30. C. IOML
31. 35 degrees caudad
32. False (15 degrees)
33. True
34. True
35. Excessive flexion of the head, or insufficient caudad CR angle
36. A. AML
37. Increase extension of the head and neck, or angle the CR. The IOML must be parallel to the film and perpendicular to the CR.
38. Reverse Waters—AP projection with cephalad angle as needed to be perpendicular to MML, and horizontal beam lateral
39. Reduce kVp to 50 to 60 range and increase mAs accordingly
40. A modified parietoacanthial (modified Waters) or a PA axial with a 30 degree caudal angle to provide a more direct view of the orbital floors and rims. (Note: the modified Waters is more commonly performed for this purpose.)

Chapter 13
Paranasal Sinuses, Mastoids, and Temporal Bones

1. 2
2. True
3. False (All communicate with each other and with nasal cavity)
4. True
5. True
6.
  A. Sphenoid sinuses
  B. Ethmoid sinuses
  C. Frontal sinuses
  D. Maxillary sinuses
  E. Frontal sinuses
  F. Ethmoid and sphenoid sinuses (superimposed)
  G. Dense petrous portion of temporal bone
  H. Maxillary sinuses
  I. Base of skull
  J. Ethmoid sinuses
  K. Sphenoid sinus
  L. Petrous portion of temporal
  M. Mastoid portion of temporal
7. Lateral masses or labyrinths
8. Sella turcica
9. Squamous portion
10. Petrous portion
11. Tympanic membrane
12. A. malleus
13. Eustachian or auditory tube
14. Auditory nerve and blood vessels
15. Epitympanic recess, mastoid
16. Encephalitis
17. C. Stapes
18. Membranous
19.
  A. Cochlea
  B. Vestibule
  C. Semicircular canals
20.
  A. Malleus
  B. Incus
  C. Stapes
  D. Internal acoustic meatus (auditory nerve)
  E. Cochlea
  F. Eustachian (auditory) tube
  G. Tympanic cavity
  H. Typanic membrane (ear drum)
  I. External acoustic meatus (canal) (EAM)
21. False. Ultrasound of the maxillary sinus can be performed
22. C. Cholesteatoma
23. True
24. A. CT
25. C. 300 to 400 mrad

26. Midway between outer canthus and EAM
27. To allow possible fluids in the sinuses to settle
28. Parietoacanthial (Waters) projection
29. To illustrate air/fluid levels without distortion
30. Insufficient angulation of the CR will lead to superimposition of the upside mastoid upon the region of interest.

31. More extension of the head is needed to eliminate superimposition of the mandible and the sinuses.
32. Additional CR angulation will project the dorsum sellae into the foramen magnum and elongate the petrous pyramids
33. Rotation of the skull
34. Approximately a 40 degree oblique will profile the downside

petrous bone. 45 degree rotation is needed for the average (mesocephalic) skull. Since there is a wider angle between petrous bone and the midsagittal plane with the brachycephalic skull, less rotation of the skull is required for the Stenvers projection.
35. Routine radiographic sinus projections or CT